Rapid Review
Biochemistry

Rapid Review Series

Series Editor
Edward F. Goljan, MD

Behavioral Science, Second Edition
Vivian M. Stevens, PhD; Susan K. Redwood, PhD; Jackie L. Neel, DO;
Richard H. Bost, PhD; Nancy W. Van Winkle, PhD; Michael H. Pollak, PhD

Biochemistry, Second Edition
John W. Pelley, PhD; Edward F. Goljan, MD

Gross and Developmental Anatomy, Second Edition
N. Anthony Moore, PhD; William A. Roy, PhD, PT

Histology and Cell Biology, Second Edition
E. Robert Burns, PhD; M. Donald Cave, PhD

Microbiology and Immunology, Second Edition
Ken S. Rosenthal, PhD; James S. Tan, MD

Neuroscience
James A. Weyhenmeyer, PhD; Eve A. Gallman, PhD

Pathology, Second Edition
Edward F. Goljan, MD

Pharmacology, Second Edition
Thomas L. Pazdernik, PhD; Laszlo Kerecsen, MD

Physiology
Thomas A. Brown, MD

USMLE Step 2
Michael W. Lawlor, MD, PhD

USMLE Step 3
David Rolston, MD; Craig Nielsen, MD

Rapid Review
Biochemistry

SECOND EDITION

John W. Pelley, PhD
Associate Professor
Department of Cell Biology and Biochemistry
Texas Tech University Health Sciences Center
School of Medicine
Lubbock, Texas

Edward F. Goljan, MD
Professor and Chair
Department of Pathology
Oklahoma State University Center for Health Sciences
College of Osteopathic Medicine
Tulsa, Oklahoma

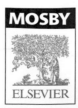

MOSBY

ELSEVIER

MOSBY
ELSEVIER

1600 John F. Kennedy Blvd.
Suite 1800
Philadelphia, PA 19103-2899

RAPID REVIEW BIOCHEMISTRY, Second Edition

NOTICE

Knowledge and best practice in this field are constantly changing. As new research and experience broaden our knowledge, changes in practice, treatment and drug therapy may become necessary or appropriate. Readers are advised to check the most current information provided (i) on procedures featured or (ii) by the manufacturer of each product to be administered, to verify the recommended dose or formula, the method and duration of administration, and contraindications. It is the responsibility of the practitioner, relying on their own experience and knowledge of the patient, to make diagnoses, to determine dosages and the best treatment for each individual patient, and to take all appropriate safety precautions. To the fullest extent of the law, neither the Publisher nor the Authors assume any liability for any injury and/or damage to persons or property arising out or related to any use of the material contained in this book.

Library of Congress Cataloging-in-Publication Data

Pelley, John W.
  Biochemistry / John W. Pelley, Edward F. Goljan.—2nd ed.
    p. ; cm.—(Rapid review series)
  ISBN-13: 978-0-323-04437-0 ISBN-10: 0-323-04437-9
    1. Biochemistry—Outlines, syllabi, etc. 2. Biochemistry—Examinations, questions, etc.
  I. Goljan, Edward F. II. Title. III. Series.
    [DNLM: 1. Metabolism—Examination Questions. 2. Biochemical Phenomena—
Examination Questions. 3. Nutrition—Examination Questions. QU 18.2 P389b 2007]
  QP518.3.P45 2007
  612'.015—dc22

                2006041850

Publishing Director: Linda Belfus
Acquisitions Editor: James Merritt
Developmental Editor: Katie DeFrancesco
Design Direction: Steven Stave

ISBN-13: 978-0-323-04437-0
ISBN-10: 0-323-04437-9

Printed in the United States of America.

Last digit is the print number: 9 8 7 6 5 4

Contributors

John A. Davis, MD, PhD
Resident
Department of Internal Medicine
Massachusetts General Hospital
Boston, Massachusetts

Çağatay H. Erşahin, MD, PhD
Resident
Department of Pathology
Loyola University Chicago
Stritch School of Medicine
Maywood, Illinois

Anna M. Szpaderska, DDS, PhD
Postdoctoral Fellow
Department of Surgery
Burn and Shock Trauma Institute
Loyola University Chicago
Stritch School of Medicine
Maywood, Illinois

Series Preface

The First Editions of the *Rapid Review Series* have received high critical acclaim from students studying for the United States Medical Licensing Examination (USMLE) Step 1 and high ratings in *First Aid for the USMLE Step 1*. The Second Editions continue to be invaluable resources for time-pressed students. As a result of reader feedback, we have improved upon an already successful formula. We have created a learning system, including a print and electronic package, that is easier to use and more concise than other review products on the market.

SPECIAL FEATURES

Book

- **Outline format:** Concise, high-yield subject matter is presented in a study-friendly format.
- **High-yield margin notes:** Key content that is most likely to appear on the exam is reinforced in the margin notes.
- **Visual elements:** Abundant two-color schematics, black and white images, and summary tables enhance your study experience.
- **Two-color design:** Colored text and headings make studying more efficient and pleasing.
- **Two practice examinations:** Two sets of 50 USMLE Step 1–type clinically oriented, multiple-choice questions (including images where necessary) and complete discussions (rationales) for all options are included.

New! Online Study and Testing Tool

- **350 USMLE Step 1–type MCQs:** Clinically oriented, multiple-choice questions that mimic the current board format are presented. These include images where necessary, and complete rationales for all answer options. All the questions from the book are included so you can study them in the most effective mode for you!
- **Test mode:** Select from randomized 50-question sets or by subject topics for an exam-like review session. This mode features a 60-minute timer to simulate the actual exam, a detailed assessment report that can be printed or saved to your hard drive, and direct links to all or only incorrect questions. The links include your answer, the correct answer, and full rationales for all answer options, so you can fully analyze your test session and learn from your mistakes.
- **Study mode:** Like the test mode, in the study mode you can select from randomized 50-question sets or by subject topics to create a dynamic study session. This mode features unlimited attempts at each question, instant feedback (either on selection of the correct answer or when using the "Show Answer" feature), complete rationales for all answer options, and a detailed progress report that can be printed or saved to your hard drive.
- **Online access:** Online access allows you to study from an internet-enabled computer wherever and whenever it is convenient. This access is activated through registration on www.studentconsult.com with the pincode printed inside the front cover.

Student Consult

- **Full online access:** You can access the complete text and illustrations of this book on www.studentconsult.com.
- **Save content to your PDA:** Through our unique Pocket Consult platform, you can clip selected text and illustrations and save them to your PDA for study on the fly!
- **Free content:** An interactive community center with a wealth of additional valuable resources is available.

Acknowledgment of Reviewers

The publisher expresses sincere thanks to the medical students who provided many useful comments and suggestions for improving the text and the questions. Our publishing program will continue to benefit from the combined insight and experience provided by your reviews. For always encouraging us to focus on our target, the USMLE Step 1, we thank the following:

Thomas A. Brown, West Virginia University School of Medicine

Patricia C. Daniel, PhD, Kansas University Medical Center

John A. Davis, PhD, Yale University School of Medicine

Daniel Egan, Mount Sinai School of Medicine

Steven J. Engman, Loyola University Chicago Stritch School of Medicine

Michael W. Lawlor, Loyola University Chicago Stritch School of Medicine

Craig Wlodarek, Rush Medical College

Acknowledgments

In a way, an author begins to work on a book long before he sits down at a word processor. Lessons learned in the past from my own teachers and mentors, discussions with colleagues and students, and daily encouragement from family and friends have contributed greatly to the writing of this book.

My wife, MJ, has been a constant source of love and support. Her sensitivity made me aware that I was ready to write this book, and she allowed me to take the time I needed to complete it.

The many caring, intelligent students whom I have taught at Texas Tech over the years have inspired me to hone my thinking, teaching, and writing skills, all of which affected the information that went into the book and the manner in which it was presented.

The editorial team at Elsevier was superb. Ruth Steyn and Sally Anderson improved the original manuscript to make my words sound better than I could alone. My highest praise and gratitude are reserved for Susan Kelly, who provided her editorial expertise and professionalism for the first edition. She has become a valued colleague and trusted friend.

My compliments to Jim Merritt, who undertook a difficult coordination effort to get all of the authors on the "same page" for this very innovative re-launch of the Rapid Review Series. He and Katie DeFrancesco are to be commended for being so helpful and professional.

John W. Pelley, PhD

The first edition of this book could not have been written and illustrated without the support of Acquisitions Editor Jason Malley and Managing Editor Susan Kelly. I also acknowledge the loving support of my wife, Joyce, who is the "wind beneath my wings."

Edward F. Goljan, MD

Contents

Carbohydrates, Lipids, and Amino Acids
Metabolic Fuels and Biosynthetic Precursors

TARGET TOPICS

- Common sugars and their derivatives that occur in metabolic pathways
- Glycosidic bond and formation of disaccharides and polysaccharides
- Fatty acids and their esterified derivatives (triacylglycerols, phospholipids, and sphingolipids)
- Major types of steroids
- Prostaglandins, thromboxanes, and leukotrienes: synthetic pathways and biological effects
- Amino acids: classification, structure, and distinguishing properties

- Weak acids and bases as buffer systems
- Clinical correlations: scurvy, cataract formation, peripheral neuropathy, retinopathy, atherosclerosis, hemolytic anemia, respiratory distress syndrome, sphingolipidoses (e.g., Tay-Sachs and Gaucher's diseases), asthma, maple syrup urine disease, phenylketonuria (PKU), glucose-6-phosphate dehydrogenase (G6PD) deficiency

---

I. Carbohydrates
- Oxidation of glucose, the most central monosaccharide in metabolism, provides a significant portion of the energy needed by cells in the fed state.
  A. Monosaccharides, the simplest carbohydrates, are aldehydes (aldoses) or ketones (ketoses) with the general molecular formula $(CH_2O)_x$, where $x = 3$ or more.
    1. Number of carbon atoms and the nature of the most oxidized group are common properties for classifying monosaccharides (Table 1-1).

Class/Sugar*	Carbonyl Group	Major Metabolic Role
Triose (3 Carbons)		
Glyceraldehyde	Aldose	Intermediate in glycolytic and pentose phosphate pathways
Dihydroxyacetone	Ketose	Reduced to glycerol (used in fat metabolism); present in glycolytic pathway
Tetrose (4 Carbons)		
Erythrose	Aldose	Intermediate in pentose phosphate pathway
Pentose (5 Carbons)		
Ribose	Aldose	Component of RNA; precursor of DNA
Ribulose	Ketose	Intermediate in pentose phosphate pathway
Hexose (6 Carbons)		
Glucose	Aldose	Absorbed from intestine with Na^+ and enters cells; starting point of glycolytic pathway; polymerized to form glycogen in liver and muscle
Fructose	Ketose	Absorbed from intestine via facilitated diffusion and enters cells; converted to intermediates in glycolytic pathway; derived from sucrose
Galactose	Aldose	Absorbed from intestine with Na^+ and enters cells; converted to glucose; derived from lactose
Heptose (7 Carbons)		
Sedoheptulose	Ketose	Intermediate in pentose phosphate pathway

*Within cells, sugars usually are phosphorylated, which prevents them from diffusing out of the cell.

- Most sugars can exist as optical isomers (D or L forms), and enzymes are specific for each isomer.
- In human metabolism, most sugars occur as D forms.

2. Pyranose sugars contain a six-membered ring (glucose and galactose), whereas furanose sugars contain a five-membered ring (fructose, ribose, and deoxyribose).

B. Monosaccharide derivatives are components of important metabolic products, and excesses of some contribute to pathogenic conditions.

1. Sugar acids
   a. Ascorbic acid (vitamin C) is required in the synthesis of collagen. Prolonged deficiency of vitamin C causes scurvy.
   b. Glucuronic acid reacts with bilirubin in the liver, forming conjugated (direct) bilirubin, which is water soluble.

Scurvy: vitamin C deficiency

Type	No. of Monomers	Examples
Monosaccharides	1	Glucose, fructose, ribose
Disaccharides	2	Lactose, sucrose, maltose
Oligosaccharides	3–10	Blood group antigens, membrane glycoproteins
Polysaccharides	>10	Starch, glycogen, glycosaminoglycans

TABLE 1-2:

Types of Carbohydrates

    c. Glucuronic acid is a component of glycosaminoglycans (GAGs), which are major constituents of the extracellular matrix.

2. Deoxy sugars: 2-deoxyribose, an essential component of DNA
3. Sugar alcohols (polyols)
    a. Glycerol derived from hydrolysis of triacylglycerol is phosphorylated to form glycerol phosphate, which is available for gluconeogenesis.
    b. Sorbitol derived from glucose is osmotically active and is responsible for damage to the lens (cataract formation), Schwann cells (peripheral neuropathy), and pericytes (retinopathy), all associated with diabetes mellitus.
    c. Galactitol derived from galactose contributes to cataract formation, which is associated with galactosemia.
4. Amino sugars: replacement of the hydroxyl group with an amino group yields glucosamine and galactosamine.
    • *N*-acetylated forms of these compounds are present in GAGs.
5. Sugar esters: sugar links with phosphate or sulfate
    • Phosphorylation of glucose after it enters cells effectively traps it as glucose-6-phosphate, which is further metabolized to meet cellular needs.

C. Larger carbohydrates are formed by condensation reactions.
1. Sugar polymers are commonly classified based on the number of sugar units (monomers) that they contain (Table 1-2).
2. A glycosidic bond linking two sugars is designated α or β.

D. Common disaccharides are hydrolyzed by digestive enzymes, and the resulting monosaccharides are absorbed into the body.
1. Maltose = glucose + glucose: starch breakdown product
2. Lactose = glucose + galactose: milk sugar
3. Sucrose = glucose + fructose: table sugar
    • Sucrose, unlike glucose, fructose, and galactose, is a nonreducing sugar.

E. Polysaccharides function to store glucose and form structural elements.
1. Starch, the primary glucose storage form in plants, has two major components, both of which can be degraded by human enzymes (e.g., amylase).
    a. Amylose has a linear structure with α-1,4 linkages.
    b. Amylopectin has a branched structure with α-1,4 linkages and α-1,6 linkages.
2. Glycogen, the primary glucose storage form in animals, has α-glycosidic linkages, similar to amylopectin, but is more highly branched (Fig. 1-1).

Sorbitol: cataracts, neuropathy, and retinopathy in diabetes mellitus

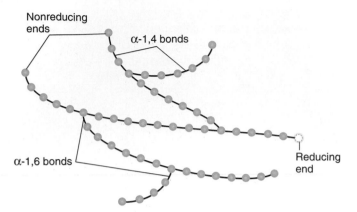

1-1: *Schematic depiction of glycogen structure. Each glycogen molecule has one reducing end (open circle) and many nonreducing ends. Because of the many branches, which are cleaved by glycogen phosphorylase one glucose unit (closed circles) at a time, glycogen can be rapidly degraded to supply glucose in response to low blood glucose.*

- Glycogen phosphorylase cleaves the α-1,4 linkages in glycogen, releasing glucose units from the nonreducing ends of the many branches when the glucose level is low.
- Liver and muscle produce glycogen from excess glucose.
  3. Cellulose, a structural polysaccharide in plants, is a glucose polymer containing β-1,4 linkages.
- Although an important source of fiber in the diet, cellulose supplies no energy because human digestive enzymes cannot hydrolyze β-1,4 linkages (insoluble fiber).
  4. Hyaluronic acid and other GAGs are negatively charged polysaccharides containing various sugar acids, amino sugars, and their sulfated derivatives.
- These structural polysaccharides form a major part of the extracellular matrix in humans.

Digestive enzymes: cleave α-glycosidic linkages in starch, not β-glycosidic bonds in cellulose (insoluble fiber)

II. Lipids
- Fatty acids, the simplest lipids, can be oxidized to generate much of the energy needed by cells in the fasting state (excluding brain cells and erythrocytes).
- Fatty acids are precursors in the synthesis of more complex cellular lipids.
- Only two fatty acids are essential and must be supplied in the diet: linoleic and linolenic.
  A. Fatty acids are composed of an unbranched hydrocarbon chain with a terminal carboxyl group.
    1. In humans, most fatty acids have an even number of carbon atoms with a chain length of 16 to 20 carbon atoms (Table 1-3).
      a. Short-chain (2 to 4 carbons) and medium-chain (6 to 10 carbons) fatty acids occur primarily as metabolic intermediates in the body.
        - These fatty acids can be directly reabsorbed in the small intestine, and they also diffuse freely into the mitochondrial matrix to be oxidized.

TABLE 1-3:
Common Fatty Acids in Humans

Common Name	Chain Length (No. of Carbon Atoms)
Palmitic	16
Stearic	18
Palmitoleic	16
Oleic	18
Linoleic (essential)	18
Linolenic (essential)	18
Arachidonic	20

TABLE 1-4:
Phospholipids

X Group	Phospholipid Type
Choline	Phosphatidylcholine (lecithin)
Ethanolamine	Phosphatidylethanolamine (cephalin)
Serine	Phosphatidylserine
Inositol	Phosphatidylinositol
Glycerol linked to a second phosphatidic acid	Cardiolipin

   b. Long-chain fatty acids (12 or more carbons) are found in triacylglycerols (fat) and structural lipids.
   • They require the carnitine shuttle to move from the cytosol into the mitochondria.
 2. Unsaturated fatty acids contain one or more double bonds.
   • Double bonds in most naturally occurring fatty acids have the *cis* (not *trans*) configuration.
   a. *Trans* fatty acids are formed in the production of margarine and other hydrogenated vegetable oils and are a risk factor for atherosclerosis.
   b. Oxidation of unsaturated fatty acids in membrane lipids yields breakdown products that cause membrane damage, which can lead to hemolytic anemia (e.g., vitamin E deficiency).
B. Triacylglycerols, a highly concentrated energy reserve, are formed by esterification of fatty acids with glycerol.
   • Excess fatty acids in the diet, as well as fatty acids synthesized from excess dietary carbohydrate and protein, are converted to triacylglycerols and stored in adipose cells.
C. Phospholipids are derivatives of phosphatidic acid (diacylglycerol with a phosphate group on the third glycerol carbon) and constitute the major component of cellular membranes.
   • They are named for the X group esterified to the phosphate (Table 1-4).
 1. Fluidity of cellular membranes correlates inversely with the melting point of the fatty acids in membrane phospholipids.
 2. Phospholipases cleave specific bonds in phospholipids.
   a. Phospholipases A_1 and A_2, which remove fatty acyl groups, play a role in remodeling and degradation of phospholipids.

Trans fatty acids: margarine, risk factor for atherosclerosis

Phospholipase A2 in cell membranes: activated by Ca^{2+}, inactivated by corticosteroids

TABLE 1-5:
Sphingolipids

X Group	Sphingolipid Type
Phosphatidylcholine	Sphingomyelin
Galactose or glucose	Cerebroside
Sialic acid–containing oligosaccharide	Ganglioside

- Increased cytosolic Ca^{2+} activates phospholipase A_2, causing cell membrane damage in tissue hypoxia.
- Corticosteroids decrease phospholipase A_2 activity, thereby decreasing the release of arachidonic acid.
  - b. Phospholipase C liberates diacylglycerol and inositol triphosphate, two potent intracellular signals.
  - c. Phospholipase D generates phosphatidic acid from various phospholipids.
3. Lung surfactant, which decreases surface tension in the alveoli, contains abundant phospholipids, especially phosphatidylcholines.

Lung surfactant: decreases surface tension, deficient in RDS

- Respiratory distress syndrome (RDS, hyaline membrane disease) is associated with insufficient lung surfactant production in premature infants or in infants of diabetic mothers, leading to partial lung collapse and impaired gas exchange.
D. Sphingolipids are derivatives of ceramide, which is formed by esterification of a fatty acid with the amino group of sphingosine.
  - Sphingolipids are localized mainly in the white matter of the central nervous system.
  - Different sphingolipids are distinguished by the moiety (X group) attached to the terminal hydroxyl group of ceramide (Table 1-5).
  - Hereditary defects in the lysosomal enzymes that degrade sphingolipids cause sphingolipidoses such as Tay-Sachs disease and Gaucher's disease.
  1. Sphingomyelins: phosphorylcholine attached to ceramide; found in nerve tissue and blood
  2. Cerebrosides: one galactose or glucose unit joined in β-glycosidic linkage to ceramide; found largely in myelin sheath

Sphingolipidoses (e.g., Tay-Sachs disease): hereditary defects in lysosomal enzymes that degrade sphingolipids

  3. Gangliosides: oligosaccharide containing at least one sialic acid (N-acetyl neuraminic acid) residue linked to ceramide; found in myelin sheath
E. Steroids are lipids containing a characteristic fused ring system with a hydroxyl or keto group on carbon 3.
  1. Cholesterol is the most abundant steroid in mammalian tissue.
    - a. Important component of cellular membranes; modulates membrane fluidity
    - b. Precursor for synthesis of steroid hormones, skin-derived vitamin D, and bile acids

Cholesterol: precursor for steroid hormones, vitamin D, and bile acids

  2. Major steroid classes differ in total number of carbons and other minor variations (Fig. 1-2).
    - a. Cholesterol: 27 carbons
    - b. Bile acids: 24 carbons (derived from cholesterol)

C₂₇ Steroids

$$CH_3$$
$$H-C-CH_2-CH_2-CH_2-C-CH_3$$
$$CH_3$$

Cholesterol

C₂₄ Steroids (bile acids)

$$CH-CH_2-CH_2-COOH$$

Cholic acid

C₂₁ Steroids (progestins/adrenocortical steroids)

Progesterone

Cortisol

Aldosterone

C₁₉ Steroids (androgens)

Testosterone

C₁₈ Steroids (estrogens)

Estradiol-17β

1-2: *Steroid structures. A characteristic four-membered fused ring with a hydroxyl or keto group on C₃ are common structural features of steroids. The five major groups of steroids differ in the total number of carbon atoms. Cholesterol (top left), obtained from the diet and synthesized in the body, is the precursor for all other steroids.*

    c. Progesterone and adrenocortical steroids: 21 carbons
    d. Androgens: 19 carbons
    e. Estrogens: 18 carbons (derived from aromatization of androgens)
  F. Eicosanoids function as short-range, short-term signaling molecules.
    • Two pathways generate three groups of eicosanoids from arachidonic acid, a 20-carbon polyunsaturated ω-6 fatty acid that is released from membrane phospholipids by phospholipase A₂ (Fig. 1-3).
    1. Prostaglandins (PGs) are formed by the action of cyclooxygenase on arachidonic acid.

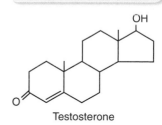
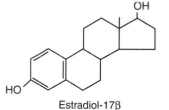
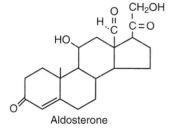

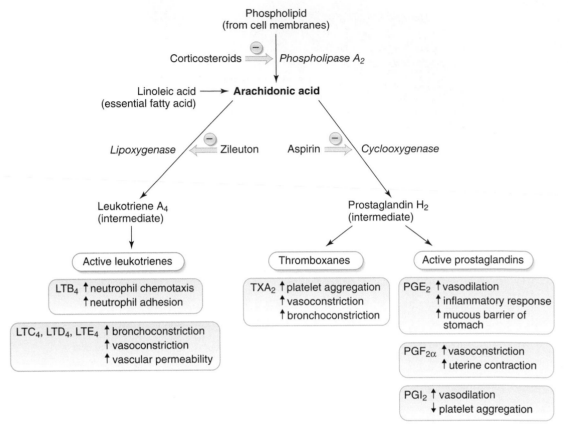

1-3: *Overview of eicosanoid biosynthesis and major effects of selected leukotrienes, thromboxanes, and prostaglandins. The active components of SRS-A (slow-reacting substance of anaphylaxis) are LTC$_4$, LTD$_4$, and LTE$_4$. PGI$_2$ is also known as prostacyclin and is synthesized in endothelial cells. The therapeutic effects of aspirin and zileuton result from their inhibition of the eicosanoid synthetic pathways. By inhibiting phospholipase A$_2$, corticosteroids inhibit the production of all the eicosanoids.*

- Prostaglandin H$_2$ (PGH$_2$), the first stable prostaglandin produced, is the precursor for other prostaglandins and for thromboxanes.
- Biological effects of prostaglandins are numerous and often related to their tissue-specific synthesis:
  a. Promote acute inflammation
  b. Stimulate or inhibit smooth muscle contraction, depending on type and tissue
  c. Promote vasodilation (e.g., afferent arterioles) or vasoconstriction (e.g., cerebral vessels), depending on type and tissue
2. Thromboxane A$_2$ (TXA$_2$) is produced in platelets by the action of thromboxane synthase on PGH$_2$.
   a. TXA$_2$ strongly promotes arteriole contraction and platelet aggregation.
   b. Dipyramidole inhibits thromboxane synthase.

    c. Aspirin and other nonsteroidal anti-inflammatory drugs (NSAIDs) acetylate and inhibit cyclooxygenase, leading to reduced synthesis of prostaglandins (anti-inflammatory effect) and of TXA_2 (antithrombotic effect due to reduced platelet aggregation).

  3. Leukotrienes (LTs) are noncyclic compounds whose synthesis begins with the hydroxylation of arachidonic acid by lipoxygenase.

    a. Leukotriene B_4 (LTB_4) is a strong chemotactic agent for neutrophils and promotes neutrophil adhesion to endothelial cells.

    b. Slow-reacting substance of anaphylaxis (SRS-A), which contains LTC_4, LTD_4, and LTE_4, is involved in allergic reactions (e.g., bronchoconstriction).

    c. Antileukotriene drugs include zileuton, which inhibits lipoxygenase, and zafirlukast and montelukast, which block leukotriene receptors on target cells.

      • These new drugs are used in the treatment of asthma, since LTC_4, LTD_4, and LTE_4 are potent bronchoconstrictors.

III. Amino Acids

  • Amino acids constitute the building blocks of proteins and also are precursors in the biosynthesis of numerous nonprotein nitrogen-containing compounds, including heme, purines, pyrimidines, and neurotransmitters (e.g., glycine and glutamate).

  • Ten of the 20 common amino acids are synthesized in the body; the others are essential and must be supplied in the diet.

  A. Basic structure of amino acids

    1. An α-carbon atom and four attached substituent groups constitute an amino acid.

      a. All amino acids possess an α-carboxyl group, α-amino group (or imino group), and hydrogen atom linked to the α-carbon.

      b. Unique side chain (R group) distinguishes one amino acid from another.

      c. The 20 common amino acids found in proteins are classified into three major groups based on the properties of their side chains: hydrophobic (nonpolar), uncharged hydrophilic (polar), or charged hydrophilic (polar).

        • Hydrophobic amino acids are most often located in the lipid portion of the cell membrane; hydrophilic amino acids are located on the outer and inner portions of the cell membrane.

      d. Asymmetry of α-carbon gives rise to two optically active isomers.

        (1) L form is unique to proteins.

        (2) D form occurs in bacterial cell walls and some antibiotics.

    2. Hydrophobic (nonpolar) amino acids have side chains that are largely insoluble in water (Table 1-6).

      a. Essential amino acids in this group are isoleucine, leucine, methionine, phenylalanine, tryptophan, and valine.

      b. Isoleucine, leucine, and valine are increased in maple syrup urine disease.

      c. Phenylalanine accumulates in phenylketonuria (PKU).

Prostaglandins: promote acute inflammation, inhibited by aspirin and NSAIDs

Isoleucine, leucine, and valine: branched-chain amino acids; increased in maple syrup urine disease

TABLE 1-6:
Hydrophobic (Nonpolar) Amino Acids

Amino Acid	Distinguishing Features
Glycine (Gly)	Smallest amino acid; inhibitory neurotransmitter of spinal cord; synthesis of heme; abundant in collagen
Alanine (Ala)	Alanine cycle during fasting; major substrate for gluconeogenesis
Valine (Val)*	Branched-chain amino acid; not degraded in liver; utilized by muscle; increased in maple syrup urine disease
Leucine (Leu)*	Branched-chain amino acid; not degraded in liver; ketogenic; utilized by muscle; increased in maple syrup urine disease
Isoleucine (Ile)*	Branched-chain amino acid; not degraded in liver; utilized by muscle; increased in maple syrup urine disease
Methionine (Met)*	Polypeptide chain initiation; methyl donor (as S-adenosyl methionine)
Proline (Pro)	Helix breaker; only amino acid with the side chain cyclized to α-amino group; hydroxylation in collagen aided by ascorbic acid; binding site for cross-bridges in collagen
Phenylalanine (Phe)*	Increased in PKU (phenylketonuria); aromatic side chains (increased in hepatic coma)
Tryptophan (Trp)*	Precursor of serotonin, niacin, and melatonin; aromatic side chains (increased in hepatic coma)

*Essential amino acids.

TABLE 1-7:
Uncharged Hydrophilic (Polar) Amino Acids

Amino Acid	Distinguishing Features
Cysteine (Cys)	Forms disulfide bonds; sensitive to oxidation; component of glutathione, an important antioxidant in RBCs
Serine (Ser)	Single-carbon donor; phosphorylated by kinases
Threonine (Thr)*	Phosphorylated by kinases
Tyrosine (Tyr)	Precursor of catecholamines, melanin, and thyroid hormones; phosphorylated by kinases; aromatic side chains (increased in hepatic coma); must be supplied in PKU (phenylketonuria); signal transduction (tyrosine kinase)
Asparagine (Asn)	Insufficiently synthesized by neoplastic cells; asparaginase used for treatment of leukemia
Glutamine (Gln)	Most abundant amino acid; major carrier of ammonia; nitrogen donor in synthesis of purines and pyrimidines; NH_3 detoxification in brain and liver; amino group carrier from skeletal muscle to other tissues in fasting state; fuel for kidney, intestine, and cells in immune system in fasting state

*Essential amino acids.

3. Uncharged hydrophilic (polar) amino acids have side chains that form hydrogen bonds (Table 1-7).
   a. Threonine is the only essential amino acid in this group.
   b. Tyrosine must be supplied in patients with PKU.
4. Charged hydrophilic (polar) amino acids have side chains that carry a net charge at or near neutral pH (Table 1-8).
   a. Essential amino acids in this group are arginine, histidine, and lysine.
   b. Arginine and histidine stimulate growth hormone and insulin and therefore are required for growth in children.
      • Both growth hormone and insulin increase amino acid uptake in muscle.

PKU: phenylalanine accumulates and tyrosine must be supplied

Arginine and histidine: stimulate growth hormone and insulin

TABLE 1-8:
Charged Hydrophilic (Polar) Amino Acids

Amino Acid	Distinguishing Features
Lysine (Lys)*	Basic; positive charge at pH 7; ketogenic; abundant in histones; hydroxylation in collagen aided by ascorbic acid; binding site for cross-bridges in collagen
Arginine (Arg)*	Basic; positive charge at pH 7; essential for growth in children; abundant in histones
Histidine (His)*	Basic; positive charge at pH 7; effective physiologic buffer; residue in hemoglobin coordinated to heme Fe^{2+}; essential for growth in children; zero charge at pH 7.40
Aspartate (Asp)	Acidic; strong negative charge at pH 7; forms oxaloacetate by transamination; important for binding properties of albumin
Glutamate (Glu)	Acidic; strong negative charge at pH 7; forms α-ketoglutarate by transamination; important for binding properties of albumin

*Essential amino acids.

B. Acid-base properties of amino acids
- Acidic groups (e.g., -COOH and $-NH_4^+$) are proton donors. Basic groups (e.g., $-COO^-$ and $-NH_3$) are proton acceptors.
- Each acidic or basic group within an amino acid has its own independent pK_a. Whether a functional group is protonated or dissociated, and to what extent, depends on its pK_a and the pH according to the Henderson-Hasselbalch equation:

$$pH = pK_a + \log \, [A^-]/[HA]$$

1. Overall charge on proteins depends primarily on the ionizable side chains of the following amino acids:
   a. Arginine and lysine (basic): positive charge at pH 7
   b. Histidine (basic): positive charge at pH 7
      - In the physiologic pH range (7.34 to 7.45), the imidazole side group ($pK_a = 6.0$) is an effective buffer (Box 1-1).
      - Histidine has a zero charge at pH 7.40.
   c. Aspartate and glutamate (acidic): negative charge at pH 7
      - Albumin has many of these acidic amino acids, which explains why it is a strong binding protein for calcium and other positively charged elements.
   d. Cysteine: negative charge at pH > 8
2. Isoelectric point (pI) is the pH value at which an amino acid (or protein) molecule has a net zero charge.
   a. When pH > pI, the net charge on molecule is negative.
   b. When pH < pI, the net charge on molecule is positive.
C. Modification of amino acid residues in proteins
- Some R groups can be modified after amino acids are incorporated into proteins.
1. Oxidation of sulfhydryl group (-SH) in cysteine forms a disulfide bond (-S-S-) with a second cysteine residue. This type of bond helps stabilize the structure of proteins, especially secreted proteins.

Physiologic pH: lysine, arginine, and histidine carry (+) charge; aspartate and glutamate carry (–) charge

BOX 1-1

BUFFERS AND THE CONTROL OF pH

Amino acids and other weak acids do not dissociate completely. Rather, they establish an equilibrium between the undissociated acid form (HA) and the dissociated conjugate base (A^-):

$$HA \rightleftharpoons H^+ + A^-$$

A mixture of a weak acid and its conjugate base acts as a buffer. Addition of acid or alkali to a buffer leads to a shift in the ratio of $[A^-]$ and $[HA]$, thereby minimizing the change in pH. The buffering ability of an acid-base pair is maximal when $pH = pK_a$, and buffering is effective within ± 1 pH unit of the pK_a. The principal buffer within the cytoplasm is the $H_2PO_4^-/HPO_4^{2-}$ conjugate pair ($pK_a = 6.7$). The pH of the blood (normally 7.37 to 7.43) is maintained mainly by the H_2CO_3/HCO_3^- buffer system; the numerator is primarily controlled by the lungs (retaining or blowing off CO_2), and the denominator is controlled by the kidneys.

- Hypoventilation causes an increase in arterial $[CO_2]$, leading to respiratory acidosis.
- Hyperventilation reduces arterial $[CO_2]$, leading to respiratory alkalosis.
- Metabolic acidosis results from conditions that cause a decrease in blood HCO_3^-, such as accumulation of lactic acid secondary to tissue hypoxia (shift to anaerobic metabolism) or of ketoacids in uncontrolled diabetes mellitus, or a loss of HCO_3^- due to fluid loss in diarrhea or to impaired kidney function (e.g., renal tubular acidosis).
- Metabolic alkalosis results from conditions that cause an increase in blood HCO_3^-, including persistent vomiting, use of thiazide diuretics with attendant loss of H^+, mineralocorticoid excess (e.g., primary aldosteronism), and ingestion of bicarbonate in antacid preparations.

2. Hydroxylation of proline and lysine yields hydroxyproline and hydroxylysine, which are important binding sites for cross-bridges in collagen.
    - Hydroxylation requires ascorbic acid.
3. Addition of sugar residues (glycosylation) to side chains of serine, threonine, and asparagine occurs during synthesis of many secreted and membrane proteins.
    - Glycosylation of proteins occurs in patients with poorly controlled diabetes mellitus (e.g., glycosylated hemoglobin and vessel basement membranes).
4. Phosphorylation of serine, threonine, or tyrosine residues modifies the activity of many proteins (e.g., inhibits glycogen synthase).

Proteins

I. Major Functions of Proteins
   A. Catalysis of biochemical reactions: enzymes
   B. Binding of molecules: antibodies, hemoglobin (Hb)
   C. Structural support: elastin, keratin, collagen
   D. Transport of molecules across cellular membranes: glucose transporters, Na^+/K^+ ATPase
   E. Signal transduction: receptor proteins, intracellular proteins (e.g., Ras)
   F. Coordinated movement of cells and cellular structures (e.g., myosin, dynein, tubulin, and actin)

II. Hierarchical Structure of Proteins
   A. Primary structure: linear sequence of amino acids composing a polypeptide or protein, which is specified by the gene encoding a complimentary RNA that is translated into a protein
      1. Peptide bond is the covalent amide linkage that joins amino acids in a protein.

2. Mutations that alter the primary structure of a protein often change its function and may change its charge, which affects its migration during protein electrophoresis.
   - Example: In hemoglobin electrophoresis, the sickle cell mutation alters the primary structure and the charge by changing glutamate to valine. This alters the migration of sickle cell hemoglobin on electrophoresis.
3. The primary structure of a protein determines its secondary (e.g., α-helices and β-sheets) and tertiary structures (overall three-dimensional structure).

B. Secondary structure: regular arrangements of portions of a polypeptide chain
   1. α-Helix is a spiral-shaped conformation of the polypeptide backbone with the side chains directed outward.
      a. Proline disrupts the α-helix because its α-imino group has no free hydrogen to contribute to the stabilizing hydrogen bonds.
      b. The leucine zipper is a supersecondary structure in which the leucine residues of one α-helix interdigitate with those of another α-helix to hold the proteins together in a dimer. Leucine zippers are commonly found in DNA-binding proteins (e.g., transcription factors).
   2. β-Sheet consists of laterally packed β-strands, which are extended regions of the polypeptide chain.
   3. Motifs are specific combinations of secondary structures that have a characteristic three-dimensional shape and occur in different proteins.
      a. These supersecondary structures often function in the binding of small ligands and ions or in protein-DNA interactions.
      b. The zinc finger is a supersecondary structure where Zn^{2+} is bound to two cysteine and two histidine residues. Zinc fingers are commonly found in receptors that have a DNA-binding domain that interacts with lipid-soluble hormones (e.g., cortisol).

C. Tertiary structure: three-dimensional folded structure of a polypeptide composed of distinct structural and functional regions, or domains; the native conformation

D. Quaternary structure: organization of multiple polypeptide chains (subunits) into functional multimeric protein
   1. Dimers containing two subunits (e.g., DNA-binding proteins) and tetramers (e.g., Hb) containing four subunits are most common.
   2. In Hb (an $\alpha_2\beta_2$ tetramer) and other proteins that exhibit cooperativity, a change in the shape of one subunit induces a change in the shape and function of an adjacent subunit, which for Hb alters its affinity for carrying O_2.

E. Disruption of stabilizing bonds (denaturation): unfolding of native conformation of a protein and loss of biological activity
   1. Secondary, tertiary, and quaternary structures are disrupted by denaturing agents, but the primary structure is not destroyed. Denaturing agents include:

Specific folding of primary structure determines the final native conformation.

Leucine zippers and zinc fingers: supersecondary structures commonly found in DNA-binding proteins

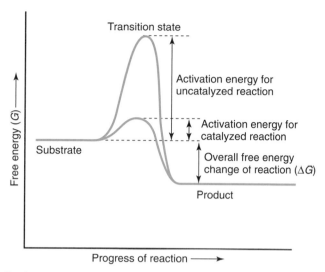

2-1: *Energy profiles for catalyzed and uncatalyzed reactions. Catalyzed reactions require less activation energy and are therefore accelerated. The equilibrium of a reaction is proportional to the overall change in free energy between substrate and product, ΔG, which must be negative for a reaction to proceed.*

    a. Extreme changes in pH or ionic strength
      • In tissue hypoxia, lactic acid accumulation in cells from anaerobic glycolysis causes denaturation of enzymes and proteins leading to coagulation necrosis.
    b. Detergents
    c. High temperature
    d. Heavy metals (arsenic, mercury, lead)
      • With heavy metal poisonings and nephrotoxic drugs (e.g., aminoglycosides), denaturation of proteins in the proximal tubules leads to coagulation necrosis (ischemic acute tubular necrosis, or ATN).
  2. Denatured polypeptide chains aggregate and become insoluble due to interactions of exposed hydrophobic side chains.
    • In glucose-6-phosphate dehydrogenase (G6PD) deficiency, increased peroxide in red blood cells (RBCs) leads to denaturation of Hb (oxidative damage) and formation of Heinz bodies.

III. Enzymes: Protein Catalysts
  A. General properties of enzymes
    1. Acceleration of reactions, the basic catalytic function of enzymes, results from their decreasing the activation energy of reactions (Fig. 2-1).
    2. High specificity of enzymes for substrates (reacting compounds) ensures that desired reactions occur in the absence of unwanted side reactions.
    3. Enzymes *do not* change the concentrations of substrates and products at equilibrium, but they do allow equilibrium to be reached more rapidly.
    4. No permanent change in enzymes occurs during the reactions they catalyze, although some undergo temporary changes.

Heavy metals, low intracellular pH: denature stabilizing bonds in proteins, causing loss of function

G6PD deficiency: increased peroxide in RBCs leads to Hb denaturation, formation of Heinz bodies

B. Coenzymes and prosthetic groups
   1. The activity of some enzymes depends on nonprotein organic molecules (e.g., coenzymes) or metal ions (e.g., cofactors) associated with the protein.
   2. Coenzymes are organic nonprotein compounds that bind reversibly to certain enzymes during a reaction and function as a cosubstrate.

   Many coenzymes are vitamin derivatives.

   a. Many coenzymes are vitamin derivatives (see Chapter 4).
   b. NAD^+ (nicotine adenine dinucleotide), a derivative of niacin, participates in many oxidation-reduction reactions (e.g., glycolytic pathway).
   c. Pyridoxal phosphate, derived from pyridoxine, functions in transamination reactions (e.g., alanine converted to pyruvic acid) and some amino acid decarboxylation reactions (e.g., histidine converted to histamine).
   d. Thiamine pyrophosphate is a coenzyme for enzymes catalyzing oxidative decarboxylation of α-keto acids (e.g., degradation of branched-chain amino acids) and for transketolase (e.g., two-carbon transfer reactions) in the pentose phosphate pathway.
   e. Tetrahydrofolate (THF), derived from folic acid, functions in one-carbon transfer reactions (e.g., conversion of serine to glycine).
   3. Prosthetic groups remain stably bound to the enzyme during the reaction.
   a. Biotin is covalently attached to enzymes that catalyze carboxylation reactions (e.g., pyruvate carboxylase).
   b. Metal ion cofactors (metalloenzymes) associate noncovalently with enzymes and may help orient substrates or function as electron carriers.
      (1) Magnesium (Mg): kinases
      (2) Zinc (Zn): carbonic anhydrase, collagenase, alcohol dehydrogenase, superoxide dismutase (neutralizes O_2 free radicals)
      (3) Copper (Cu): oxidases (e.g., lysyl oxidase for cross-bridging in collagen synthesis), ferroxidase (converts Fe^{3+} to Fe^{2+} to bind to transferrin)
      (4) Iron (Fe): cytochromes
      (5) Selenium (Se): glutathione peroxidase

Metal ion cofactors: Mg, Zn, Cu, Fe, Se

C. Active site
   1. In the native conformation of an enzyme, amino acid residues that are widely separated in the primary structure are brought into proximity to form the three-dimensional active site, which binds and activates substrates.
   2. Substrate binding often causes a conformational change in the enzyme (induced fit) that strengthens binding.
   3. Transition state represents an activated form of the substrate that immediately precedes formation of product (see Fig. 2-1).
   4. Precise orientation of amino acid side chains in the active site of an enzyme depends on the amino acid sequence, pH, temperature, and ionic strength. Mutations or nonphysiologic conditions that alter the active site cause a change in enzyme activity.

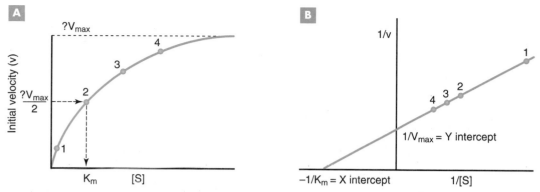

2-2: *Enzyme kinetic curves.* **A,** *Initial velocity (v) versus substrate concentration [S] at constant enzyme concentration for an enzymatic reaction with Michaelis-Menten kinetics.* **B,** *Lineweaver-Burk double reciprocal plot obtained from data points in* **A** *(1, 2, 3, 4).* K_m *and* V_{max} *are determined accurately from the intersection of the resulting straight line with the axes (horizontal and vertical axes, respectively).*

D. Enzyme kinetics
1. Reaction velocity (v), measured as the rate of product formation, always refers to the initial velocity after substrate is added to the enzyme.
2. Michaelis-Menten model involves a single substrate (S). Binding of substrate to enzyme (E) forms an enzyme-substrate complex (ES), which may react to form product (P) or dissociate without reacting:

$$E + S \rightleftharpoons ES \rightarrow E + P$$

3. Plot of initial velocity at different substrate concentrations, [S], (constant enzyme concentration) produces a rectangular hyperbola for reactions that fit the Michaelis-Menten model (Fig. 2-2A).
    a. Maximal velocity, V_{max}, is reached when the enzyme is fully saturated with substrate (i.e., all of the enzyme exists as ES).
        (1) In a zero-order reaction, velocity is independent of [S].
        (2) In a first-order reaction, velocity is proportional to [S].
    b. K_m, the substrate concentration at which the reaction velocity equals one-half of V_{max}, reflects the affinity of enzyme for substrate.
        (1) Low K_m enzymes have a high affinity for S (e.g., hexokinase).
        (2) High K_m enzymes have a low affinity for S (e.g., glucokinase).
4. Lineweaver-Burk plot, a double reciprocal plot of 1/v versus 1/[S], produces a straight line (Fig. 2-2B).
    a. Y intercept equals $1/V_{max}$.
    b. X intercept equals $1/K_m$.
5. Temperature and pH affect the velocity of enzyme-catalyzed reactions.
    a. Velocity increases as the temperature increases until a maximum (optimal) temperature is reached; then velocity decreases due to irreversible denaturation and loss of enzymatic activity.
    b. Changes in pH affect velocity by altering the ionization of residues at the active site and in the substrate.
        • Extremes of either high or low pH may cause denaturation.

Low K_m: high affinity of enzyme for substrate (e.g., hexokinase); high K_m: low affinity of enzyme for substrate (e.g., glucokinase)

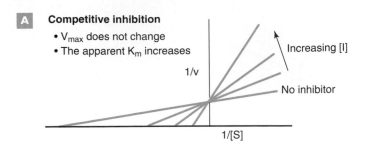

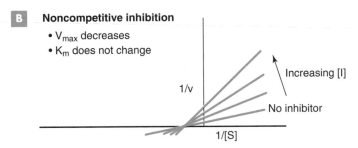

2-3: *Effect of competitive and noncompetitive inhibitors (I) on Lineweaver-Burk plots. Note that competitive inhibitor plots (**A**) intersect on the vertical axis (V$_{max}$ the same), whereas noncompetitive inhibitor plots (**B**) intersect on the horizontal axis (K$_m$ the same).*

     c. Velocity also increases with an increase in enzyme and substrate concentrations.

E. Enzyme inhibition

    1. Some drugs and toxins can reduce the catalytic activity of enzymes. Such inhibition is *not* part of the normal physiologic mechanism for regulating enzyme activity.

Competitive inhibition: ↑ K$_m$, V$_{max}$ unchanged; ↑ substrate reverses inhibition

    2. Competitive inhibitors are substrate analogues that compete with normal substrate for binding to the active site, forming an unreactive enzyme-inhibitor (EI) complex (Fig. 2-3A).

     a. K$_m$ is increased (X intercept in Lineweaver-Burk plot has smaller absolute value).

     b. V$_{max}$ is unchanged (Y intercept in Lineweaver-Burk plot is unaffected).

     c. Examples of competitive inhibitors

      (1) Methanol and ethylene glycol (antifreeze) compete with ethanol for binding sites to alcohol dehydrogenase. Infusing ethanol decreases the metabolism of methanol and ethylene glycol to toxic compounds.

      (2) Methotrexate, whose structure is similar to folic acid, competitively inhibits dihydrofolate reductase, preventing regeneration of tetrahydrofolate from dihydrofolate.

     d. High substrate concentration reverses competitive inhibition by saturating enzyme with substrate.

3. Noncompetitive inhibitors bind reversibly away from the active site, forming unreactive enzyme-inhibitor and enzyme-substrate-inhibitor complexes (Fig. 2-3B).
   a. K_m is unchanged (X intercept in Lineweaver-Burk plot is not affected).
   b. V_{max} is decreased (Y intercept in Lineweaver-Burk plot is larger).
   c. Examples of noncompetitive inhibitors
      (1) Physostigmine, a cholinesterase inhibitor used in the treatment of glaucoma
      (2) Captopril, an angiotensin-converting enzyme inhibitor used in the treatment of hypertension
      (3) Allopurinol, a noncompetitive inhibitor of xanthine oxidase, reduces formation of uric acid and is used in the treatment of gout.
   d. High substrate concentration does not reverse noncompetitive inhibition because inhibitor binding reduces the effective concentration of active enzyme.

Noncompetitive inhibition: ↓ V_{max}, K_m unchanged; ↑ substrate does not reverse inhibition

4. Irreversible inhibitors permanently inactivate enzymes.
   a. Heavy metals (often complexed to organic compounds) inhibit by binding tightly to sulfhydryl groups in enzymes and other proteins, causing widespread detrimental effects in the body.
   b. Aspirin acetylates the active site of cyclooxygenase, irreversibly inhibiting the enzyme and reducing the synthesis of prostaglandins and thromboxanes (see Fig. 1-3).
   c. Fluorouracil binds to thymidylate synthase like a normal substrate, but forms an intermediate that permanently blocks the enzyme's catalytic activity.
   d. Organophosphates in pesticides irreversibly inhibit cholinesterase.

Irreversible enzyme inhibitors: heavy metals, aspirin, fluorouracil, and organophosphates

5. Overcoming enzyme inhibition
   a. Effects of competitive and noncompetitive inhibitors dissipate as the inhibitor is inactivated in the liver or eliminated by the kidneys.
   b. Effects of irreversible inhibitors, which cause permanent enzyme inactivation, are only overcome by synthesis of a new enzyme.

F. Allosteric enzymes
1. Some enzymes and other proteins (e.g., Hb) exhibit changes in activity as the result of binding normal ligands.
2. Cooperativity, exhibited by many multimeric enzymes, occurs when binding of substrate (or other ligand) to one subunit increases binding of the same substrate to other subunits (homotropic effect).
   a. Enzymes shift from the less active T (tense) form to the more active R (relaxed) form as additional substrate molecules are bound.
   b. Sigmoidal shape of the plot of velocity versus [S] characterizes cooperativity.
3. Allosterism occurs when binding of one ligand by a protein increases or decreases its affinity for a different ligand (heterotropic effect).
   a. Allosteric effectors of enzymes are nonsubstrate molecules that bind to sites other than the active site and cause a change in conformation and activity.

b. Positive effectors stabilize the more active form so that the apparent K_m decreases (higher affinity for substrate). The velocity-versus-[S] curve is displaced to the left.

c. Negative effectors stabilize the less active form so that the apparent K_m increases (lower affinity for substrate). The velocity-versus-[S] curve is displaced to the right.

4. Examples of allosteric enzymes in the glycolytic pathway are glucokinase, phosphofructokinase, and pyruvate kinase.
   a. The enzymes can be inhibited or enhanced.
   b. These enzymes catalyze one-way reactions since they release so much energy; different enzymes are therefore required for gluconeogenesis.

5. Regulated enzymes generally catalyze rate-limiting steps at the beginning of metabolic pathways (e.g., aminolevulinic acid, or ALA, synthase at the beginning of heme synthesis).
   - The end-product of a regulated pathway is often an allosteric inhibitor of an enzyme near the beginning of the pathway (e.g., carbamyl phosphate synthetase II is inhibited by uridine triphosphate end-product, and ALA synthase is inhibited by heme, the end-product of porphyrin metabolism).

G. Cellular strategies for regulating metabolic pathways
   1. Compartmentation of enzymes within specific organelles can permanently separate competing metabolic pathways and control access of enzymes to substrates.
      - Example: Enzymes that synthesize fatty acids are located in the cytosol, whereas those that oxidize fatty acids are located in the mitochondrial matrix.
      - Other examples: alkaline phosphatase (cell membranes), aspartate aminotransferase (mitochondria), γ-glutamyl transferase (smooth endoplasmic reticulum), and myeloperoxidase (lysosomes)
   2. Change in gene expression leading to increased or decreased enzyme synthesis (i.e., induction or repression) can provide long-term regulation but has relatively slow response time (hours to days).
      - Example: Synthesis of fat-metabolizing enzymes in skeletal muscle is induced in response to aerobic exercise conditioning.

Feedback inhibition (allosteric regulation): end-product of a pathway inhibits starting enzyme

   3. Allosteric regulation can rapidly (seconds to minutes) increase or decrease operation of a metabolic pathway.
      - Example: Cytidine triphosphate, the end-product of the pyrimidine biosynthetic pathway, inhibits aspartate transcarbamoylase, the first enzyme in this pathway (feedback inhibition).
   4. Reversible phosphorylation and dephosphorylation is a common mechanism by which hormones regulate enzyme activity.
      a. Kinases phosphorylate serine, threonine, or tyrosine residues in regulated enzymes; phosphatases remove the phosphate groups (dephosphorylation).
      b. Reversible phosphorylation and dephosphorylation, often under hormonal control (e.g., glucagon), increases or decreases the activity of key enzymes.

- Example: Glycogen phosphorylase is activated by phosphorylation (protein kinase A), whereas glycogen synthase is inhibited.

5. Enzyme cascades, in which a series of enzymes sequentially activate each other, can amplify a small initial signal, leading to a large response.
    - Example: Binding of glucagon to its cell surface receptor on liver cells triggers a cascade that ultimately activates many glycogen phosphorylase molecules, which each catalyze production of numerous glucose molecules. This leads to a rapid increase in blood glucose.

6. Proenzymes (zymogens) are inactive storage forms that are activated as needed by proteolytic removal of an inhibitory fragment.
    a. Digestive proteases, such as pepsin and trypsin, are initially synthesized as proenzymes (e.g., pepsinogen, chymotrypsinogen) that are activated after their release into the stomach or small intestine.
    b. In acute pancreatitis, activation of zymogens (e.g., alcohol, hypercalcemia) leads to autodigestion of the pancreas.

H. Isoenzymes
1. Some multimeric enzymes have alternative forms, called isoenzymes, that differ in their subunit composition (derive from different genes) and can be separated by electrophoresis.
2. Different isoenzymes may be produced in different tissues.
    a. Creatine kinases: CK-MM predominates in skeletal muscle; CK-MB in cardiac muscle; and CK-BB in brain, smooth muscle, and the lungs.
    b. Of the five isoenzymes of lactate dehydrogenase, LDH_1 predominates in cardiac muscle and RBCs, and LDH_5 predominates in skeletal muscle and the liver.
3. Different isoenzymes may be localized to different cellular compartments.
    - Example: The cytosolic and mitochondrial forms of isocitrate dehydrogenase
4. Isoforms are subtypes of the individual isoenzymes (e.g., CK-MM isoforms).

I. Diagnostic enzymology
1. Plasma in normal patients contains few active enzymes (e.g., clotting factors).
2. Because tissue necrosis causes the release of enzymes into serum, the appearance of tissue-specific enzymes or isoenzymes in the serum is useful in diagnosing some disorders and estimating the extent of damage (Table 2-1).

IV. Hemoglobin and Myoglobin: O_2 Binding Proteins
A. Structure of Hb and myoglobin
1. Adult hemoglobin (HbA) is a tetrameric protein composed of two α-globin subunits and two β-globin subunits.
    a. A different globin gene encodes each type of subunit.
    b. All globins have a largely α-helical secondary structure and are folded into a compact, spherical tertiary structure.

Proenzymes, or zymogens: inactive storage forms activated as needed (e.g., digestive proteases)

Serum enzyme markers: used for diagnosis; few active enzymes in normal plasma

TABLE 2-1:

Serum Enzyme Markers Useful in Diagnosis

Serum Enzyme	Major Diagnostic Use
Alanine aminotransferase (ALT)	Viral hepatitis (ALT > AST)
Aspartate aminotransferase (AST)	Alcoholic hepatitis (AST > ALT)
	Myocardial infarction (AST only)
Alkaline phosphatase	Osteoblastic bone disease (e.g., fracture repair, Paget's disease, metastatic prostate cancer), obstructive liver disease
Amylase	Acute pancreatitis, mumps (parotitis)
Creatine kinase (CK)	Myocardial infarction (CK-MB)
	Duchenne muscular dystrophy (CK-MM)
γ-Glutamyl transferase (GGT)	Obstructive liver disease, increased in alcoholics
Lactate dehydrogenase (LDH, type I)	Myocardial infarction
Lipase	Acute pancreatitis (more specific than amylase)

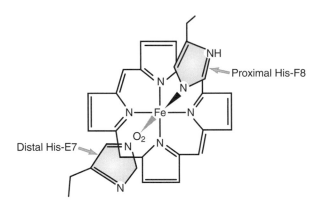

2-4: *Structure of heme showing its relation to two histidines (shaded) in the globin chain. Heme is located within a crevice in the globin chains. Reduced ferrous iron (Fe2+) forms four coordination bonds to the pyrrole rings of heme and one to the proximal histidine of globin. The sixth coordination bond position is used to bind O₂ or is unoccupied. The side chains attached to the porphyrin ring are omitted.*

2. One heme prosthetic group is located within a hydrophobic pocket in each subunit of Hb (total of four heme groups).
   a. The heme molecule is an iron-containing porphyrin ring (Fig. 2-4).
      • Defects in heme synthesis cause porphyria and sideroblastic anemias (e.g., lead poisoning).
   b. Iron normally is in reduced form (Fe^{2+}), which binds O_2.
   c. In methemoglobin, iron is in oxidized form (Fe^{3+}), which cannot bind O_2.
      • An increase in methemoglobin causes cyanosis since heme groups cannot bind to O_2, which decreases the O_2 saturation.
3. Myoglobin is a monomeric heme-containing protein whose tertiary structure is very similar to that of α-globin or β-globin.

B. Functional differences between Hb and myoglobin
   1. Differences in the functional properties of hemoglobin (four heme groups) and myoglobin (one heme group) are largely due to the presence or absence of the quaternary structure in these proteins (Table 2-2).

Hb has four heme groups to bind O₂; myoglobin has one heme group.

TABLE 2-2:

Comparison of Hemoglobin and Myoglobin

Characteristic	Hemoglobin	Myoglobin
Function	O_2 transport	O_2 storage
Location	In RBCs	In skeletal muscle
Amount of O_2 bound at P_{O_2} in lungs	High	High
Amount of O_2 bound at P_{O_2} in tissues	Low	High
Quaternary structure	Yes (tetramer)	No (monomer)
Binding curve (% saturation vs P_{O_2})	Sigmoidal (cooperative binding of multiple ligand molecules)	Hyperbolic (binding of one ligand molecule in reversible equilibrium)
Number of heme groups	Four	One

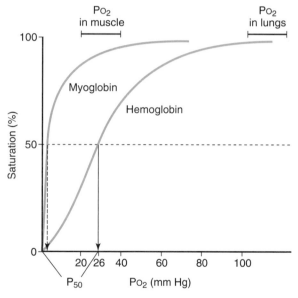

2-5: O_2 binding curve for hemoglobin and myoglobin. P_{50}, the P_{O_2} corresponding to 50% saturation, is equivalent to K_m for an enzymatic reaction. The lower the value of P_{50}, the greater the affinity for O_2. The very low P_{50} for myoglobin ensures that O_2 remains bound, except under hypoxic conditions. Note the sigmoidal shape of the Hb curve, which is indicative of multiple subunits and cooperative binding. The myoglobin curve is hyperbolic, indicating noncooperative binding of O_2.

2. Sigmoidal O_2 binding curve for Hb indicates that binding (and dissociation) is cooperative (Fig. 2-5).
   a. Binding of O_2 to the first subunit of deoxyhemoglobin increases the affinity for O_2 of other subunits.
   b. During successive oxygenation of subunits, their conformation changes from the deoxygenated T form (low O_2 affinity, right shift of the O_2-binding curve) to the oxygenated R form (high O_2 affinity, left shift of the O_2-binding curve).

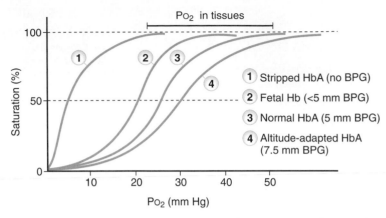

2-6: *Effect of 2,3-BPG on O_2 binding by Hb. In HbA stripped of 2,3-BPG, the O_2 affinity is so high that Hb would remain nearly saturated at Po_2 values typical of tissues.*

    c. Hb has high O_2 affinity at high Po_2 (in lungs) and low O_2 affinity at low Po_2 (in tissues), making it a good O_2 transport protein.

3. Hyperbolic O_2 binding curve for myoglobin indicates that it lacks cooperativity (as expected for a monomeric protein).
   - Myoglobin is saturated at normal Po_2 in skeletal muscle and releases O_2 only when tissue becomes hypoxic, making it a good O_2 storage protein.

4. Carbon monoxide (CO)
   a. Hb and myoglobin have a 200-fold greater affinity for CO than for O_2.
   b. CO binds at the same sites as O_2 so that relatively small amounts rapidly cause hypoxia due to a decrease in O_2 saturation of Hb (fewer heme groups occupied by O_2).
   c. CO poisoning produces cherry red discoloration of the skin and organs. It is treated with 100% O_2 or hyperbaric O_2.

C. Factors affecting O_2 binding by Hb
   1. Shift in O_2 binding curve indicates a change in Hb affinity for O_2.
      a. Left shift = increased affinity, which promotes O_2 loading.
      b. Right shift = decreased affinity, which promotes O_2 unloading.
   2. Binding of 2,3-bisphosphoglycerate (2,3-BPG), H^+ ions, or CO_2 to Hb stabilizes the T form and reduces affinity for O_2.
      a. 2,3-BPG, a normal product of glycolysis in erythrocytes, is critical to the release of O_2 from Hb at Po_2 values found in tissues (Fig. 2-6).
         - 1,3-BPG in glycolysis is converted into 2,3-BPG by a mutase.
      b. Elevated levels of H^+ and CO_2 (acidotic conditions) within erythrocytes in tissues also promote unloading of O_2.
         (1) The acidotic environment in tissue causes a right shift of the O_2 binding curve, thus ensuring release of O_2 to tissue.
         (2) Bohr effect is the decrease in the affinity of Hb for O_2 as the pH drops (increased acidity).
      c. Chronic hypoxia at high altitude increases synthesis of 2,3-BPG, causing a right shift of the O_2 binding curve.

Both CO and methemoglobin (Fe^{3+}) decrease O_2 saturation of blood.

A

In systemic capillaries
High CO_2 pressure
Low O_2 pressure

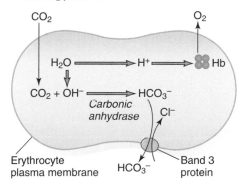

B

In pulmonary capillaries
Low CO_2 pressure
High O_2 pressure

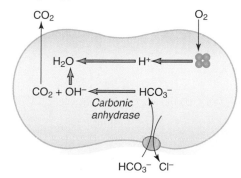

2-7: *Interrelation between the transport of CO_2 and O_2 in the blood.* **A,** *Most of the CO_2 that enters erythrocytes in peripheral capillaries is converted to HCO_3^- and H^+. The resulting decrease in intracellular pH leads to protonation of histidine residue in Hb, reducing its O_2 affinity and promoting O_2 release. HCO_3^- exits the cell in exchange for Cl^- (chloride shift) via an ion-exchange protein (band 3 protein), shifting the equilibrium so that more CO_2 can enter.* **B,** *Within the lungs, reversal of these reactions leads to release of CO_2 and uptake of O_2.*

    d. Increase in temperature decreases O_2 affinity and promotes O_2 unloading from Hb during the accelerated metabolism that accompanies a fever.
      • Reduction of fever with antipyretics may be harmful since neutrophils require molecular O_2 in the O_2-dependent myeloperoxidase system to kill bacteria.

   3. The following factors all promote increased O_2 affinity of Hb and cause a left shift of the O_2 binding curve:
    a. Decreased 2,3-BPG
    b. Carbon monoxide
    c. Methemoglobin
    d. Hypothermia
    e. Alkalosis
    f. Fetal hemoglobin (HbF)

D. Role of Hb and bicarbonate (HCO_3^-) in CO_2 transport
   1. CO_2 produced in tissues diffuses into RBCs and either combines with Hb or is converted to HCO_3^-.
   2. About 20% of the CO_2 in blood is transported as carbamino Hb.
    • CO_2 reacts with the N-terminal amino group of globin chains, forming carbamate derivative.
   3. About 70% of the CO_2 in blood is in the form of HCO_3^- (Fig. 2-7).
    • Carbonic anhydrase within RBCs rapidly converts CO_2 from tissues to HCO_3^-, which exits the cell in exchange for Cl^- (chloride shift). In the lungs, the process reverses.
   4. About 10% of the CO_2 in blood is dissolved in plasma.

Right shift of O_2-binding curve: ↑ 2,3-BPG, acidotic state, high altitude, fever promote O_2 unloading from Hb to tissues

Left shift of O_2-binding curve: ↓ 2,3-BPG, CO, methemoglobin, hypothermia, alkalosis, HbF promote increased O_2 affinity of Hb

HCO_3^-: major vehicle for carrying CO_2 in blood

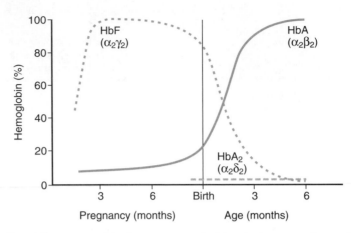

2-8: *Hb profile at different stages of development. In normal adults, HbA (consisting of two α-chains and two β-chains) constitutes >95% of total Hb; HbA$_2$ (two α-chains and two δ-chains) and HbF (two α-chains and two γ-chains), each approximately 1% or 2%. Note that β-chain production does not occur until after birth. HbA$_{1c}$, a glycosylated form of HbA, constitutes approximately 5% of the total Hb in normal adults but is elevated in diabetics. HbA$_{1c}$ is an excellent marker for long-term glycemic control.*

E. Other normal Hbs
   1. Several normal types of Hb are produced in humans at different developmental stages (Fig. 2-8).
   2. HbA$_{1c}$, a type of glycosylated Hb, is formed by a spontaneous binding (nonenzymatic glycosylation) of blood glucose to the terminal amino group of the β subunits in HbA.
      a. In normal adults, HbA$_{1c}$ constitutes about 5% of total Hb (HbA accounts for more than 95%).
      b. Uncontrolled diabetes mellitus (elevated blood glucose) is associated with elevated HbA$_{1c}$ concentration.
         • HbA$_{1c}$ concentration indicates the levels of blood glucose over the previous 4 to 8 weeks, or roughly the lifespan of an RBC, and serves as a marker for long-term glycemic control.
   3. HbF has higher affinity for O$_2$ than HbA, permitting O$_2$ to flow from maternal circulation to fetal circulation in the placenta.
      • Greater O$_2$ affinity of HbF results from its weaker binding of the negative allosteric effector 2,3-BPG compared to HbA (see Fig. 2-6).
F. Hemoglobinopathies due to structural alterations in globin chains
   1. Sickle cell hemoglobin (HbS) results from a mutation that replaces glutamic acid with valine at residue 6 in β-globin (β6 Glu → Val) and primarily affects individuals of African American descent.
      a. Deoxygenated HbS forms large linear polymers, causing normally flexible erythrocytes to become stiff and sickle shaped. Sickled cells plug venules, preventing capillaries from draining.
      b. Sickle cell anemia: homozygous condition
         (1) Sickle cell anemia is an autosomal recessive (AR) disorder.

HbA$_{1c}$: marker for long-term glycemic control

      (2) Hb profile: 85% to 95% HbS; small amounts of HbF and HbA_2 (no HbA)

      (3) Marked by severe hemolytic anemia, multiorgan pain due to microvascular occlusion, autosplenectomy, periodic attacks of acute symptoms (sickle cell crises), and osteomyelitis *(Salmonella)* and *Streptococcus pneumoniae* sepsis.

      (4) HbF inhibits sickling; hence, increased levels of HbF reduce the number of crises.

      (5) Hydroxyurea increases synthesis of HbF.

   c. Sickle cell trait: heterozygous condition

      (1) Hb profile: 55% to 60% HbA; 40% to 45% HbS; small amounts of HbA_{1c}, HbF, and HbA_2

      (2) Usually asymptomatic, except in the renal medulla, where O_2 tensions are low enough to induce sickling and renal damage (e.g., renal papillary necrosis)

> Deoxygenated sickled RBCs: block circulation; HbF inhibits sickling.

2. Hemoglobin C (HbC) results from substitution of lysine for glutamate at position 6 in β-globin (β6 Glu → Lys).

   • Although HbC and HbS are mutated at the same site, HbC is associated only with a mild chronic anemia in homozygotes.

3. Hereditary methemoglobinemia results from any one of several single amino acid substitutions that stabilize heme iron in the oxidized form (HbM).

   a. Characterized by slate-gray cyanosis in early infancy without pulmonary or cardiac disease

   b. Exhibits autosomal dominant (AD) inheritance

4. Acquired methemoglobinemia results from exposure to nitrate and nitrite compounds, sulfonamides, and aniline dyes. These chemicals convert Hb to methemoglobin (heme Fe^{3+}), which does not bind O_2 (low O_2 saturation).

   a. Symptoms such as cyanosis, headache, and dizziness occur.

   b. Intravenous methylene blue (primary treatment) and ascorbic acid (ancillary treatment) help reduce Fe^{3+} to the Fe^{2+} state.

G. Hemoglobinopathies due to altered rates of globin synthesis

  1. A group of microcytic anemias are caused by mutations that lead to the absence or reduced production of α-globin or β-globin.

  2. β-Thalassemias (ARs) result from mutation in the single β-globin gene on chromosome 11 and are most prevalent in Mediterranean and African American populations.

   a. Thalassemia major (homozygous), also known as Cooley's anemia, is lethal by adulthood.

      (1) HbF and HbA2 are produced, but there is little or no HbA.

      (2) As HbF production decreases following birth, progressively severe anemia develops with bone distortions, splenomegaly, and hemosiderosis (iron overload from blood transfusions).

   b. Thalassemia minor (heterozygous condition) is characterized by mild anemia, with a slight decrease in HbA (decrease in β-globin chains) and an increase in both HbA2 and HbF.

> Mild β-thalassemia (microcytic anemia): slightly decreased HbA, increased HbA_2 and HbF

3. ARs result from deletion of one or more of the four α-globin genes on chromosome 16 and are most prevalent in Asian and African American populations.

    a. Since two copies (alleles) of each α-globin gene are present, four mutant phenotypes are possible, depending on the number of alleles that are affected.

    b. Deletion of all four α-globin genes (homozygous condition) is incompatible with life and results in intrauterine death (called Hb Bart's disease).
- Hb Bart's hemoglobin consists of four γ-globin chains.

    c. Deletion of one to three α-globin genes (heterozygous condition) results in progressively more severe microcytic anemia.
- Deletion of three alleles is called HbH disease (HbH hemoglobin consists of four β-globin chains).

    d. Hb electrophoresis in mild α-thalassemia (one or two gene deletions) is normal since HbA, HbA2, and HbF all require α-globin chains and all are equally decreased.

Mild α-thalassemia (microcytic anemia): normal Hb electrophoresis

V. Collagen: Prototypical Fibrous Protein

  A. Collagen, the most abundant protein in the body, is the major fibrous component of connective tissue (e.g., bone, cartilage).
- Fibrous proteins (e.g., collagen, keratin, elastin) provide structural support for cells and tissues.

  B. Tropocollagen, the basic structural unit of collagen, is a right-handed triple helix of α-chains (Fig. 2-9A).

    1. α-Chains, the individual polypeptides composing tropocollagen, consist largely of -Gly-X-Y- repeats.

      a. Proline and hydroxyproline (or hydroxylysine) are often present in the X and Y positions, respectively.

      b. Hydroxylation of proline and lysine in α-chains occurs in the rough endoplasmic reticulum (RER) in a reaction that requires ascorbic acid (vitamin C).

    2. Procollagen triple helix assembles spontaneously from hydroxylated and glycosylated helical α-chains in the RER.

    3. Extracellular peptidases remove terminal propeptides from procollagen after it is secreted, yielding tropocollagen.

  C. Collagen fibrils form spontaneously from tropocollagen and are stabilized by covalent cross-links between lysine and hydroxylysine residues on adjacent chains (Fig. 2-9B).

Ascorbic acid: hydroxylation of proline and lysine in collagen synthesis; promotes cross-bridging

    1. Lysyl oxidase, an extracellular Cu^{2+}-containing enzyme, oxidizes the lysine side chain to reactive aldehydes (site of proline and lysine hydroxylation) that spontaneously form cross-links, which increase the tensile strength of collagen.

    2. Cross-link formation continues throughout life, causing collagen to stiffen with age.
- Increased cross-linking associated with aging decreases the elasticity of skin and joints.

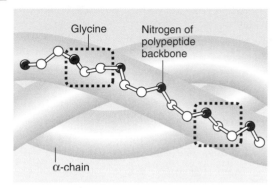

A   **Tropocollagen triple helix**

Glycine

Nitrogen of
polypeptide
backbone

α-chain

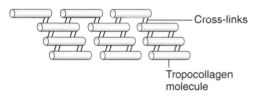

B   **Collagen fibril**

Cross-links

Tropocollagen
molecule

2-9: *Collagen structure.* **A,** *Triple-stranded helix of tropocollagen, the structural unit of collagen. In all α-chains, much of the sequence contains glycine at every third position (boxes). Proline and hydroxyproline (or hydroxylysine) commonly occupy the other two positions in the -Gly-X-Y- repeats.* **B,** *Note the typical staggered array of linked tropocollagen molecules in fibrils of fibrous collagen. The cross-links increase the tensile strength of collagen.*

    3. Deficient cross-linking reduces the tensile strength of collagen fibers.

  D. Different collagen types contain α-chains that vary slightly in amino acid composition.

    1. Fibrous collagens, which constitute about 70% of the total, have fibrillar structure (see Fig. 2-9B).

      a. Type I: skin, bone, tendons, cornea

      b. Type II: cartilage, intervertebral disks

      c. Type III: blood vessels, lymph nodes, dermis, early phases of wound repair

      d. Type X: epiphyseal plates

    2. Type IV collagen forms flexible, sheetlike networks and is present within all basement membranes.

      • In Goodpasture's syndrome, antibodies are directed against the basement membrane of pulmonary and glomerular capillaries.

  E. Collagen disorders may result from mutations in α-chain genes or defects in the synthetic pathway.

    1. Ehlers-Danlos syndrome (multiple types of Mendelian defects) is associated with hyperextensive joints, hyperelasticity of skin, dissecting aortic aneurysms, rupture of the colon, and vessel instability resulting in skin hemorrhages.

Ehlers-Danlos syndrome:
loose joints, hyperelastic
skin, dissecting aortic
aneurysms, colon
rupture, collagen defects

a. Ehlers-Danlos syndrome is caused by mutations in α-chains resulting in abnormalities in collagen structure, synthesis, secretion, or degradation.

b. Types I and III collagen are most often affected.

Osteogenesis imperfecta: decreased synthesis of type I collagen; pathologic fractures, blue sclera

2. Osteogenesis imperfecta (brittle bone disease) results from a deficiency in the synthesis of type I collagen and is marked by multiple fractures, retarded wound healing, hearing loss, and blue sclera.

a. Blue sclera is due to a thinning of the sclera from loss of collagen, allowing visualization of the underlying choroidal veins.

b. Osteogenesis imperfecta is predominantly an AD disorder.

Alport's syndrome: defective type IV collagen; nephritis, hearing loss, ocular defects

3. Alport's syndrome, an X-linked dominant disease caused by defective type IV collagen, is characterized by glomerulonephritis, sensorineural hearing loss, and ocular defects.

4. Scurvy is caused by prolonged deficiency of vitamin C, which is needed for hydroxylation of proline and lysine residues in collagen.

a. Hemorrhages in the skin, bleeding gums leading to loosened teeth, bone pain, hemarthroses (vessel instability), perifollicular hemorrhage, and a painful tongue (glossitis) eventually develop.

Scurvy: tensile strength of collagen weakened due to lack of cross-bridges

b. The tensile strength of collagen is decreased due to lack of cross-bridging.

3 CHAPTER

Membrane Biochemistry and Signal Transduction

I. Membrane Function
   A. Separation of cell contents from external environment (plasma membrane)
   B. Compartmentalization of intracellular enzyme systems (organelle membranes)
   C. Catalytic activity due to membrane-associated enzymes (e.g., phospholipases, adenylate cyclase)
   D. Regulation of intracellular environment by action of membrane transport proteins that confer selective permeability (e.g., Na^+/K^+ ATPase channel)
   E. Cell-cell communication mediated by receptor proteins linked to intracellular signal transduction pathways (e.g., G protein-associated receptors)

II. Basic Properties of Membranes
   A. Membrane components

1. Cell membrane lipids are arranged in two monolayers, or leaflets, to form the lipid bilayer, the basic structural unit of cellular membranes.
   a. Lipid composition differs within membranes of the same cell type, but phospholipids are the major lipid component of most membranes.
      • In membranes, the hydrophilic portion of the phospholipids is oriented facing outward toward the surrounding aqueous environment, and the hydrophobic portion is oriented facing inward toward the center of the bilayer.
   b. Cholesterol is present in both the inner and the outer leaflets.
   c. Phosphatidylcholine and sphingomyelin are found predominantly in the outer leaflet of the erythrocyte plasma membrane.
   d. Phosphatidylserine and phosphatidylethanolamine are found predominantly in the inner leaflet of the erythrocyte plasma membrane.

Cholesterol: present in inner and outer leaflets of cell membrane

2. Proteins constitute 40% to 50% by weight of most cellular membranes.
   • The particular proteins associated with each type of cellular membrane are largely responsible for its unique functional properties.
3. Carbohydrates in membranes are present only as extracellular moieties covalently linked to some membrane lipids (glycolipids) and proteins (glycoproteins).

B. Association of membrane proteins with the lipid bilayer
   1. Integral (intrinsic) proteins that span the entire bilayer, called transmembrane proteins, interface with the cytosol and the external environment.
      • Examples: Transport proteins (e.g., glucose transporters), receptors for water-soluble extracellular signaling molecules (e.g., peptide hormones), and energy-transducing proteins (e.g., adenosine triphosphate [ATP] synthase)
   2. Peripheral (extrinsic) proteins are loosely associated with the surface of either side of the membrane.
      • Examples: Protein kinase C on the cytosolic side and certain extracellular matrix proteins on the external side
   3. Lipid-anchored proteins are tethered to the inner or outer membrane leaflet by a covalently attached lipid group (e.g., isoprenyl group to RAS molecule).
      a. Alkaline phosphatase is anchored to the outer leaflet.
      b. RAS and other G proteins (key signal-transducing proteins) are anchored to the inner leaflet.

RAS and other G proteins (key signal-transducing proteins): anchored to inner leaflet of cell membrane

C. Fluid properties of membranes
   1. Membrane fluidity is controlled by several factors:
      a. Long-chain saturated fatty acids interact strongly with each other and decrease fluidity.
      b. *Cis* unsaturated fatty acids disrupt the interaction of fatty acyl chains and increase fluidity.
      c. Cholesterol prevents the movement of fatty acyl chains and decreases fluidity.

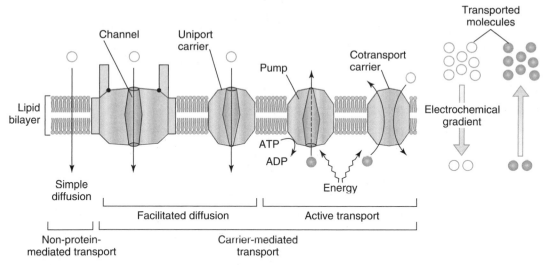

3-1: *Overview of various types of membrane transport mechanisms. Open circles represent molecules that are moving down their electrochemical gradient by simple or facilitated diffusion. Shaded circles represent molecules that are moving against their electrochemical gradient, which requires an input of cellular energy by active transport. Primary active transport is unidirectional and utilizes pumps, whereas secondary active transport takes place via cotransport carrier proteins.*

        d. Higher temperatures favor a disordered state of fatty acids and increase fluidity.

    2. Lateral movement is restricted by the presence of cell-cell junctions in the membrane or by interactions between membrane proteins and the extracellular matrix.

III. Movement of Molecules and Ions across Membranes (Fig. 3-1 and Table 3-1)

    A. Simple diffusion of molecules or ions down the concentration gradient requires no additional energy and occurs without aid of a membrane protein.

        1. A limited number of substances cross membranes by simple diffusion.

            a. Gases (O_2, CO_2, nitric oxide)

            b. Small uncharged polar molecules (water, ethanol, short-chain neutral fatty acids)

            c. Lipophilic molecules (steroids)

        2. Transport in either direction occurs, with net transport depending only on the direction of the gradient.

        3. Rate of diffusion depends on the size of the transported molecule and gradient steepness.

            a. Smaller molecules diffuse faster than larger molecules.

            b. A steep concentration gradient produces faster diffusion than a shallow gradient.

    B. Facilitated diffusion requires the aid of specialized membrane proteins that move molecules across the membrane down the concentration gradient without input of cellular energy.

Passive transport: movement of molecules across membrane down concentration gradient by simple or facilitated diffusion

TABLE 3-1:

Mechanisms for Transporting Small Molecules and Ions across Biomembranes

Property	Passive Diffusion	Facilitated Diffusion	Primary Active Transport	Secondary Active Transport
Requires transport protein	−	+	+	+
Works against gradient	−	−	+	+
Coupled to ATP hydrolysis	−	−	+ (directly)	− (indirectly)
Powered by movement of cotransported ion	−	−	−	+
Examples of transported molecules	O_2, CO_2, many drugs, steroid hormones	Glucose and amino acids (most cells); Cl^- and HCO_3^- exchange (RBCs)	Na^+/K^+, Ca^{2+}	Glucose and amino acids (intestine and kidney tubule); Ca^{2+} (cardiac muscle)

1. Ion channels are protein-lined passageways through which ions flow at a high rate when the channel is open.
   a. Many channels, which are usually closed, open in response to specific signals.
   b. Nicotinic acetylcholine (ACh) receptor in the plasma membrane of skeletal muscle is a Na^+K^+ channel that opens on binding of an ACh.
2. Uniport carrier proteins facilitate diffusion of a single substance (e.g., glucose, particular amino acid).
   a. Na^+-independent glucose transporters (GLUTs) are uniporters that passively transport glucose, galactose, and/or fructose from the blood into most cell types down a steep concentration gradient (Table 3-2).
   b. Cycling of the uniporter between alternative conformations allows binding and release of transported molecule (Fig. 3-2).
   c. Direction of transport by the uniporter depends on the direction of the concentration gradient for the transported molecule.
3. Cotransport carrier proteins mediate movement of two different substances at the same time via facilitated diffusion or secondary active transport.
   a. The direction of transport depends on the direction of the gradients for the transported molecules (similar to uniporters).
   b. Symporters move both transported substances in the same direction.
   c. Antiporters move the transported substances in opposite directions.
   • Example: Cl^-/HCO_3^- exchange protein (band 3 protein) in erythrocyte membrane, an antiporter that facilitates diffusion of Cl^- and HCO_3^-, functions in the transport of CO_2 from tissues to the lungs (see Fig. 2-7).

Primary active transport: energy-requiring movement of molecules across membrane against concentration gradient, coupled directly to ATP hydrolysis

TABLE 3-2:

Hexose Transport Proteins

Transporter	Primary Tissue Location	Specificity/Physiologic Functions
GLUT1	Most cell types (e.g., brain, erythrocytes, endothelial cells, fetal tissues) but *not* kidney and small intestinal epithelial cells	Transports glucose (high affinity) and galactose but not fructose; mediates basal glucose uptake
GLUT2	Hepatocytes, pancreatic β cells, epithelial cells of small intestine and kidney tubules (basolateral surface)	Transports glucose (low affinity), galactose, and fructose; mediates high-capacity glucose uptake by liver at high blood glucose levels; serves as "glucose sensor" for β cells (insulin independent); exports glucose into blood after its uptake from lumen of intestine and kidney tubules
GLUT3	Neurons, placenta, testes	Transports glucose (high affinity) and galactose but not fructose; mediates basal glucose uptake
GLUT4	Skeletal and cardiac muscle, adipocytes	Mediates uptake of glucose (high affinity) in response to insulin stimulation, which induces translocation of GLUT4 transporters from the Golgi apparatus to the cell surface
GLUT5	Small intestine, sperm, kidney, brain, muscle, adipocytes	Transports fructose (high affinity) but not glucose or galactose
GLUT7	Membrane of endoplasmic reticulum (ER) in hepatocytes	Transports free glucose produced in ER by glucose-6-phosphatase to cytosol for release into blood by GLUT2
SGLUT1 (Na^+/K^+ symporter)	Epithelial cells of small intestine and kidney tubules (apical surface)	Cotransports glucose or galactose (but not fructose) and Na^+ in same direction; mediates uptake of sugar from lumen against its concentration gradient powered by coupled transport of Na^+ down its gradient

C. Primary active transport pumps move molecules or ions against the concentration gradient with energy supplied by coupled ATP hydrolysis.
  1. Pumps mediate unidirectional movement of each molecule transported.
  2. Na^+/K^+ ATPase pump, located in the plasma membrane of every cell, maintains low intracellular Na^+ and high intracellular K^+ concentrations relative to the external environment.
     a. Hydrolysis of 1 ATP is coupled to the translocation of 3 Na^+ outward and 2 K^+ inward against their concentration gradients.
     b. Cardiotonic steroids, including digitalis and ouabain, specifically inhibit the Na^+/K^+ ATPase pump.
     c. Albuterol enhances the pump and drives K^+ from the extracellular compartment into the cell.

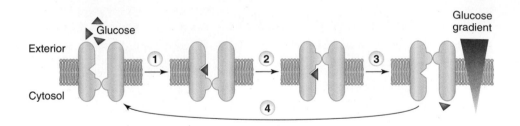

1. Glucose binds to outward-facing binding site
2. Conformational change generates inward-facing binding site
3. Glucose dissociates from inward-facing binding site
4. Reverse conformational change restores outward-facing binding site

3-2: *Facilitated diffusion of glucose by the Na⁺-independent glucose transporter (GLUT). In most cells, GLUT operates to import glucose delivered in the blood, as illustrated. The imported glucose is rapidly metabolized within cells, thereby maintaining the inward glucose gradient. However, all steps in the transport process are reversible; if the glucose gradient is reversed, GLUT can transport glucose from the cytosol to the extracellular space, as occurs in the liver during fasting.*

3. Ca^{2+} ATPase pumps maintain low cytosolic Ca^{2+} concentration.
   a. Plasma membrane Ca^{2+} ATPase, present in most cells, transports Ca^{2+} out of cell.
   b. Muscle Ca^{2+} ATPase, located in the sarcoplasmic reticulum (SR) of skeletal muscle, transports Ca^{2+} from the cytosol to the SR lumen.
      (1) Release of stored Ca^{2+} from SR to cytosol triggers muscle contraction.
      (2) Rapid removal of Ca^{2+} by the ATPase pump and restoration of a low cytosolic level permits relaxation.
   c. In tissue hypoxia, the decrease in ATP production affects the Ca^{2+} ATPase pump and allows Ca^{2+} into the cell, where it activates various enzymes (e.g., phospholipases, caspases [pro-apoptotic enzymes]), leading to irreversible cell damage.

D. Secondary active transport by cotransport carrier proteins moves one substance against its concentration gradient with energy supplied by the coupled movement of a second substance (usually Na^+ or H^+) down its gradient.

Secondary active transport: molecule moves against its concentration gradient with energy from movement of cotransported ion down its gradient

   1. Na^+-linked symporters transport glucose and amino acids against a concentration gradient from the lumen into the epithelial cells lining the small intestine and renal tubules.
      a. Symporter in apical membrane couples movement of 1 or 2 Na^+ into the cell, down the concentration gradient with energetically unfavorable import of a second molecule (glucose or amino acid).
         (1) Absorption of glucose by epithelial cells of kidney tubules and intestine occurs against a steep glucose gradient by secondary active transport mediated by Na^+/glucose symporter (SGLUT1).

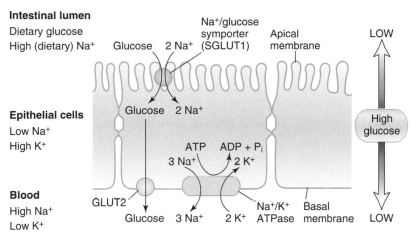

3-3: Transport of glucose from the intestinal lumen to the blood. Three different membrane transport proteins participate in this process. Glucose moves across the apical membrane into an epithelial cell against its gradient via a Na⁺/glucose symporter, also designated SGLUT1 (secondary active transport). Glucose exits from the basal surface via a GLUT2 uniporter (facilitated diffusion). Na⁺/K⁺ ATPase pumps Na⁺ out of the cell (primary active transport), maintaining the low intracellular Na⁺ level needed for operation of the symporter.

(2) For Na^+ to be reabsorbed in the small bowel, glucose must be present. In patients with cholera, it is important to orally replenish Na^+.

    b. Na^+/K^+ ATPase pump in the basal membrane maintains an Na^+ gradient necessary for the operation of Na^+-linked symporters (Fig. 3-3).

  2. Na^+-linked Ca^{2+} antiporter in the plasma membrane of cardiac muscle cells is primarily responsible for maintaining low cytosolic Ca^{2+}.

    a. Coupled movement of 3 Na^+ into the cell down the concentration gradient powers the export of 1 Ca^{2+}.

    b. Operation of antiporter is indirectly inhibited by digitalis, accounting for its cardiotonic effect (Fig. 3-4).

  E. Hereditary defects in transport proteins cause diseases such as cystic fibrosis (Box 3-1).

IV. Receptors and Signal Transduction Cascades

  A. Sequence of events in cell-cell signaling

    1. Release of signal molecules from the signaling cell normally occurs in response to a specific stimulus (e.g., increased blood glucose stimulates pancreatic β cells to release insulin).

     • Hormones, growth factors, neurotransmitters, and cytokines are the most common types of extracellular signals.

    2. Binding of the signal to its specific receptor causes receptor activation.

     a. A cell can respond only to those signal molecules whose specific receptor proteins it expresses.

Cystic fibrosis, cystinuria, Hartnup's disease: caused by hereditary defects in transport proteins

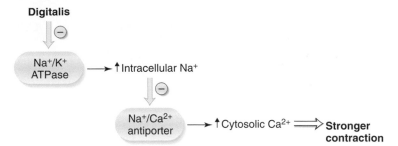

3-4: *Mechanism of action of digitalis on cardiac muscle. The cardiotonic effect of digitalis stems from its inhibition of Na^+/K^+ ATPase, leading to a rise in intracellular Na^+ and a secondary inhibition of the Na^+/Ca^{2+} antiporter. Increased cytosolic Ca^{2+} results in an increase in cardiac muscle contraction. In skeletal muscle, control of the cytosolic Ca^{2+} level is effected by Na^+-independent Ca^{2+} pumps; hence, digitalis does not affect skeletal muscle.*

BOX 3-1

DISORDERS CAUSED BY DEFECTIVE TRANSPORTERS

Cystic fibrosis is caused by an autosomal recessive (AR) defect in CFTR (cystic fibrosis transmembrane regulator) on chromosome 7. CFTR is a Cl^- ATPase pump in epithelial cells of the lungs, pancreas, intestines, and skin. The resulting dysfunction in exocrine glands leads to high Na^+ and Cl^- in sweat (the basis of the sweat test) and production of highly viscous mucus, which obstructs the airways and the pancreatic and bile ducts. Common symptoms include failure to thrive, malabsorption (atrophy of pancreatic exocrine glands), and recurrent respiratory infections due to *Pseudomonas aeruginosa*, which are the usual causes of death.

Cystinuria results from a hereditary defect (AR) in the carrier protein that mediates reabsorption of dibasic amino acids (cystine, arginine, lysine, and ornithine) from renal tubules. Formation of cystine kidney stones and excessive urinary excretion of dibasic amino acids are common clinical features. Cystine is a hexagonal-shaped crystal in urine.

Hartnup's disease is caused by an AR defect in the carrier protein that mediates intestinal and renal tubular absorption of neutral amino acids. Clinically, it is marked by pellagra-like symptoms (diarrhea, dermatitis, and dementia) due to impaired absorption of tryptophan, which reduces the synthesis of niacin.

Familial hypercholesterolemia is an autosomal dominant disease characterized by a lack of functional receptors for low-density lipoprotein. The resulting high blood levels of cholesterol contribute to premature atherosclerosis and susceptibility to acute myocardial infarctions and stroke at an early age.

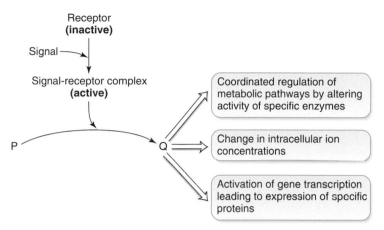

3-5: *Generalized signal transduction cascade. Binding of an extracellular signal to its receptor activates the receptor. The activated receptor transduces the signal by binding to a molecule within the cell (P) and converting it into another molecule (Q). Q can then act as a signal (often with intervening transducing molecules), leading to three major types of effects. Amplification of the signal occurs at every step after signal receptor binding. For example, one active receptor molecule can interact with many molecules of P, yielding many Q molecules.*

        b. Because of different downstream proteins, hormones may have different actions in different cells, even if they express the same receptor.

    3. Activated receptor-signal complex in turn functions as a signal, triggering an intracellular signal transduction cascade that ultimately leads to specific cellular responses (Fig. 3-5).

  B. General properties of cell surface receptors

    1. Receptors located on the exterior surface of the cell bind peptide hormones and other extracellular signals that are hydrophilic and cannot penetrate the cell membrane.

      • Steroid hormones, thyroxine, and retinoic acid, on the other hand, are lipophilic and diffuse through the plasma membrane to receptors in the cytosol (steroid hormones) or nucleus (thyroxine, retinoic acid).

    2. Binding interaction between the receptor and the hormone demonstrates reversibility (like enzyme-substrate interactions) and inhibition by antagonists (either competitive or noncompetitive).

    3. Cellular response to a hormone may be positive or negative (even in the same tissue), depending on the particular receptors present.

    4. Signal amplification by a transduction cascade means that binding and activation of only a small fraction of receptors generates an effective response.

    5. Receptor-hormone dissociation constants correlate with physiologic concentrations of hormones.

  C. Common features of G protein-coupled receptors (GPCRs) and the signal transduction cascades associated with them

TABLE 3-3:
Major Trimeric G Proteins

G$_\alpha$ Type	Function*	Coupled Receptors
G$_s$	Stimulates adenylate cyclase (↑ cAMP)	Dopamine (D$_1$), epinephrine (β$_1$, β$_2$), glucagon histamine (H$_2$), vasopressin (V$_2$)
G$_i$	Inhibits adenylate cyclase (↓ cAMP)	Dopamine (D$_2$), epinephrine (α$_2$)
G$_q$	Stimulates phospholipase C (↑ IP$_3$, DAG)	Angiotensin II epinephrine (α$_1$), oxytocin vasopressin (V$_1$)
G$_t$ (transducin)	Stimulates cGMP phosphodiesterase (↑ cGMP)	Rhodopsin (light sensitive)

*In some signaling pathways, G$_s$ and G$_i$ are associated with ion channels, which open or close in response to hormone binding.
DAG, diacylglycerol; IP$_3$, inositol triphosphate.

1. GPCRs are monomeric proteins (single polypeptide chain) containing seven transmembrane α-helices.
   a. The extracellular domain contains a hormone binding site.
   b. The cytosolic domain interacts with trimeric G protein consisting of three subunits (a, β, and γ).
2. Trimeric G proteins alternate between an active state with bound guanosine triphosphate (GTP) and an inactive state with bound guanosine diphosphate (GDP).
   • In the active state, which is generated by the hormone binding to the coupled receptor, the α subunit (G$_\alpha$) interacts with and either stimulates or inhibits an associated effector protein.
3. Second messengers, generated by stimulated effector proteins, are small intracellular signal molecules that regulate the activity of various cellular proteins.
4. Multiple G proteins are coupled to different receptors and transduce signals to different effector proteins, leading to a wide range of responses (Table 3-3).

D. Cyclic AMP (cAMP) pathway
   1. Receptors for glucagon, epinephrine (β receptors), and other hormones coupled to G$_s$ protein transmit a hormonal signal via the second messenger cAMP (Fig. 3-6).
   2. Hormone binding to the appropriate receptor causes a conformational change in the intracellular domain, allowing the receptor to interact with the G$_s$ protein.
   3. Hormone-induced elevation of cAMP produces a variety of effects in different tissues (Table 3-4).
   4. β-Adrenergic receptors undergo accommodation (reduction in physiologic response upon repeated stimulation) when exposed to sustained, constant concentration of epinephrine (e.g., pheochromocytoma).
      a. Phosphorylation of receptor by β-adrenergic receptor kinase prevents the hormone-receptor complex from interacting with G$_s$ protein, thus attenuating the response to epinephrine.

G protein-coupled receptors often transduce signals through second messengers: cyclic AMP (cAMP pathway), IP$_3$, and DAG (phosphoinositide pathway)

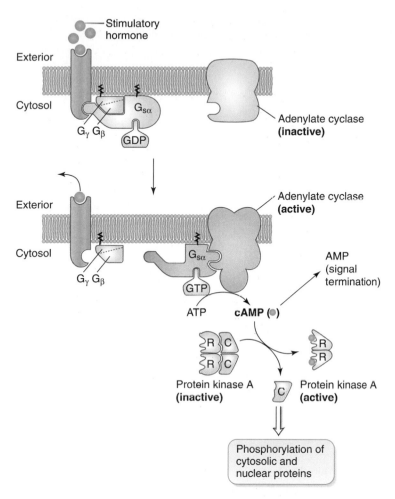

3-6: *Cyclic adenosine monophosphate (cAMP) pathway. Following hormone binding, coupled G protein exchanges bound guanosine diphosphate (GDP) for guanosine triphosphate (GTP). Active $G_{s\alpha}$-GTP diffuses in the membrane and binds to membrane-bound adenylate cyclase, stimulating it to produce cAMP. Binding of cAMP to the regulatory subunits (R) of protein kinase A releases the active catalytic (C) subunits, which mediate various cellular responses.*

    b. The concentration of hormone must increase to generate new active
       hormone-receptor complexes.

E. Phosphoinositide pathway

  1. Receptors coupled to G_q protein transmit signals from hormones such as
     oxytocin, angiotensin II, and vasopressin (V_1 receptor) via several second
     messengers (Fig. 3-7, top).

  2. Phospholipase C is stimulated by active $G_{q\alpha}$ subunit (similar to
     stimulation of adenylate cyclase by $G_{s\alpha}$) and cleaves PIP_2 (phosphatidyl
     inositol 4,5-bisphosphate) to yield two second messengers:

Binding of epinephrine (β receptors) or glucagon leads to phosphorylation inside cell via cAMP pathway; stored energy mobilized

TABLE 3-4:
Effects of Elevated cAMP in Various Tissues

Tissue/Cell Type	Hormone Increasing cAMP	Major Cellular Response
Adipose tissue	Epinephrine, adrenocorticotropic hormone (ACTH)	↑ Hydrolysis of triglycerides
Adrenal cortex	ACTH	Hormone secretion
Cardiac muscle	Epinephrine, norepinephrine	↑ Contraction rate
Intestinal mucosa	Vasoactive intestinal peptide, epinephrine	Secretion of water and electrolytes
Kidney tubules	Vasopressin (V_2 receptor)	Resorption of water
Liver	Glucagon, epinephrine	↑ Glycogen degradation ↑ Glucose synthesis
Platelets	Prostacyclin	Inhibition of aggregation
Skeletal muscle	Epinephrine	↑ Glycogen degradation
Smooth muscle (vascular and bronchial)	Epinephrine	Relaxation (bronchial) Contraction (arterioles)
Thyroid gland	Thyroid-stimulating hormone	Synthesis and secretion of thyroxine

IP$_3$ increases cytosolic Ca^{2+} concentrations by stimulating release of stored Ca^{2+} from ER.

DAG: required for activation of protein kinase C

   a. IP$_3$ (inositol 1,4,5-triphosphate), which can diffuse in the cytosol
   b. DAG (diacylglycerol), which remains associated with the plasma membrane
3. IP$_3$, a second messenger in the phosphoinositide pathway, causes a rapid release of Ca^{2+} from the endoplasmic reticulum (ER) by opening Ca^{2+} channels in the ER membrane.
   a. Ca^{2+} is a potent enzyme activator, and its access to the cytoplasm is tightly regulated. Free Ca^{2+} concentrations in the cytosol are normally about 100 nM, whereas extracellular concentrations of calcium are 10,000-fold higher.
   b. Calmodulin binds cytosolic Ca^{2+}, forming the Ca^{2+}-calmodulin complex that activates Ca^{2+}-calmodulin-dependent protein kinases.
      • Phosphorylation of target proteins by these kinases regulates their activity, leading to various cellular responses.
   c. Hormone-induced contraction of smooth muscle results from activation of myosin light-chain (MLC) kinase by Ca^{2+}-calmodulin (Fig. 3-7, bottom).
4. DAG activates protein kinase C, which regulates various target proteins by phosphorylation.
      • Elevated cytosolic Ca^{2+} promotes the interaction of inactive protein kinase C with the plasma membrane, where it can be activated by DAG.
F. Receptor tyrosine kinases
   1. Receptors in this class contain a single transmembrane α-helix, an extracellular hormone-binding domain, and a cytosolic domain with tyrosine kinase catalytic activity.
   2. Hormone binding (e.g., insulin) activates tyrosine kinase activity, leading to autophosphorylation of the receptor.

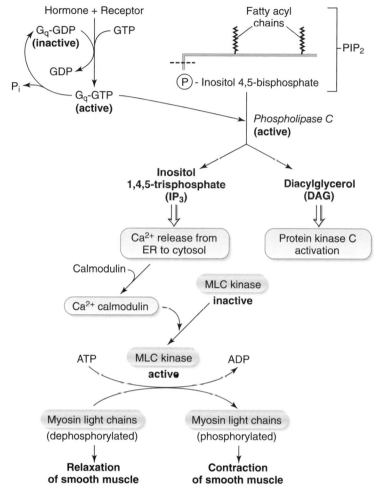

3-7: *Phosphoinositide pathway linked to G_q-coupled receptor. Top, The two fatty acyl chains of PIP_2 (phosphatidylinositol 4,5-bisphosphate) are embedded in the plasma membrane with the polar phosphorylated inositol group extending into the cytosol. Hydrolysis of PIP_2 (dashed line) produces DAG, which remains associated with the membrane, and IP_3, which is released into the cytosol. Bottom, Contraction of smooth muscle induced by hormones such as epinephrine (a_1 receptor), oxytocin, and vasopressin (V_1 receptor) results from the IP_3-stimulated increase in cytosolic Ca^{2+}, which forms a Ca^{2+}-calmodulin complex that activates myosin light-chain (MLC) kinase. MLC kinase phosphorylates myosin light chains, leading to muscle contractions. ER, endoplasmic reticulum.*

3. RAS, another type of G protein, functions in the signaling pathway from receptors for growth factors such as epidermal growth factor and platelet-derived growth factor receptor.
   a. These monomeric receptors aggregate on binding of hormone, usually forming dimers.
   b. Hormonal signal is transmitted from activated receptor via adapter proteins to membrane-bound RAS, converting it to the active GTP-bound form.

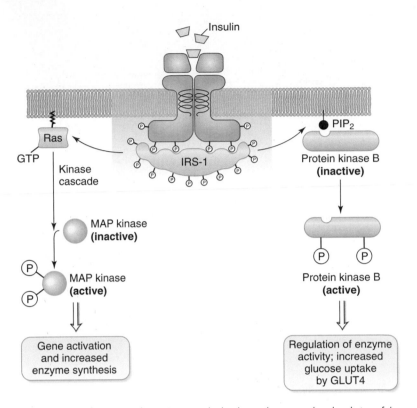

3-8: *Signal transduction from an insulin receptor. Insulin binding induces autophosphorylation of the cytosolic domain. IRS-1 (insulin receptor substrate) then binds and is phosphorylated by the receptor's tyrosine kinase activity. Long-term effects of insulin, such as increased synthesis of glucokinase in the liver, are mediated via the RAS pathway, which is activated by MAP (mitogen-activated protein) kinase (left). Two adapter proteins transmit the signal from IRS-1 to RAS, converting it to the active form. Short-term effects of insulin, such as increased activity of glycogen synthase in the liver, are mediated by the protein kinase B (PKB) pathway (right). A kinase that binds to IRS-1 converts phosphatidylinositol in the membrane to PIP_2 (phosphatidylinositol 4,5-bisphosphate), which binds cytosolic PKB and localizes it to the membrane. Membrane-bound kinases then phosphorylate and activate PKB.*

    c. Kinase cascade triggered by RAS-GTP culminates in activation of MAP (mitogen-activated protein) kinase, which translocates to the nucleus and regulates the activity of transcription factors, leading to changes in gene expression.
- Signaling pathways that regulate gene expression take hours to days to produce cellular responses, whereas those that control the activity of existing proteins produce cellular responses much more quickly (seconds to minutes).

4. Insulin receptor is a disulfide-bonded tetrameric receptor tyrosine kinase (RTK) that uses insulin receptor substrate 1 (IRS-1) to transduce insulin signal via two pathways (Fig. 3-8).

    a. RAS-dependent pathway, similar to that used by growth factor RTKs, mediates the long-term effects of insulin (e.g., increased synthesis of glucokinase in liver).

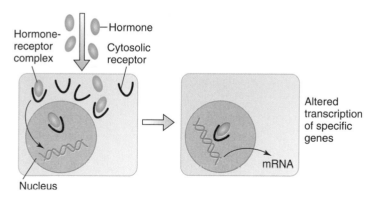

Hormone-receptor complex

Hormone

Cytosolic receptor

Altered transcription of specific genes

mRNA

Nucleus

3-9: *Signaling by hormones with intracellular receptors. Steroid hormones (e.g., cortisol) bind to their receptors in the cytosol, and the hormone-receptor complex moves to the nucleus. In contrast, the receptors for thyroid hormone and retinoic acid are located only in the nucleus. Binding of the hormone-receptor complex to regulatory sites in DNA activates gene transcription.*

  b. RAS-independent pathway, which leads to activation of protein kinase B, mediates the short-term effects of insulin (e.g., increased glucose uptake by muscle and adipocytes, increased activity of glycogen synthase).

G. Intracellular receptors for lipophilic hormones (Fig. 3-9)

 1. Lipophilic hormones, such as steroid hormones (e.g., cortisol), thyroid hormone, and retinoic acid, have receptors that are located in the cytosol or nucleus.

  a. Steroid hormones bind to their receptors in the cytosol, and the hormone-receptor complexes move to the nucleus.

  b. Thyroxine and retinoic acid have receptors only in the nucleus.

   • These receptors contain a hormone-binding domain and DNA-binding domain.

 2. Hormone-receptor complexes function as transcription factors, which regulate the expression of specific target genes.

H. Clinical aspects of cell-cell signaling

 1. Cholera, enterotoxigenic *Escherichia coli,* and pertussis toxins catalyze ADP ribosylation of the α subunit of G proteins.

  a. Cholera toxin produced by *Vibrio cholerae* and the toxin produced by enterotoxigenic *E. coli* permanently activate G_s protein (by ADP ribosylation of G_s protein), which activates adenylate cyclase.

   • The resulting increase in cAMP in the intestinal mucosa produces a massive secretory diarrhea with a loss of isotonic fluid (approximately the same tonicity as plasma).

  b. Pertussis toxin, produced by *Bordetella pertussis,* permanently inactivates G_i protein (by ADP ribosylation of G_i protein), which activates adenylate cyclase.

   • The resulting increase in cAMP causes increased mucus secretion in the respiratory tract (whooping cough).

Cholera and enterotoxigenic *E. coli* toxin permanently activate G_s and pertussis toxin permanently inactivates G_i by ADP ribosylation.

Graves' disease: IgG antibodies against TSH receptors produce hyperthyroidism.

2. Graves' disease results from inappropriate stimulation of thyroid-stimulating hormone (TSH) receptors by IgG autoantibodies.
   a. Manifestations include thyromegaly, exophthalmos, and signs of hyperthyroidism, which include weight loss, fatigue, heat intolerance, diarrhea, and hand tremors.
   b. Autoantibodies against receptors are type II hypersensitivity reactions.
3. Mutant RAS protein encoded by the *ras* oncogene, which has undergone a point mutation, has a very low GTPase activity and thus is permanently in the active state.
   a. Cell responds as if high levels of hormone were present, leading to increased cell proliferation.
   b. Mutation of *ras* protooncogene to *ras* oncogene has been implicated in the development of various types of cancer (e.g., pancreatic, colon, endometrial, and thyroid cancers).

Ras oncogene encodes a mutant RAS protein that leads to cancer (e.g., pancreas, colon).

4. Many drugs bind to receptors and either stimulate or inhibit intracellular signaling.
   a. Agonists activate receptors and thus mimic the action of normal signal molecules. Examples:
      (1) Ephedrine, a general agonist of α_1 adrenergic receptors; produces vasoconstriction (nasal decongestant)
      (2) Albuterol and terbutaline, which are relatively selective for α_2 receptors; produce smooth muscle relaxation (bronchodilator for asthma)
   b. Antagonists inhibit the action of normal signal molecules by blocking access to receptor. Examples:
      (1) β-Blockers, which may be nonselective (propranolol, timolol) or β_1 selective (metoprolol, atenolol); decrease blood pressure, may precipitate asthma
      (2) Losartan, which blocks angiotensin II receptors; decreases blood pressure
      (3) Antipsychotics, such as chlorpromazine and haloperidol, which block dopamine D_2 receptors

4

Nutrition

I. Nutrient and Energy Requirements in Humans
- The normal diet provides fuel for energy, precursors (e.g., essential fatty acids and amino acids), and micronutrients (e.g., vitamins, minerals, trace elements).
  A. Dietary requirements for protein, vitamins, minerals, and trace elements are specified in terms of the recommended daily allowance (RDA).

  RDA: optimal dietary intake of nutrients

  1. RDA represents an optimal dietary intake of nutrients that under ordinary conditions will maintain a healthy general population.
  2. RDA varies with sex, age, body weight, diet, and physiologic status.
     - Example: RDAs for nutrients increase during childhood, pregnancy, and lactation.

Daily energy
expenditure: BMR +
thermic effect foods +
physical activity

B. Daily energy expenditure depends on the basal metabolic rate (BMR), thermic effect of foods, and the degree of physical activity.
  1. BMR accounts for ~60% of daily energy expenditure and refers to the energy consumption of an individual at rest.
     a. BMR reflects the energy involved in normal body functions (e.g., cardiac function, maintaining ion pumps) and primarily depends on body weight.
        • An estimate of BMR is obtained by multiplying the body weight in kilograms times 24 (1 kg equals 2.2 pounds):

$$BMR = 24 \times \text{weight in kilograms}$$

BMR: 24 × body weight
in kg

     b. Other factors affecting BMR
        (1) Gender: Males have a higher BMR than females
        (2) Age: Children have a higher BMR than adults
        (3) Fever: BMR increased
        (4) Thyroid function: BMR increased in hyperthyroidism, decreased in hypothyroidism
  2. Thermic effect of foods accounts for ~10% of daily energy expenditure and represents the energy used in digestion, absorption, and distribution of nutrients.
  3. Physical activity is variable and is expressed as an activity factor, which when multiplied by the BMR equals the daily energy expenditure.
     • The activity factor for a sedentary person is 1.3, for a moderately active person 1.5, and for a very active person (e.g., marathon runner) 1.7.
  4. Sample calculations: Calculate the BMR and daily energy expenditure for a 220-pound man (patient A) with sedentary habits and a 110-pound woman (patient B) who runs 10 miles a day and is an aerobic exercise instructor at night.
     a. Patient A: 220 pounds = 220/2.2 = 100 kg
        BMR: 24 × 100 = 2400 kcal/day
        Daily energy expenditure: 2400 × 1.3 = 3120 kcal/day
     b. Patient B: 110 pounds = 110/2.2 = 50 kg
        BMR: 24 × 50 = 1200 kcal/day
        Daily energy expenditure: 1200 × 1.7 = 2040 kcal/day

II. Dietary Fuels
  A. Energy-yielding dietary carbohydrates are digested, absorbed, and metabolized in the body (see Chapter 1).
     1. Carbohydrates include
        a. Polysaccharides (e.g., starch)
        b. Disaccharides (e.g., lactose, sucrose, maltose)
        c. Monosaccharides (e.g., glucose, galactose, fructose)
        d. Insoluble fiber (e.g., cellulose, lignin)
        e. Soluble fiber (e.g., pectins, hemicellulose)
     2. α-Amylase, which is found in saliva in the mouth and in pancreatic secretions in the small intestine, cleaves the α-1,4 linkages in starch, producing smaller molecules (e.g., oligosaccharides and disaccharides).

BOX 4-1

LACTOSE INTOLERANCE

Lactose intolerance, the most common type of digestive enzyme deficiency, is caused by insufficient lactase activity. It may result from an inherited decrease in lactase production or from damage to mucosal cells due to drugs, diarrhea, or protein deficiency (e.g., kwashiorkor). The incidence of lactose intolerance is much higher (up to 90%) in those of Asian and African descent than in those of northern European descent (<10%).

The signs and symptoms of lactose intolerance result from the inability to digest lactose, a disaccharide that is present in dairy products. Unabsorbed lactose is osmotically active, causing retention of water in the gastrointestinal tract and production of a watery diarrhea. Bacterial degradation of lactose produces lactic acid and gases (i.e., hydrogen, carbon dioxide, and methane), which cause abdominal bloating, cramps, and flatulence. The stool has an acid pH. Elimination of dairy products from the diet is the most effective treatment.

---

3. Intestinal brush border enzymes (e.g., lactase, sucrase, maltase) hydrolyze dietary disaccharides into the monosaccharides glucose, galactose, and fructose, which are reabsorbed into the portal circulation by carrier proteins in intestinal epithelial cells (see Chapter 3).
   a. Glucose is the predominant sugar in human blood.
   b. Glucose is stored as glycogen, which is primarily located in liver and muscle.
   c. Complete oxidation of carbohydrates to CO_2 and H_2O in the body produces 4 kcal/g.
   d. Lactose intolerance due to lactase deficiency is discussed in Box 4-1.   Carbohydrate: 4 kcal/g
4. Insoluble and soluble dietary fiber supply no energy, but they serve important functions in the body.
   • Insoluble fiber has β-1,4 glycosidic linkages, which cannot be hydrolyzed by amylase.
   a. Fiber increases intestinal motility, which results in less contact of bowel mucosa with potential carcinogens (e.g., lithocholic acid).
      • Fiber reduces the risk for colorectal cancer by absorbing lithocholic acid and reducing its contact with intestinal mucosa.
   b. Fiber softens stool, which alleviates constipation and reduces the incidence of diverticulosis of the sigmoid colon.
   c. Fiber reduces absorption of cholesterol (decreasing blood cholesterol), fat-soluble vitamins, and some minerals (e.g., zinc).
      • Soluble fiber (e.g., oat bran, psyllium seeds) has a greater cholesterol-lowering effect than insoluble fiber (e.g., wheat bran).

B. Triacylglycerols are the major dietary lipids, although phospholipids and cholesterol are also consumed in the diet.

1. Triacylglycerols provide the major source of energy to cells, with the exception of red blood cells (RBCs) and the brain.

2. Dietary fats contain essential fatty acids and are required for the reabsorption of fat-soluble vitamins.

3. The composition of dietary triacylglycerols, which contain long chains of fatty acids, varies in plants and animals.

   a. Plants primarily contain unsaturated fats, but a few are saturated.
      (1) Monounsaturated fats (one double bond) are present in olive oil and canola oil.
      (2) Polyunsaturated fats (two or more double bonds) are present in soybean oil and corn oil.
      (3) Saturated fats (no double bonds) are present in coconut oil and palm oil.

   b. Animal fats are primarily saturated and include butter, lard, red meats, and cheeses.

4. Essential fatty acids are required in the diet and include the polyunsaturated fatty acids linoleic (ω6) and linolenic (ω3) acids.

   a. Functions of essential fatty acids
      (1) Help maintain fluidity of cellular membranes
      (2) Synthesize arachidonic acid (linoleic acid), from which the eicosanoids (e.g., prostaglandins) are derived
      (3) Prevent platelet aggregation (linolenic acid), which reduces the incidence of strokes and myocardial infarctions

   b. Essential fatty acids are present in high concentration in fish oils, canola oil, and walnuts.

   c. Deficiency results in scaly dermatitis, poor wound healing, and hair loss.

5. Dietary triacylglycerols are digested primarily in the small intestine (Fig. 4-1).

   a. Pancreatic lipase (aided by colipase) degrades triacylglycerol into 2-monoacylglycerol and free fatty acids.

   b. Pancreatic cholesterol esterase hydrolyzes cholesteryl esters and releases free cholesterol.

   c. 2-Monoacylglycerol, free fatty acids, and cholesterol, along with fat-soluble vitamins and phospholipids, are micellarized by bile salts, which emulsify and make them soluble in aqueous solution. The tiny globules, or micelles, are reabsorbed into intestinal mucosal cells by passive diffusion.
      (1) Resynthesis of triacylglycerols and of cholesteryl esters occurs within mucosal cells.
      (2) Short- and medium-chain fatty acids are directly reabsorbed and released into the portal circulation; they also bypass the carnitine cycle and are used directly by the mitochondria.

   d. Nascent chylomicrons are assembled in mucosal cells and contain triacylglycerols (~85%), cholesteryl esters (~3%), phospholipids, the

Essential fatty acids: linoleic (ω6), linolenic (ω3)

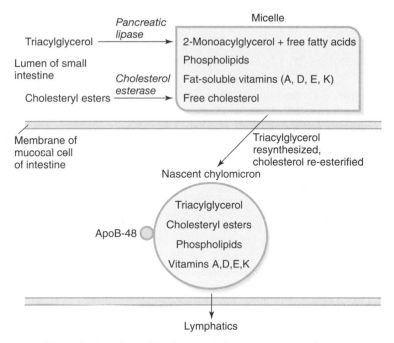

4-1: *Digestion of dietary lipids and assembly of nascent chylomicrons. Pancreatic lipase acts on triacylglycerol to produce 2-monoacylglycerol and free fatty acids, and pancreatic cholesterol esterase hydrolyzes cholesteryl esters to free cholesterol. These degradation products, as well as phospholipids and fat-soluble vitamins, are micellarized by bile salts and absorbed into intestinal cells by passive diffusion. Triacylglycerols are resynthesized, cholesterol is re-esterified, and all components are packaged into nascent chylomicrons with apolipoprotein (Apo) B-48 on their surfaces. ApoB-48 is required for secretion of chylomicrons into the lymphatics and bloodstream.*

fat-soluble vitamins (A, D, E, and K), and apolipoprotein B-48, which is necessary for secretion of chylomicrons into the lymphatics.

- When discharged into the lymphatic vessels, lipoproteins rich in triacylglycerols ultimately enter the bloodstream and circulate to deliver fatty acids to tissues (see Chapter 7).

  e. Complete oxidation of fats to CO_2 and H_2O in the body produces 9 kcal/g.

Dietary triacylglycerol: 9 kcal/g

6. The pathophysiology of lipid malabsorption is discussed in Box 4-2.
C. Dietary proteins provide amino acids for degradation into carbon skeletons to synthesize glucose for energy and amino acids for the synthesis of other proteins (e.g., enzymes, structural components).
   1. The biological value of a dietary protein is determined by its content of essential amino acids (see Chapter 1).
      a. Plant proteins (e.g., rice, wheat, corn, beans) are of low biological value individually.
         - Combining plant proteins from different sources (e.g., rice, beans) ensures a more complete complement of essential amino acids.
      b. Animal proteins (e.g., eggs, meat, poultry, fish, dairy products) are of high biological value because they contain all the essential amino acids.

BOX 4-2

PATHOGENESIS OF MALABSORPTION

Malabsorption is a general term referring to increased fecal excretion of fat, called steatorrhea, with concurrent deficiencies of vitamins (particularly fat-soluble vitamins), minerals, carbohydrates, and proteins. The pathophysiology of malabsorption is classified into three major categories: pancreatic insufficiency, bile salt deficiency, and small bowel disease.

Pancreatic insufficiency causes a maldigestion of fats due to diminished lipase activity, resulting in the presence of undigested neutral fats and fat droplets in stool. There is also a maldigestion of proteins due to diminished trypsin, leading to undigested meat fibers in stool. Carbohydrate digestion is not affected because of the presence of amylase in salivary glands and disaccharidases in brush border enzymes. Chronic pancreatitis due to alcoholism is the most common cause of pancreatic insufficiency in adults; chronic pancreatitis due to cystic fibrosis is the most common cause in children.

Bile salt deficiency results in defective micellarization of fats, which is necessary for their absorption by small intestinal villi. Causes of bile salt deficiency include cirrhosis (inadequate production of bile salts and acids from cholesterol), intrahepatic or extrahepatic blockage of bile (e.g., calculus in common bile duct), bacterial overgrowth in the small bowel with destruction of bile salts, excess binding of bile salts (e.g., use of cholestyramine), and terminal ileal disease (inability to recycle bile salts and acids).

Small bowel disease associated with a loss of the villous surface leads to a malassimilation of fats, proteins, and carbohydrates. Celiac disease, or sprue, an autoimmune disease caused by antibodies directed against gluten in wheat, and Crohn's disease, an inflammatory bowel disease involving the terminal ileum, commonly produce malabsorption.

Characteristic clinical findings in malabsorption include weight loss, anemia, chronic diarrhea, and malnutrition. The signs and symptoms associated with multiple fat-soluble vitamin deficiencies are usually present. Night blindness (vitamin A deficiency), rickets (vitamin D deficiency), and a hemorrhagic diathesis with ecchymoses and gastrointestinal bleeding (vitamin K deficiency) are the usual findings.

    c. The dietary RDA for high-quality protein is 0.8 g/kg for men and women, which is equivalent to ~60 g/day for men and ~50 g/day for women.

2. Digestion of dietary proteins begins in the stomach, where the low pH denatures proteins, making them more susceptible to enzymatic hydrolysis.

    a. In the stomach, pepsin secreted by gastric chief cells converts proteins to smaller polypeptides.

  b. Pancreatic proteases (e.g., trypsin) and peptidases secreted by intestinal epithelial cells act on the partially digested material delivered from the stomach and release amino acids.

  c. Uptake of amino acids from the intestinal lumen and their release into the portal circulation by carrier proteins in the intestinal epithelial cells are driven by the hydrolysis of ATP.

  d. Complete oxidation of proteins to CO_2 and H_2O produces 4 kcal/g.

Proteins: 4 kcal/g

3. Proteins are in a constant state of degradation and resynthesis.

  a. When amino acids are oxidized, their nitrogen atoms are fed into the urea cycle in the liver and excreted as urea in the urine (primary route), feces, and sweat (see Chapter 8).

  • Other nitrogenous excretory products include uric acid, creatinine, and ammonia.

  b. Nitrogen balance is the difference in the amount of nitrogen (protein) consumed and the amount of nitrogen excreted in the urine, sweat, and feces.

  (1) Healthy adults are normally in zero nitrogen balance (nitrogen intake equals nitrogen loss).

  (2) A positive nitrogen balance (nitrogen intake is greater than nitrogen loss) indicates active synthesis of new protein.

  • It is associated with pregnancy and lactation, growth in children, and recovery from surgery, trauma, or extreme starvation.

  (3) A negative nitrogen balance (nitrogen loss is greater than nitrogen intake) indicates breakdown of tissue proteins.

  • It is associated with diets containing protein of low biological value and with physiologic stress (e.g., third-degree burns).

4. Carbohydrates have a protein-sparing effect.

  a. An adequate intake of carbohydrate provides the glucose that is necessary for complete oxidation into CO_2 and H_2O via glycolysis and the citric acid cycle.

  b. An inadequate intake of carbohydrate (e.g., <150 g/day) causes degradation of skeletal muscle with the release of amino acids that are deaminated and converted into substrates (e.g., pyruvate) for gluconeogenesis (see Chapter 9).

5. Protein-energy malnutrition results from inadequate intake of protein and/or calories.

  a. Marasmus is caused by a diet deficient in both protein and calories (e.g., total calorie deprivation).

Marasmus: total calorie deprivation

  (1) Marasmus is marked by extreme muscle wasting ("broomstick extremities") due to breakdown of muscle protein for energy, as well as growth retardation.

  (2) It occurs primarily during the first year of life.

  b. Kwashiorkor is caused by a diet inadequate in protein in the presence of an adequate caloric intake consisting primarily of carbohydrates.

Kwashiorkor: inadequate protein intake

  (1) Marked by pitting edema and ascites (loss of the oncotic effect of albumin), enlarged fatty liver (decreased apolipoproteins), anemia,

diarrhea (loss of brush border enzymes), and defects in cellular immunity

(2) Less extreme muscle wasting than occurs in marasmus due to the protein-sparing effect of carbohydrates

III. Dietary Recommendations

A. The body mass index (BMI) is primarily used to determine whether an individual's body weight is in the acceptable range for his or her height.

1. BMI = weight in kg/height in m^2

2. Acceptable BMI is 20 to $25 \, kg/m^2$; 25 to $29.9 \, kg/m^2$ is overweight; 30 to $39.9 \, kg/m^2$ is obese; and $>40 \, kg/m^2$ is considered morbidly obese.

B. The recommended distribution of total caloric intake in a diet is 50% to 60% from carbohydrates, no more than 30% from fats (ideal is <25%), and 10% to 20% from proteins.

1. The BMI should be in the acceptable range of 20 to $25 \, kg/m^2$.

2. Fat distribution should be 10% monounsaturated fats, 10% polyunsaturated fats, and 10% saturated fats.

3. Cholesterol intake should be less than 300 mg/day.

4. Protein intake should be 0.8 g/kg/day.

C. To lose weight, the total calories expended must be greater than the total intake of calories.

1. When primarily drawing on adipose tissue to meet energy needs, to lose ~1 pound, a person must expend 3500 calories more than are consumed.

2. Sample calculations using two patients, A and B:

a. Patient A consumes 3600 kcal/day consisting of 168 g of fat, 108 g of protein, and 414 g of carbohydrates. Calculate the percentage of each of the nutrients. Is the patient gaining, maintaining, or losing weight?

(1) Fat kcal: 168 g × 9 kcal/g = 1512 kcal/day; fat percentage = 1512/3600 = 42% (exceedingly high)

(2) Protein kcal: 108 g × 4 kcal/g = 432 kcal/day; protein percentage = 432/3600 = 12% (normal)

(3) Carbohydrate kcal: 414 g × 4 kcal/g = 1656 kcal/day; carbohydrate percentage = 1656/3600 = 46% (slightly decreased)

(4) Since the patient's calculated daily energy expenditure is 3120 kcal/day (see calculation I B), the patient is consuming more calories (3600 kcal/day) than are being expended. A net gain of 480 kcal/day results in a gain of 1 pound in ~7 days (3500/480 = 7.3).

b. Patient B consumes 2000 kcal/day consisting of 67 g of fat, 60 g of protein, and 290 g of carbohydrates. Calculate the percentage of each of the nutrients. Is the patient gaining, maintaining, or losing weight?

(1) Fat kcal: 67 g × 9 kcal/g = 603 kcal/day; fat percentage = 603/2000 = 30% (normal)

(2) Protein kcal: 60 g × 4 kcal/g = 240 kcal/day; protein percentage = 240/2000 = 12% (normal)

(3) Carbohydrate kcal: 290 g × 4 kcal/g = 1160 kcal/day; carbohydrate percentage = 1160/2000 = 58% (normal)

BMI: weight in kg/height in m^2

Recommended caloric intake: carbohydrate 50% to 60%; fat <30%; protein 10% to 20%

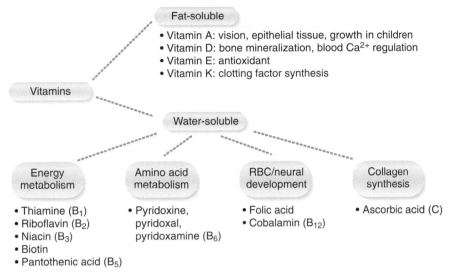

4-2: *Classification and functions of the vitamins.*

(4) Since the patient's calculated daily energy expenditure is 2040 kcal/day (see I), the patient is consuming almost the same number of calories (2000 kcal/day) as are being expended, so the current weight will likely be maintained.

IV. Water-Soluble Vitamins (Fig. 4-2 and Table 4-1)
- Water-soluble vitamins, which generally function as cofactors in enzyme reactions, are readily excreted in the urine and rarely reach toxic levels.

A. Thiamine (vitamin B_1)

1. Sources of thiamine include enriched and whole-grain cereals, brewer's yeast, meats, legumes, and nuts.
2. Thiamine pyrophosphate is the active form of the vitamin.
3. It is a cofactor for dehydrogenases in oxidative decarboxylation of α-keto acids (e.g., pyruvate dehydrogenase conversion of pyruvate into acetyl cofactor A [CoA]) and for transketolase (two-carbon transfer reactions) in the pentose phosphate pathway.
4. Thiamine deficiency most commonly occurs in alcoholics or malnourished individuals.
   a. The majority of the clinical findings in thiamine deficiency are due to loss of ATP from dysfunction of the pyruvate and α-ketoglutarate dehydrogenase reactions, which normally gain 2 NADH (6 ATP).
   b. Intravenous infusion of a glucose-containing fluid may precipitate acute thiamine deficiency in alcoholics (depleted by the pyruvate dehydrogenase reaction); deficiency is manifested by Wernicke-Korsakoff syndrome.
   c. Clinical findings associated with thiamine deficiency (see Table 4-1)

Thiamine (B_1) deficiency: causes beriberi

TABLE 4-1:
Water-Soluble Vitamins: Signs and Symptoms of Deficiency

Vitamin	Signs and Symptoms of Deficiency
Thiamine (vitamin B_1)	Wernicke-Korsakoff syndrome (confusion, ataxia, nystagmus, ophthalmoplegia, antegrade and retrograde amnesia, precipitated by giving thiamine with glucose in intravenous solution); peripheral neuropathy (dry beriberi); congestive cardiomyopathy (wet beriberi)
Riboflavin (vitamin B_2)	Corneal neovascularization; glossitis; cheilosis; angular stomatitis
Niacin (vitamin B_3)	Pellagra, with diarrhea, dermatitis, dementia
Pantothenic acid (vitamin B_5)	None identified
Pyridoxine (vitamin B_6)	Sideroblastic anemia; peripheral neuropathy; convulsions
Cobalamin (vitamin B_{12})	Macrocytic (megaloblastic) anemia; neutropenia and thrombocytopenia; hypersegmented neutrophils; glossitis; subacute combined degeneration; dementia; achlorhydria, atrophic gastritis body and fundus, aa serum gastrin (only in pernicious anemia); amino acid plasma homocysteine; amino acid urine methylmalonic acid
Folic acid	Same as vitamin B_{12} deficiency with the following exceptions: no neurologic dysfunction and normal urine methylmalonic acid
Biotin	Dermatitis, alopecia, glossitis, lactic acidosis
Ascorbic acid (vitamin C)	Bleeding diathesis (ecchymoses, hemarthroses, bleeding gums, perifollicular hemorrhages); loosened teeth; poor wound healing; glossitis

B. Riboflavin (vitamin B_2)
  1. Sources of riboflavin include milk, eggs, meats, poultry, fish, and green leafy vegetables.
  2. Flavin adenine dinucleotide (FAD) and flavin mononucleotide (FMN) are the active forms of riboflavin.
    a. FAD is a cofactor associated with succinate dehydrogenase, which converts succinate to fumarate in the citric acid cycle.
    b. FMN is a component of the electron transport chain and accepts two hydrogen atoms (becomes $FMNH_2$) from NADH in a reaction catalyzed by NADH dehydrogenase.
  3. Riboflavin deficiency is usually seen in severely malnourished individuals or pure vegans, who lack intake of dairy products.
    • Clinical findings associated with riboflavin deficiency (see Table 4-1)
C. Niacin (vitamin B_3, or nicotinic acid)
  1. Sources of niacin include meat, enriched and whole-grain cereals, and synthesis from tryptophan-containing foods, such as milk and eggs.
  2. The two active forms of niacin are NAD^+ and $NADP^+$.
    a. Excess tryptophan is metabolized to niacin and supplies ~10% of the niacin RDA.
    b. NAD^+ and $NADP^+$ are important cofactors in redox reactions.
      (1) NAD^+ reactions are primarily catabolic (e.g., glycolysis).
      (2) $NADP^+$ reactions are primarily anabolic (e.g., fatty acid synthesis).

3. Niacin deficiency, known as pellagra, primarily occurs in individuals whose diets are deficient in both niacin and tryptophan or in conditions in which tryptophan is lost in urine and feces (e.g., Hartnup's disease) or excessively utilized (e.g., carcinoid syndrome).

    a. Individuals who consume corn-based diets are particularly prone to pellagra since maize protein has a low tryptophan content and niacin is in a bound form that cannot be reabsorbed (treating corn with lime, or calcium carbonate, releases bound niacin).

    b. Hartnup's disease is an autosomal recessive disease with a defect in the intestinal and renal reabsorption of neutral amino acids (e.g., tryptophan).

    c. In carcinoid syndrome, tryptophan is used to synthesize serotonin, which produces the flushing and diarrhea associated with the syndrome.

    d. Clinical findings associated with pellagra (see Table 4-1)

4. Excessive intake of niacin leads to flushing due to vasodilatation.

D. Pantothenic acid (vitamin B_5)

    1. Pantothenic acid is present in a wide variety of foods.

    2. It is a component of CoA and the fatty acid synthase complex, which is involved in fatty acid synthesis.

    3. Pantothenic acid deficiency is uncommon.

E. Pyridoxine (vitamin B_6)

    1. Sources of pyridoxine include whole-grain cereals, eggs, meats, fish, soybeans, and nuts.

    2. Pyridoxal phosphate is the active form of the vitamin.

    3. Functions of pyridoxine

        a. Pyridoxine is involved in transamination reactions (reversible conversion of amino acids to α-keto acids), which are catalyzed by the transaminases alanine aminotransferase (ALT) and aspartate aminotransferase (AST).

        b. It is a cofactor for δ-aminolevulinic acid (ALA) synthase, which catalyzes the rate-limiting reaction that converts succinyl CoA + glycine into δ-ALA in heme synthesis.

        c. Pyridoxine is involved in the synthesis of neurotransmitters such as γ-aminobutyrate, serotonin, and norepinephrine.

        d. It is a cofactor in decarboxylation reactions (e.g., conversion of histidine to histamine), glycogenolysis (e.g., glycogen phosphorylase), deamination reactions (e.g., conversion of serine to pyruvate and ammonia), and conversion of tryptophan to niacin.

    4. Pyridoxine deficiency is most commonly seen in alcoholics and in patients receiving isoniazid therapy for tuberculosis.

      • Pyridoxine deficiency is also found in individuals who consume unfortified goat's milk.

    5. Clinical findings associated with pyridoxine deficiency (see Table 4-1)

F. Cobalamin (vitamin B_{12}; contains cobalt)

    1. Sources of cobalamin include meats, shellfish, poultry, eggs, and dairy products only.

Niacin (B_3) deficiency: causes pellagra, with diarrhea, dermatitis, dementia

Pyridoxine (B_6) deficiency: caused by isoniazid therapy

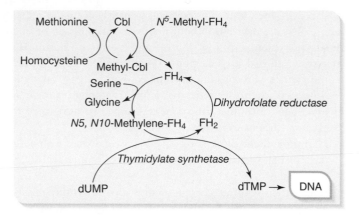

4-3: *Vitamin B$_{12}$ (cobalamin) and folic acid in DNA synthesis. Cobalamin (Cbl) is important in the demethylation of N^5-methyltetrahydrofolate (N^5-methyl-FH$_4$) and methylation of homocysteine to form methionine. Tetrahydrofolate (FH$_4$) receives a methylene group (-CH$_2$-) from serine to produce N^5,N^{10}-methylene-FH$_4$, which transfers the methylene group to deoxyuridine monophosphate (dUMP) to produce deoxythymidine monophosphate (dTMP).*

a. Pure vegans lack vitamin B$_{12}$, whereas ovolactovegetarians obtain adequate sources of vitamin B$_{12}$ from eggs and dairy products.

b. Pure vegans who are pregnant or who are breast-feeding require vitamin B$_{12}$ supplements to prevent anemia from developing in the infant.

2. Functions of cobalamin (Fig. 4-3)

a. Cobalamin removes the methyl group from N^5-methyltetrahydrofolate (N^5-methyl-FH$_4$) to form tetrahydrofolate (FH$_4$), which is used to synthesize deoxythymidine monophosphate (dTMP) from deoxyuridine monophosphate (dUMP) for DNA synthesis.

b. It transfers methyl groups to homocysteine to form methionine.
- A deficiency of either vitamin B$_{12}$ or folic acid leads to an increase in plasma homocysteine levels, which damages vessels and poses a risk for vessel thrombosis.

c. Cobalamin is involved in odd-chain fatty acid metabolism.
(1) Propionyl CoA, the end-product of odd-chain fatty acid metabolism, is converted into methylmalonyl CoA.
(2) Cobalamin is a cofactor for methylmalonyl CoA mutase, which converts methylmalonyl CoA into succinyl CoA.
(3) Vitamin B$_{12}$ deficiency results in an accumulation of methylmalonyl CoA (proximal to the enzyme block), which is converted into methylmalonic acid.

3. Vitamin B$_{12}$ metabolism
a. Vitamin B$_{12}$ complexes with the R factor in saliva.
b. Intrinsic factor (IF) is synthesized in parietal cells located in the body and fundus of the stomach.
- Vitamin B$_{12}$ requires IF for reabsorption in the terminal ileum.

Cobalamin function: converts homocysteine to methionine; odd-chain fatty acid metabolism

    c. Pancreatic enzymes cleave off R factor, which allows vitamin B_{12} to complex with IF.

    d. The vitamin B_{12}-IF complex is reabsorbed in the terminal ileum.

    e. After reabsorption, vitamin B_{12} is bound to transcobalamin in the plasma and is delivered to metabolically active cells or stored in the liver (6- to 9-year supply).

4. Vitamin B_{12} deficiency is most commonly caused by autoimmune destruction of parietal cells, called pernicious anemia.

5. Other causes of deficiency

    a. Pure vegan diet

    b. Chronic pancreatitis: cannot cleave off R factor

    c. Bacterial overgrowth: vitamin B_{12}-IF complex destroyed

    d. Fish tapeworm

    e. Terminal ileal disease (e.g., Crohn's disease)

6. Clinical findings associated with vitamin B_{12} deficiency (see Table 4-1)

G. Folic acid

1. Sources of folic acid include green leafy vegetables, liver, legumes, whole-grain cereals, and yeast.

2. Functions of folic acid (see Fig. 4-3)

    a. Tetrahydrofolate (FH_4) receives a methylene group ($-CH_2-$), an example of a one-carbon transfer reaction, from serine to produce N^5,N^{10}-methylene-tetrahydrofolate. The methylene group is then transferred by thymidylate synthase to dUMP to produce dTMP for DNA synthesis.

       (1) Folic acid deficiency impairs DNA replication due to the shortage of purine nucleotides and thymine.

       (2) Fluorouracil, a chemotherapeutic drug, is converted to a compound that binds to thymidylate synthase, inactivating it.

    b. Two hydrogens from FH_4 are utilized in the formation of dTMP, resulting in the formation of dihydrofolate (FH_2).

    c. FH_2 is reduced to FH_4 by dihydrofolate reductase.

       • Methotrexate and trimethoprim, also chemotherapeutic drugs, inhibit dihydrofolate reductase, causing folic acid deficiency and a macrocytic anemia.

3. Folic acid metabolism

    a. Folic acid is ingested in a polyglutamate form.

    b. Polyglutamates are converted into monoglutamates in the jejunum by intestinal conjugase.

       • The enzyme is inhibited by phenytoin, which causes folic acid deficiency.

    c. Monoglutamate is reabsorbed in the jejunum.

       • Its reabsorption is blocked by alcohol and by oral contraceptives, leading to folic acid deficiency.

    d. Folic acid circulates and is measured in the blood as methyltetrahydrofolate.

    e. Only a 3- or 4-month supply of folic acid is stored in the liver.

Vitamin B_{12} (cobalamin) deficiency: caused by pernicious anemia; causes macrocytic anemia

Folic acid function: DNA synthesis; deficiency causes macrocytic anemia

Drugs and folic acid deficiency: methotrexate, trimethoprim, alcohol, phenytoin, oral contraceptives

4. Folic acid deficiency is most commonly caused by alcoholism. Other causes:
   a. Diet lacking fruits and vegetables
   b. Drugs: methotrexate, phenytoin, oral contraceptives
   c. Pregnancy: Women must have adequate levels of folate prior to becoming pregnant to prevent failure of the neural tube to close between the 23rd and the 28th day of embryogenesis.
   d. Rapidly growing cancers (e.g., leukemia): Malignant cells utilize folic acid.
   e. Small bowel malabsorption (e.g., celiac disease)
   f. Unfortified goat's milk

Folic acid supplementation before pregnancy: reduces risk for neural tube defects

5. Clinical and laboratory findings are similar to vitamin B_{12} deficiency except for the absence of neurologic deficits and normal levels of methylmalonic acid (see Table 4-1).

H. Biotin
   1. Most of the daily requirement of biotin is supplied by bacterial synthesis in the intestine.
   2. It is a cofactor in carboxylase reactions (e.g., pyruvate carboxylase, acetyl CoA carboxylase, propionyl CoA carboxylase).
   3. Biotin deficiency is caused by eating raw eggs (egg whites contain avidin, which binds biotin) and by taking broad-spectrum antibiotics, which prevent bacterial synthesis of the vitamin.
   4. Clinical findings associated with biotin deficiency (see Table 4-1)

I. Ascorbic acid (vitamin C)
   1. Sources of vitamin C include citrus fruits, potatoes, green and red peppers, broccoli, tomatoes, spinach, and strawberries.
   2. Functions of vitamin C
      a. Hydroxylation of lysine and proline residues during collagen synthesis
      b. Antioxidant activity (sequesters free radicals)
      c. Reduces non-heme iron (Fe^{3+}) from plants to the ferrous (Fe^{2+}) state for reabsorption in the duodenum
      d. Keeps FH_4 in its reduced form
      e. Cofactor in the conversion of dopamine to norepinephrine in catecholamine synthesis

Ascorbic acid deficiency: causes scurvy

   3. Causes of vitamin C deficiency (scurvy) include diets lacking fruits and vegetables ("tea and toast" diet) and smoking cigarettes.
   4. Excess intake of vitamin C may result in the formation of renal calculi.
   5. Clinical findings associated with vitamin C deficiency (see Table 4-1)

V. Fat-Soluble Vitamins
   • The fat-soluble vitamins A, D, E, and K function as hormones, cofactors, hemostatic agents, and antioxidants. They are absorbed with fats, transported in chylomicrons, and stored in the liver and adipose tissue; toxicity can occur.
   A. Vitamin A (retinol)
      1. Sources of vitamin A include cod liver oil, dairy products, and egg yolk.

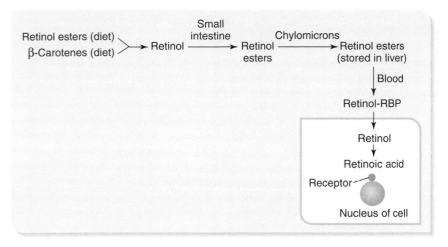

4-4: *Vitamin A absorption and transport. Ingested retinol esters and β-carotenes are converted to retinol, the key absorption and transport form of vitamin A. In the small intestine, retinol is converted to retinol esters, the key storage form of vitamin A. When needed, retinol is released from the liver into the bloodstream, where it complexes with retinol-binding protein (RBP). Within cells, retinol is irreversibly oxidized to retinoic acid, which binds to nuclear receptors and activates gene transcription.*

2. Retinol (alcohol), retinal (aldehyde), and retinoic acid are the active forms of vitamin A (Fig. 4-4).
   a. β-Carotenes (provitamin A) found in dark green leafy and yellow vegetables (e.g., spinach, carrots) and retinol esters in the diet are converted into retinol, which is esterified (forming retinol esters) in the enterocytes of the small intestine.
      • An excess of β-carotenes in the diet turns the skin yellow, but the sclera remains white (unlike in jaundice).
   b. Retinol esters are packaged into chylomicrons and transported to the liver for storage.
   c. Retinol is released from the liver, complexes with retinol-binding protein, and is delivered to target tissues throughout the body (except heart and skeletal muscle).
   d. In the cytosol, retinol is irreversibly oxidized to retinoic acid.
   e. Retinoic acid (similar to steroid hormones and vitamin D) binds to nuclear receptors, forming a complex that activates gene transcription of protein products.
3. Functions of vitamin A
   a. A component of the visual pigments within rod and cone cells of the retina
   b. Important in normal cell differentiation and prevents epithelial cells from undergoing squamous metaplasia
   c. Important in normal bone and tooth development
   d. Supports spermatogenesis and placental development
   e. Drugs used in the treatment of skin disorders and acute promyelocytic leukemia

TABLE 4-2:
Fat-Soluble Vitamins: Signs and Symptoms of Deficiency and Excess

Vitamin	Signs and Symptoms of Deficiency	Signs and Symptoms of Excess
Vitamin A	Night blindness; eye abnormalities (dry eyes, blindness); skin abnormalities (follicular hyperkeratosis, dry skin); lung abnormalities (bronchitis, pneumonia, possibly lung cancer); growth retardation; poor wound healing	Increased intracranial pressure (papilledema, convulsions); liver toxicity; bone pain
Vitamin D	Rickets in children and osteomalacia in adults; findings in both conditions—pathologic fractures, excess osteoid, bowed legs; findings in rickets only—craniotabes, skeletal deformities, rachitic rosary, defective epiphyseal plates with growth retardation	Hypercalcemia, renal calculi
Vitamin E	Hemolytic anemia; peripheral neuropathy; posterior column degeneration (poor joint sensation and absent vibratory sensation); retinal degeneration; myopathy	Decreased synthesis of vitamin K—dependent coagulation factors (enhances anticoagulation effect of coumarin derivatives)
Vitamin K	Bleeding diathesis (gastrointestinal bleeding, ecchymoses); prolonged prothrombin time	Hemolytic anemia and jaundice in newborns if mother receives excess vitamin K

Oral isotretinoin: severe cystic acne; teratogenic

All-*trans*-retinoic acid: treatment for acute promyelocytic leukemia

  (1) Topical tretinoin (all-*trans*-retinoic acid) is used in the treatment of psoriasis and mild acne.
  (2) Oral isotretinoin is used to treat severe cystic acne; however, because it is teratogenic, women must have a pregnancy test before the drug is prescribed.
  (3) All-*trans*-retinoic acid is used to treat acute promyelocytic leukemia (hypergranular M3) and is thought to induce maturation of the leukemic cells.
 4. Causes of vitamin A deficiency include a diet poor in dark green leafy and yellow vegetables and individuals with fat malabsorption (e.g., celiac disease).
 5. Causes of vitamin A excess include eating polar bear liver and isotretinoin therapy.
 6. Clinical findings associated with vitamin A deficiency and excess (Table 4-2)
B. Vitamin D
 1. Sources of vitamin D include liver, egg yolk, saltwater fish, and vitamin D-fortified foods.
 2. Synthesis of calcitriol (1,25-dihydroxycholecalciferol), the active form of vitamin D, occurs in the following sequence (Fig. 4-5).

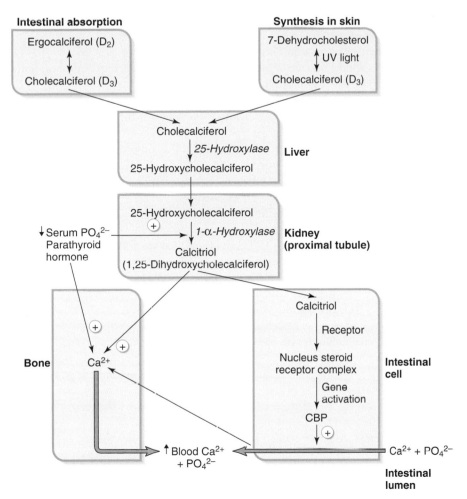

4-5: *Formation of calcitriol, the active form of vitamin D, and its action in calcium homeostasis. Note that the key functions of calcitriol are to mineralize bone using calcium and phosphorus and, in combination with parathyroid hormone (PTH), to maintain serum calcium levels. CBP, calcium-binding protein.*

   a. Preformed vitamin D in the diet consists of cholecalciferol (vitamin D_3) and ergocalciferol (vitamin D_2, found in plants), which is interconvertible with vitamin D_3.

   b. Endogenous vitamin D is produced by photoconversion of 7-dehydrocholesterol to vitamin D_3 in sun-exposed skin (most important source of vitamin D).

   c. The first hydroxylation, which produces 25-hydroxycholecalciferol, occurs in the liver within the cytochrome P450 system.

   d. The second hydroxylation, by 1-α-hydroxylase, produces 1,25-dihydroxycholecalciferol (calcitriol) and occurs in the proximal tubules of the kidneys.

     • The activity of 1-α-hydroxylase in the kidneys is enhanced by parathyroid hormone (PTH) and low serum phosphorus levels.

e. Receptors for vitamin D are located in the intestine, kidneys, and on osteoblasts in bone.

3. Functions of vitamin D

a. Vitamin D increases intestinal reabsorption of calcium and phosphorus and renal reabsorption of calcium.

(1) Reabsorption of calcium and phosphorus provides an adequate solubility product (calcium × phosphorus) for vitamin D to mineralize bone.

- Hydroxyapatite, $Ca_{10}(PO_4)_6(OH)_2$, is the crystalline salt deposited in bone.

(2) When vitamin D interacts with its receptors on osteoblasts, alkaline phosphatase is released.

- Vitamin D hydrolyzes pyrophosphate, an inhibitor of bone mineralization.

b. In combination with PTH, vitamin D has the following effects.

(1) It increases the mobilization of calcium from bone by stimulating the conversion of macrophage stem cells in the bone marrow into osteoclasts.

(2) It maintains the serum calcium concentration.

PTH and vitamin D: maintain ionized calcium level

4. Causes of vitamin D deficiency

a. Renal failure (most common cause): due to deficiency of 1-α-hydroxylase enzyme

b. Fat malabsorption: cannot reabsorb fat-soluble vitamins (e.g., celiac disease)

c. Chronic liver disease: cannot carry out the first hydroxylation of vitamin D_3

d. Enhanced liver cytochrome P450 system (e.g., alcohol, phenytoin, barbiturates): increased metabolism of 25-hydroxycholecalciferol

e. Inadequate exposure to sunlight: decreased synthesis of cholecalciferol (vitamin D_3)

f. Primary hypoparathyroidism: PTH is required for enhancing the activity of 1-α-hydroxylase

g. Type I vitamin D-dependent rickets: deficiency of 1-α-hydroxylase

h. Type II vitamin D-dependent rickets: deficiency of vitamin D receptors in target tissue

5. Patients taking megadoses of vitamin D may develop vitamin D toxicity.

6. Clinical findings associated with vitamin D deficiency and excess (see Table 4-2)

C. Vitamin E

1. α-Tocopherol has the highest biological activity of the naturally occurring tocopherols that constitute vitamin E and is abundant in fruits, vegetables, and grains.

2. Vitamin E is an antioxidant and scavenger of free radicals that protects polyunsaturated fats and fatty acids in cell membranes from lipid peroxidation and also protects low-density lipoprotein (LDL) from oxidation.

a. Oxidized LDL is more likely than nonoxidized LDL to cause atherosclerosis.

b. Vitamin E protects erythrocytes from oxidative damage that leads to hemolysis.

3. Vitamin E deficiency is uncommon and primarily occurs in children with malabsorption secondary to cystic fibrosis and in abetalipoproteinemia (see Chapter 7).

4. Patients taking megadoses of vitamin E may develop vitamin E toxicity.

5. Clinical findings associated with vitamin E deficiency and excess (see Table 4-2)

D. Vitamin K

1. Sources of vitamin K include green leafy vegetables (which supply vitamin K_1, phylloquinone) and bacterial synthesis in the colon (which supplies vitamin K_2, or menaquinone).

a. After reabsorption in the bowel, vitamin K is oxidized to form an inactive epoxide.

b. To be catalytically active, vitamin K must be reduced by epoxide reductase.

2. Vitamin K δ-carboxylates glutamate residues in the vitamin K-dependent coagulation factors, which are factors II (prothrombin), VII, IX, X, and proteins C and S.

a. The vitamin K-dependent coagulation factors are all synthesized in the liver in a nonfunctional state.

b. When γ-carboxylated in the liver by vitamin K and released into the circulation, these coagulation factors are able to bind to calcium, which is essential to the formation of a clot.

c. The prothrombin time is a coagulation test that evaluates all of the vitamin K-dependent factors, except factor IX and proteins C and S.

d. Coumarin derivatives act as anticoagulants by inhibiting the activity of epoxide reductase; hence, the vitamin K-dependent coagulation factors are rendered nonfunctional by their inability to bind to calcium.

  • Coumarin derivatives are present in rat poison, which is a common cause of poisoning in children.

3. Vitamin K deficiency is rare but can be caused by the use of broad-spectrum antibiotics, which destroy colonic bacterial synthesis of the vitamin.

4. Other causes of vitamin K deficiency

a. Therapy with coumarin derivatives: inhibits hepatic epoxide reductase

b. Fat malabsorption: cannot reabsorb fat-soluble vitamins (e.g., celiac disease)

c. Newborns: lack bacterial colonization of the bowel and must receive an intramuscular vitamin K injection at birth to prevent hemorrhagic disease of the newborn

d. Breast milk: inadequate supply of vitamin K

5. Excessive intake of vitamin K leading to toxicity is uncommon.

6. Clinical findings associated with vitamin K deficiency and excess (see Table 4-2)

Vitamin E: protects erythrocytes from oxidative damage leading to hemolysis

Vitamin K: γ-carboxylates liver-derived vitamin K-dependent coagulation factors

Coumarin derivative: anticoagulant that inhibits hepatic epoxide reductase

VI. Minerals and Electrolytes
- Minerals (RDA > 100 mg/day), trace elements (RDA < 100 mg/day), and vitamins are micronutrients that are required in the normal diet. Most minerals are found in the body fluids as electrolyte solutions.

A. Calcium
1. Sources of calcium include dairy products, leafy green vegetables, legumes, nuts, and whole grains.
2. Functions of calcium
   a. Bone formation and teeth
   b. Nerve conduction
   c. Skeletal, cardiac, smooth muscle contraction
   d. Binds to vitamin K-dependent coagulation factors and activates factor XIII to cross-link fibrin strands
   e. Calcium-calmodulin complex activates many enzymes.
3. Regulation of calcium
   a. Parathyroid hormone increases reabsorption in the early distal tubule of the kidneys and mobilizes calcium from bone.
   b. Vitamin D (calcitriol) increases calcium reabsorption in the intestine and kidneys.
   c. Calcitonin, which is synthesized by C cells in the thyroid gland, inhibits osteoclasts, thereby inhibiting the release of calcium from bones.
   d. Approximately 40% of calcium is bound to albumin; 13% is bound to phosphorus and citrates; and 47% circulates as free, ionized calcium, which is metabolically active.
      (1) Alkalotic conditions decrease ionized calcium levels by increasing the amount of calcium bound to albumin.
         - An alkalotic state increases the number of negative charges on albumin (fewer hydrogen ions); therefore, proportionately more calcium is bound to albumin at the expense of the ionized calcium level.
      (2) Hypoalbuminemia decreases the total serum calcium without altering the ionized calcium level.
4. Causes of hypocalcemia
   a. Hypoalbuminemia: most common nonpathologic cause
   b. Hypomagnesemia: most common pathologic cause
   c. Vitamin D deficiency
   d. Primary hypoparathyroidism
5. Causes of hypercalcemia
   a. Primary hyperparathyroidism: most common cause in the ambulatory population
   b. Malignancy: most common cause in a hospitalized patient
   c. Sarcoidosis: granuloma synthesis of vitamin D
6. Clinical findings associated with hypocalcemia and hypercalcemia (Table 4-3)

B. Phosphate (phosphorus)
- Phosphate is the most abundant intracellular anion.

Alkalotic state: lowers ionized calcium, causing tetany

TABLE 4-3:
Minerals: Signs and Symptoms of Deficiency and Excess

Mineral	Signs and Symptoms of Deficiency	Signs and Symptoms of Excess
Calcium	Tetany (signs of tetany: carpopedal spasm, Chvostek's sign, muscle twitching); osteoporosis	Renal calculi; metastatic calcification; polyuria
Phosphorus (phosphate)	Muscle weakness; rhabdomyolysis with myoglobinuria (due to low ATP); hemolytic anemia (due to low ATP)	Hypocalcemia; hypovitaminosis D (inhibits activity of 1-α-hydroxylase)
Sodium	Mental status abnormalities (cerebral edema); convulsions	Mental status abnormalities; convulsions
Chloride	No specific signs and symptoms	No specific signs and symptoms
Potassium	Muscle weakness; polyuria	Heart stops in diastole
Magnesium	Hypocalcemia with tetany; tachycardia	Neuromuscular depression; bradycardia

1. Sources of phosphate include most foods.
2. Functions of phosphate
   a. Mineralization of bones and teeth
   b. Component of DNA and RNA
   c. Component of phosphorylated vitamins (e.g., thiamine, pyridoxine) and ATP
   d. Traps monosaccharides in cells (e.g., phosphorylation of glucose in glycolysis)
   e. Activates enzymes (e.g., protein kinase) and deactivates enzymes (e.g., glycogen synthase)
   f. Maintains pH: protons secreted into the renal tubule lumen react with dibasic phosphate (HPO_4^{2-}) to form monobasic phosphate ($H_2PO_4^-$), which is called titratable acidity.
3. Control of phosphate
   a. Parathyroid hormone has a phosphaturic effect.
   b. Vitamin D (calcitriol) increases reabsorption of phosphate in the small bowel.
4. Causes of hypophosphatemia
   a. Respiratory and metabolic alkalosis: most common cause; alkalosis enhances glycolysis and phosphorylation of glucose
   b. Hypovitaminosis D due to malabsorption: decreased intestinal reabsorption of phosphate
   c. Primary hyperparathyroidism: increased loss of phosphate in urine
5. Causes of hyperphosphatemia
   a. Renal failure: most common cause; decreased renal excretion
   b. Primary hypoparathyroidism
   c. Normal children: higher levels of phosphate help drive calcium into bone
6. Clinical findings associated with hypophosphatemia and hyperphosphatemia (see Table 4-3)

Phosphate: component of ATP

C. Sodium
- Sodium is the most abundant cation in extracellular fluid.
1. It is primarily found in table salt.
2. Functions of sodium
   a. Regulation of pH, osmotic pressure, and water movement in body fluids
      - The serum sodium concentration is the primary determinant of water movements by osmosis between the extracellular and intracellular fluid compartments.
   b. Maintains muscle and nerve excitability
   c. Active transport of glucose, galactose, and amino acids in the small intestine
   d. Maintains the diffusion potential of membranes
3. Control of sodium
   a. Diet
   b. Aldosterone: controls renal reabsorption (when present) and excretion (when absent)
   c. Atrial natriuretic peptide: decreases reabsorption in the kidneys
4. Causes of hyponatremia
   a. Thiazide and loop diuretics: most common cause; increase renal excretion
   b. Inappropriate secretion of antidiuretic hormone: dilutional effect in plasma of excess water reabsorption from the collecting tubules of the kidneys
   c. Congestive heart failure and chronic liver disease: dilutional effect in plasma of excess water reabsorbed from the kidneys
5. Causes of hypernatremia
   a. Osmotic diuresis: most common cause; loss of a hypotonic salt solution in the kidneys due to glucosuria, excess urea, or mannitol (treatment of cerebral edema)
   b. Diabetes insipidus: loss of water due to deficiency or dysfunction of antidiuretic hormone
6. Clinical findings associated with hyponatremia and hypernatremia (see Table 4-3)

D. Chloride
- Chloride is the most abundant anion in extracellular fluid.
1. It is primarily found in table salt.
2. Functions of chloride
   a. Regulation of pH and osmotic pressure
   b. Regulates neuromuscular excitability and muscle contraction
3. Control of chloride
   a. Diet
   b. Aldosterone: controls renal reabsorption (when present) and excretion (when absent)
4. Causes of hypochloremia
   a. Thiazide and loop diuretics: increase renal excretion
   b. Vomiting

Sodium: controls water movement between extracellular and intracellular fluid compartments

5. Causes of hyperchloremia
   a. Mineralocorticoid excess: increases both sodium and chloride reabsorption
   b. Renal tubular acidosis and diarrhea: loss of bicarbonate causes increase in chloride to offset the loss of negative charges

E. Potassium
   - Potassium is the most abundant intracellular cation.
   1. Sources of potassium include meats, vegetables, fruits, nuts, and legumes.
   2. Functions of potassium
      a. Regulation of pH and osmotic pressure
      b. Regulation of neuromuscular excitability and muscle contraction
      c. Regulates insulin secretion: hypokalemia inhibits insulin; hyperkalemia stimulates insulin secretion
   3. Control of potassium
      a. Aldosterone: controls renal reabsorption (when absent) and excretion (when present)
      b. Arterial pH
         (1) Alkalotic conditions cause hydrogen ions to move out of the cell (provides protons) and potassium to move into the cell (leads to hypokalemia) to maintain electroneutrality.
         (2) Acidotic conditions cause hydrogen ions to move into cells (for buffering) in exchange for potassium (leads to hyperkalemia).
   4. Causes of hypokalemia
      a. Thiazide and loop diuretics: increase renal excretion
      b. Vomiting and diarrhea: lost in the body fluids
      c. Aldosterone excess: increased renal excretion
   5. Causes of hyperkalemia
      a. Renal failure: decreased excretion of potassium
      b. Addison's disease: due to loss of aldosterone
   6. Clinical findings associated with hypokalemia and hyperkalemia (see Table 4-3)

F. Magnesium
   1. Sources of magnesium include green vegetables, nuts, and legumes.
   2. Functions of magnesium
      a. Calcium metabolism
         (1) Cofactor of adenylate cyclase involved in the activation of PTH
         (2) Increases PTH synthesis and release
      b. Component of bone
      c. Muscle contraction: modulates the vasoconstrictive effects of intracellular calcium
      d. Nerve impulse propagation
      e. Cofactor in ATPases (e.g., Na^{2+}/K^+ ATPase, Ca^{2+} ATPase)
   3. Causes of hypomagnesemia
      a. Alcoholism: most common cause; increased renal loss
      b. Diuretics: increased renal loss
      c. Drugs (e.g., aminoglycosides, cisplatinum): increased renal loss

Potassium: major intracellular cation

Magnesium: important in function of PTH

4. Causes of hypermagnesemia
   a. Renal failure: decreased excretion
   b. Treatment of eclampsia with magnesium sulfate
5. Clinical findings associated with hypomagnesemia and hypermagnesemia (see Table 4-3)

VII. Trace Elements
   A. Iron
      1. Primary sources of iron include meat, eggs, vegetables, and fortified cereals.
      2. Iron is the structural component of heme in hemoglobin, myoglobin, and the cytochrome oxidase system. It is also an important cofactor for enzymes (e.g., catalase).
         a. Meat contains heme iron, which is ferrous (Fe^{2+}) and available for reabsorption in the duodenum.
            (1) Once reabsorbed by duodenal enterocytes, heme is enzymatically degraded to release iron.
            (2) Most of the iron is diverted to storage as apoferritin in the enterocyte, whereas a small amount is delivered to plasma transferrin, the circulating binding protein of iron.
         b. Plants contain non-heme iron, which is in the ferric state (Fe^{3+}); hence, reabsorption of non-heme iron is more complex and involves a number of different binding proteins before it is transferred to transferrin.
         c. Ferritin, a soluble iron-protein complex, is the storage form of iron in the intestinal mucosa, liver, spleen, and bone marrow.
            (1) Serum ferritin levels reflect iron stores in the bone marrow.
            (2) Serum ferritin is the best screening test for iron deficiency and iron overload disorders (e.g., hemochromatosis).
         d. Hemosiderin is an insoluble storage product of ferritin degradation.
            (1) Hemosiderosis is an acquired accumulation of hemosiderin in macrophages in tissues throughout the body.
               • Alcoholics and patients with chronic illnesses who require ongoing transfusions are at risk for hemosiderosis.
            (2) Hemochromatosis is an autosomal recessive disease characterized by unrestricted reabsorption of iron from the duodenum, leading to an accumulation of iron in liver, heart, pancreas, skin, and other tissues.
               • Hemochromatosis causes cirrhosis of the liver, bronze skin color, diabetes mellitus, malabsorption, and heart failure.
         e. Transferrin, the primary binding protein for iron, is synthesized in the liver and transports iron to macrophages in the bone marrow for storage or to the developing RBCs for hemoglobin synthesis.
            (1) When iron stores in the bone marrow macrophages are decreased (e.g., iron deficiency), liver synthesis of transferrin increases, which increases total iron-binding capacity.
            (2) When iron stores in the bone marrow macrophages are increased (e.g., hemochromatosis), transferrin synthesis is decreased, which decreases the total iron-binding capacity.

Serum ferritin: low in iron deficiency, high in hemochromatosis

TABLE 4-4:

Trace Elements: Signs and Symptoms of Deficiency

Trace Element	Signs and Symptoms of Deficiency
Iron	Microcytic anemia; low serum ferritin, low serum iron, high total iron-binding capacity (correlates with increased transferrin synthesis); Plummer-Vinson syndrome (esophageal webs, glossitis, spoon nails, achlorhydria); excessive fatigue
Zinc	Poor wound healing; dysgeusia (inability to taste); anosmia (inability to smell); perioral rash; hypogonadism; growth retardation
Copper	Microcytic anemia (decreased ferroxidase activity); aortic dissection; poor wound healing
Iodine	Goiter (due to relative or absolute deficiency of thyroid hormones)
Chromium	Impaired glucose tolerance; peripheral neuropathy
Selenium	Muscle pain and weakness; cardiomyopathy
Fluoride	Dental caries

3. Causes of iron deficiency vary by age.
   a. Newborn: bleeding Meckel's diverticulum
   b. Child: bleeding Meckel's diverticulum, milk diet
   c. Woman younger than 50 years of age: menorrhagia
   d. Man younger than 50 years of age: peptic ulcer disease
   e. Men and women older than 50 years of age: colon polyps or cancer
4. Causes of excess serum iron
   a. Iron poisoning: common in children; causes hemorrhagic gastritis and liver necrosis
   b. Iron overload diseases: hemochromatosis; hemosiderosis; sideroblastic anemia (due to pyridoxine deficiency, lead poisoning, alcoholism)
     (1) Sideroblastic anemias are associated with excess iron accumulation in mitochondria resulting from difficulties in heme synthesis.
     (2) Excess iron in mitochondria produces ringed sideroblasts (mitochondria are located around the nucleus of immature RBCs).
5. Clinical findings associated with iron deficiency (Table 4-4)
B. Zinc
  1. Primary sources of zinc include meat, liver, eggs, and oysters.
  2. Zinc primarily serves as a cofactor for metalloenzymes.
   a. Superoxide dismutase
   b. Collagenase: important in remodeling of a wound and replacing type III collagen with type I collagen to increase tensile strength
   c. Alcohol dehydrogenase: converts alcohol into acetaldehyde
   d. Alkaline phosphatase: important in bone mineralization; marker of obstruction to bile flow in the liver or common bile duct
  3. Zinc is also important in spermatogenesis and in growth in children.
  4. Causes of zinc deficiency
   a. Diseases: alcoholism, rheumatoid arthritis, acute and chronic inflammatory diseases, chronic diarrhea

b. Acrodermatitis enteropathica: autosomal recessive disease associated with dermatitis, diarrhea, growth retardation in children, decreased spermatogenesis, and poor wound healing

5. Clinical findings associated with zinc deficiency (see Table 4-4)

C. Copper

1. Sources of copper include shellfish, organ meats, poultry, cereal, fruits, and dried beans.

2. Copper primarily serves as a cofactor for metalloenzymes.

   a. Ferroxidase: binds iron to transferrin; causes iron deficiency if deficient

   b. Lysyl oxidase: cross-linking of collagen and elastic tissue

   c. Superoxide dismutase: neutralizes superoxide, an O_2 free radical

   d. Tyrosinase: important in melanin synthesis; deficient in albinism

   e. Cytochrome c oxidase: component of the electron-transport chain

3. Ceruloplasmin is a copper-binding plasma protein that is synthesized in the liver and is involved in copper transport and regulation.

4. Copper deficiency (hypocupremia) is most often due to total parenteral nutrition (TPN).

5. An excess of free copper (hypercupremia) is present in Wilson's disease, an autosomal recessive disease associated with a defect in secreting copper into bile.

   • Characteristic findings include chronic liver disease, deposition of free copper into the eye (Kayser-Fleischer ring) and lenticular nuclei (dementia, movement disorder), low serum ceruloplasmin, and high free copper levels in blood and urine.

6. Clinical findings associated with copper deficiency (see Table 4-4)

D. Iodine

1. Sources of iodine include iodized table salt and seafood.

2. Iodine is used in the synthesis of thyroid hormones.

3. Iodine deficiency is due primarily to an inadequate intake of seafood or iodized table salt.

4. Clinical findings associated with iodine deficiency (see Table 4-4)

E. Chromium

1. Sources of chromium include wheat germ, liver, and brewer's yeast.

2. Chromium is a component of glucose tolerance factor, which facilitates insulin action through postreceptor effects.

3. Chromium deficiency primarily occurs in patients receiving TPN.

4. Clinical findings associated with chromium deficiency (see Table 4-4)

F. Selenium

1. Sources of selenium include seafood and liver.

2. Selenium is a component of glutathione peroxidase.

   • Glutathione is a potent antioxidant that neutralizes peroxide and peroxide free radicals (see Chapter 6).

3. Selenium deficiency occurs primarily in patients receiving TPN.

4. Clinical findings associated with selenium deficiency (see Table 4-4)

G. Fluoride

1. Sources of fluoride include tea and fluoridated water.

Zinc deficiency: poor wound healing, loss of taste and smell

Wilson's disease: copper accumulates in liver, brain, and eyes

Iodine deficiency: produces goiter

Selenium: antioxidant

2. Fluoride is a structural component of calcium hydroxyapatite in bone and teeth.
3. Deficiency of fluoride is primarily due to inadequate intake of fluoridated water.
4. An excess in fluoride is due primarily to an excess of fluoride in drinking water.
   - Fluorosis is associated with chalky deposits on the teeth, calcification of ligaments, and an increased risk for bone fractures.
5. Clinical findings associated with fluoride deficiency (see Table 4-4)

Fluoride deficiency: dental caries

Generation of Energy from Dietary Fuels

TARGET TOPICS

- Free-energy change (ΔG) and the direction of metabolic pathways
- ATP as the cell's energy currency
- Redox coenzymes (NAD^+, FAD, NADPH) as the cell's electron carriers
- Structural-functional compartments of the mitochondrion
- Citric acid cycle: role in energy metabolism,
- regulation, interface with other pathways
- Components of the electron transport chain and their role in ATP synthesis
- Clinical correlations: Leber's hereditary optic neuropathy, mitochondrial myopathies, electron transport blockers and uncouplers of mitochondrial ATP production

I. Energetics of Metabolic Pathways
   A. Free-energy change (ΔG) for a biochemical reaction indicates its tendency to proceed and the amount of free energy it will release or require.
   B. Coupled reactions share a common intermediate. For example, the common intermediate **D** couples the two reactions below:

$$A + B \rightleftarrows C + \mathbf{D}$$
$$\mathbf{D} + E \rightleftarrows F + G$$

   1. Overall coupled reaction ($A + B \rightleftarrows F + G$) proceeds spontaneously in a forward direction if the sum of ΔG values of the individual reactions is negative.
   2. Metabolic pathways consist of a series of coupled reactions linked by common intermediates (Fig. 5-1).
      a. ΔG values are additive for all pathway reactions.
         - An energetically favorable reaction (e.g., hydrolysis of ATP) drives an energetically unfavorable coupled reaction in the forward direction.
      b. If ΔG for consecutive reactions is negative, the reactions operate spontaneously in the forward direction.

Negative ΔG: allows coupled reactions to proceed spontaneously in a forward direction

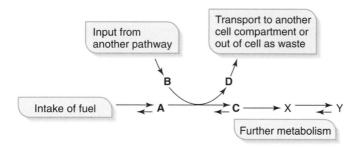

5-1: *Processes that affect flow through metabolic pathways. In the absence of such processes, individual reversible reactions eventually reach equilibrium and the flow of metabolites through a pathway ceases. For example, a genetic defect or inhibitor that reduces production of B also decreases operation of the pathway from fuel →A →Y.*

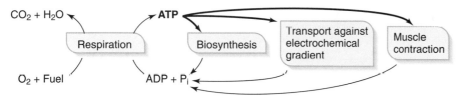

5-2: *ATP-ADP cycle. Energy stored in reduced fuel molecules is extracted during oxidative metabolism (respiration) and converted to ATP. Hydrolysis of ATP releases energy that cells use for major types of energy-requiring processes (thick arrows).*

C. ATP-ADP cycle is the most common mechanism of energy exchange in biological systems (Fig. 5-2).
  1. Hydrolysis of high-energy bonds in ATP has a large $-\Delta G°$ of approximately 7 kcal/mol.
  2. Hydrolysis of other nucleoside triphosphates and other high-energy compounds provides energy for some metabolic processes. For example:
     a. GTP during ribosomal steps of protein synthesis
     b. CTP during lipid synthesis
     c. UTP during polysaccharide synthesis
     d. Phosphocreatine in muscle replenishes ATP
D. Redox coenzymes serve as carrier molecules for hydrogen and electrons during biological oxidation-reduction reactions (Fig. 5-3).
  1. Nicotinamide adenine dinucleotide (NAD^+) and flavin adenine dinucleotide (FAD) are the major electron acceptors in the catabolism of fuel molecules.
     • Reduced forms of NAD^+ and FAD (i.e., NADH and $FADH_2$) ultimately transfer electrons to O_2 with the coupled formation of ATP (oxidative phosphorylation).
  2. NADPH (a phosphorylated derivative of NADH) is the primary electron donor in reductive biosynthetic reactions (e.g., synthesis of fatty acids, cholesterol, and steroids).

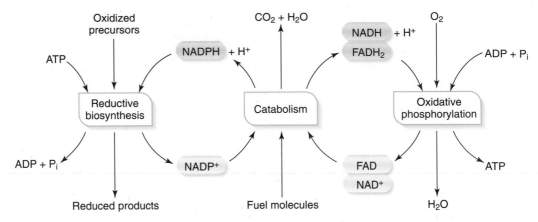

5-3: *Role of redox coenzymes as electron carriers. Oxidized coenzymes (light shading) are reduced during catabolism. Reduced coenzymes (dark shading) are used in reductive biosynthesis (left) or in oxidative phosphorylation to generate ATP (right).*

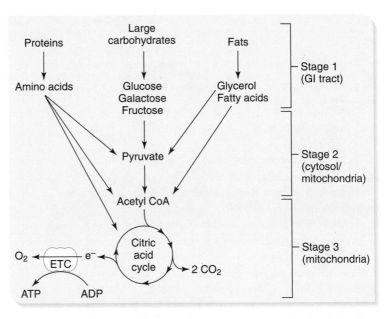

5-4: *Three stages in catabolism of the energy-yielding major nutrients. Note the central role of pyruvate and acetyl CoA. Oxidative phosphorylation, the formation of ATP coupled to the flow of electrons (e^-) through the electron-transport chain (ETC), generates most of the ATP resulting from catabolism.*

II. Introduction to Intermediary Metabolism

    A. Catabolism of foodstuffs to generate ATP occurs in three stages (Fig. 5-4).

        1. Breakdown of large dietary constituents (carbohydrates, fats, and proteins) to their small building blocks by digestive enzymes

        2. Formation of acetyl CoA by degradation of the products of digestion (e.g., glucose, fatty acids, glycerol, and amino acids)

3. Oxidation of acetyl CoA in the citric acid cycle and the flow of electrons through the electron transport chain with coupled formation of ATP (oxidative phosphorylation)

B. Metabolic pathways are localized to particular cellular sites.
1. Mitochondria
    a. Matrix: production of acetyl CoA, citric acid cycle, β-oxidation of fatty acids, ketogenesis
    b. Inner membrane: oxidative phosphorylation
2. Cytosol: glycolysis, glycogenesis, glycogenolysis, pentose phosphate shunt, fatty acid synthesis, steroid synthesis (smooth endoplasmic reticulum), protein synthesis (rough endoplasmic reticulum)
3. Mitochondria and cytosol: gluconeogenesis, urea cycle, heme synthesis
4. Nucleus and mitochondria: DNA and RNA synthesis

C. Four common perspectives, applicable to various metabolic pathways, provide a consistent framework for learning intermediary metabolism.
1. Individual reaction characteristics: Each reaction in a pathway has unique characteristics regarding substrates, products, enzymes, cofactors, and inhibitors.
2. Regulated steps: At least one step in a metabolic pathway is generally regulated by hormones and/or metabolites that restrict or accelerate the flow of metabolites through the pathway.
3. Interface with other pathways: Many intermediates within one pathway are substrates for other pathways, providing a means for different pathways to interact.
4. Pathway malfunction: Significant reduction in the activity of an enzyme catalyzing one step in a pathway, due to a genetic defect or inhibitor, leads to accumulation of some metabolites and reduced levels of others, often with pathologic consequences.

Metabolic pathways occur in specific cellular sites (e.g., glycolysis in cytosol, citric acid cycle and oxidative phosphorylation in mitochondria)

III. Citric Acid Cycle
A. In the citric acid cycle (also known as the Krebs cycle and tricarboxylic, or TCA, cycle), acetyl CoA is oxidized to CO_2, producing reduced coenzymes and GTP (Fig. 5-5).
   • All of the enzymes catalyzing the citric acid cycle are located in the matrix or inner membrane of mitochondria, which are contained in all human cells, except mature red blood cells and platelets.

B. Individual reaction characteristics of the citric acid cycle (Fig. 5-6)
1. Condensation of acetyl CoA with oxaloacetate to form six-carbon citrate begins the cycle.
2. Two oxidative decarboxylation reactions release acetyl carbons as CO_2 and produce 2 NADH (6 ATP).
3. Conversion of succinyl CoA to malate occurs in three steps that also yield 1 GTP (energetically equivalent to 1 ATP) and 1 $FADH_2$ (2 ATP).
4. Regeneration of oxaloacetate produces a third molecule of NADH (3 ATP).
5. A total of 24 ATP per glucose molecule is generated by the citric acid cycle.

Citric acid cycle revolution produces: 3 NADH (9 ATP), 1 GTP (1 ATP), 1 $FADH_2$ (2 ATP)

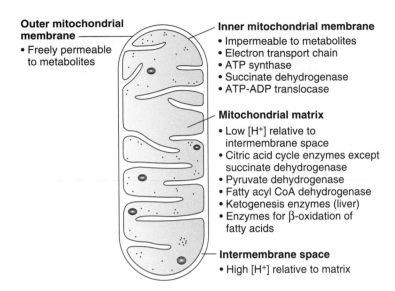

Outer mitochondrial membrane
- Freely permeable to metabolites

Inner mitochondrial membrane
- Impermeable to metabolites
- Electron transport chain
- ATP synthase
- Succinate dehydrogenase
- ATP-ADP translocase

Mitochondrial matrix
- Low [H$^+$] relative to intermembrane space
- Citric acid cycle enzymes except succinate dehydrogenase
- Pyruvate dehydrogenase
- Fatty acyl CoA dehydrogenase
- Ketogenesis enzymes (liver)
- Enzymes for β-oxidation of fatty acids

Intermembrane space
- High [H$^+$] relative to matrix

5-5: *Schematic diagram of a mitochondrion showing the location of key enzymes.*

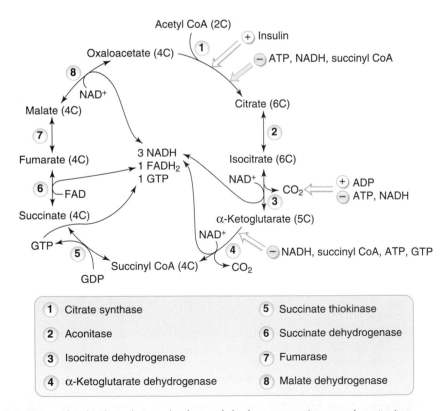

1	Citrate synthase	**5**	Succinate thiokinase
2	Aconitase	**6**	Succinate dehydrogenase
3	Isocitrate dehydrogenase	**7**	Fumarase
4	α-Ketoglutarate dehydrogenase	**8**	Malate dehydrogenase

5-6: *Citric acid cycle. The cycle is regulated primarily by three enzymes (citrate synthase, isocitrate dehydrogenase, and α-ketoglutarate dehydrogenase), which are inhibited (–) or activated (+) by the indicated metabolites.*

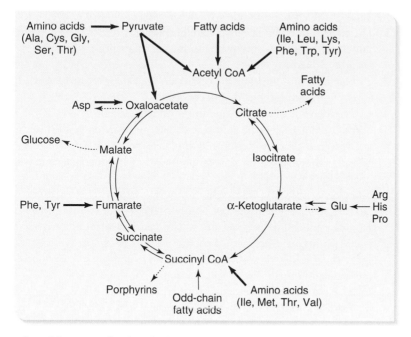

5-7: *Interface of the citric acid cycle with other pathways. Note that many amino acids produce cycle intermediates (thick arrows). Cycle intermediates also take part in synthetic pathways leading to glucose, fatty acids, porphyrins, and amino acids (dashed arrows).*

C. Regulated steps of citric acid cycle
  1. Three regulated enzymes in the cycle control the flow of substrates largely in response to the cell's need for ATP (see Fig. 5-6): citrate synthase, isocitrate dehydrogenase, and α-ketoglutarate dehydrogenase.
  2. Citrate synthase is inhibited by ATP, NADH, and succinyl CoA, and it is stimulated by insulin.
  3. Isocitrate dehydrogenase, the cycle's "pacemaker," is stimulated by ADP and inhibited by ATP and NADH.
  4. α-Ketoglutarate dehydrogenase is inhibited by two of its products, NADH and succinyl CoA, as well as by ATP and GTP.
D. Overall features and unique aspects of the citric acid cycle
  1. Energy yield of the citric acid cycle is equivalent to 12 ATP per acetyl CoA oxidized.
  2. Replenishing reactions restore cycle intermediates that are drained off to biosynthetic pathways or needed in greater amounts.
    a. Pyruvate carboxylase, which forms oxaloacetate by carboxylation of pyruvate, is allosterically activated by acetyl CoA.
    b. Various amino acids are converted to acetyl CoA, α-ketoglutarate, succinyl CoA, fumarate, or oxaloacetate (Fig. 5-7).
      • Example: glutamate is converted to α-ketoglutarate, methionine is converted to succinyl CoA, and aspartate is converted to oxaloacetate.

E. Interface of the citric acid cycle with other pathways (see Fig. 5-7)
   1. The citric acid cycle accepts metabolites generated in catabolic pathways and contributes cycle intermediates for use in anabolic pathways, including gluconeogenesis.
   2. Carbons entering the cycle as acetyl CoA are always oxidized to CO_2 and never contribute carbons to gluconeogenesis.
      • Acetyl CoA is not a substrate for gluconeogenesis.
   3. Carbons from glucogenic amino acids and pyruvate enter the cycle as intermediates that are convertible to malate, which is exported to the cytosol and converted to oxaloacetate to enter the gluconeogenic pathway (see Chapter 6).

F. Malfunction of the citric acid cycle
   1. Fluoroacetate, a potent poison, is converted to fluorocitrate, which inhibits aconitase, blocking operation of the citric acid cycle and its energy output.
   2. Five vitamins are precursors of coenzymes that participate in the citric acid cycle. A deficiency of any of these vitamins negatively impacts operation of the cycle and impairs energy production.

Coenzyme-vitamin precursor relationships in citric acid cycle: NAD^+-niacin, FAD-riboflavin (B_2), thiamine pyrophosphate-thiamine (B_1), CoA-pantothenate, succinyl CoA-vitamin B_{12}

      a. Niacin $\rightarrow NAD^+$ (see steps 3, 4, and 8 in Fig. 5-6)
      b. Riboflavin (vitamin B_2) $\rightarrow$ FAD (see step 6 in Fig. 5-6)
      c. Thiamine (vitamin B_1) $\rightarrow$ thiamine pyrophosphate (see step 4 in Fig. 5-6)
      d. Pantothenate $\rightarrow$ coenzyme A
      e. Vitamin B_{12} (cobalamin) $\rightarrow$ succinyl CoA via odd-chain fatty acid metabolism

IV. Electron Transport and Oxidative Phosphorylation
   A. Most of the ATP generated by aerobic metabolism of fuel molecules is produced by oxidative phosphorylation, the synthesis of ATP coupled to the stepwise flow of electrons from NADH (donates 2 hydrogen atoms [$2e^- + 2H^+$]) and $FADH_2$ to O_2 in the electron transport chain.
   B. The electron transport chain consists of a series of four large multiprotein complexes (I-IV) located in the inner mitochondrial membrane (Fig. 5-8).
      1. Coenzyme Q (CoQ) and cytochrome c, two smaller carriers, shuttle electrons between the large complexes.
      2. Prosthetic groups in each complex reversibly accept and release electrons.
         a. FMN and FAD (riboflavin derivative): complexes I and II
         b. Heme groups: complexes III and IV
         c. Copper ions: complex IV

Cytochrome oxidase: inhibited by CO and CN^-

            • Cytochrome oxidase (complex IV) is inhibited by carbon monoxide (CO) and cyanide (CN^-), which stop electron transport.
         d. O_2: electron acceptor
            (1) Hypoxia, or inadequate concentration of O_2, has its main effect on oxidative phosphorylation and the synthesis of ATP.
            (2) In tissue hypoxia, cells utilize anaerobic glycolysis to obtain ATP (2 ATP per glucose molecule).

O_2: electron acceptor in oxidative phosphorylation

      3. Decrease in free energy as electrons move through electron transport complexes favors electron flow from NADH and $FADH_2$ to O_2.

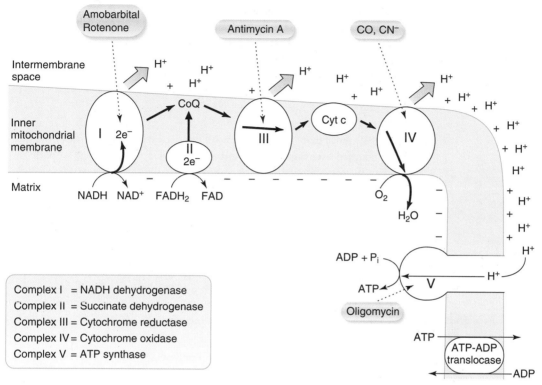

5-8: *Overview of oxidative phosphorylation in the inner mitochondrial membrane. Electron flow (thick arrows) through complexes I, III, and IV provides energy to pump H+ ions from the matrix to the intermembrane space (shaded wide arrows) against the proton electrochemical gradient. The "downhill" movement of H+ ions back into the matrix provides the energy for ATP synthesis by complex V. Preferential export of ATP from the matrix by ATP-ADP translocase (an antiport) maintains a high ADP:ATP ratio in the matrix. Inhibitors block electron flow through the indicated complexes (dashed arrows); as a result, ATP synthesis also ceases. CN⁻,cyanide; CO, carbon monoxide.*

C. ATP formation is driven by a proton gradient across the inner mitochondrial membrane, a process called chemiosmotic coupling (see Fig. 5-8).
  1. Proton gradient is established by complexes I, III, and IV, which pump H^+ ions from the mitochondrial matrix to the intermembrane space.
  2. ATP synthase is inhibited by oligomycin.
  3. ATP yield from oxidative phosphorylation accounts for approximately 85% of the maximal 38 ATP generated in complete oxidation of glucose to CO_2.
    a. 1 NADH → 3 ATP
    b. 1 $FADH_2$ → 2 ATP
D. ADP level controls the rate of oxidative phosphorylation.
  1. Tight coupling of electron flow and ATP synthesis in mitochondria ensures that O_2 consumption depends on availability of ADP, a phenomenon termed respiratory control.

Mitochondrial DNA disorders: maternal transmission to all children; no paternal transmission

2. Low ADP (high ATP) decreases the flow of electrons, which decreases O_2 consumption.
3. High ADP (low ATP) increases the flow of electrons, which increases O_2 consumption.
E. Mutations in mitochondrial DNA affect electron transport and ATP synthesis (Box 5-1).

V. Mitochondrial Transport Systems
   A. ATP-ADP translocase in the inner mitochondrial membrane carries out the tightly coupled exchange of ATP and ADP (see Fig. 5-8).
      • The outer mitochondrial membrane is permeable to most small metabolites, whereas the inner membrane is not.
   B. Shuttle mechanisms transport electrons from cytosolic NADH into the mitochondria.

BOX 5-1

HEREDITARY MITOCHONDRIAL DISEASES

Most mitochondrial diseases are caused by mutations in mitochondrial DNA (mtDNA), which has a higher mutation rate than nuclear DNA. Since all mitochondria in the zygote come from the ovum, these diseases exhibit maternal inheritance, where affected mothers transmit the disease to all their children. Affected males do not transmit mitochondrial diseases because the tail of the sperm, which contains the mitochondria, falls off following fertilization. Because mtDNA-encoded proteins are associated with electron transport and ATP synthesis, tissues with a very high oxygen demand are most affected by mitochondrial dysfunction.

• Leber's hereditary optic neuropathy: progressive loss of central vision and eventual blindness due to degeneration of the optic nerve. Caused by a defect in NADH dehydrogenase (complex I), this disease affects more males than females, with onset most common in the third decade.

Other defects in mtDNA produce several syndromes known as mitochondrial myopathies:

• Kearns-Sayre syndrome: degeneration of retinal pigments, ophthalmoplegia, pain in the eyes, and cardiac conduction defects, which may cause death. Muscle biopsy reveals ragged red fibers marked by an irregular contour and structurally abnormal mitochondria that stain red. Onset occurs before age 20.
• MELAS syndrome: mitochondrial encephalomyopathy, lactic acidosis, and stroke-like episodes
• MERRF syndrome: myoclonus epilepsy with ragged red fibers

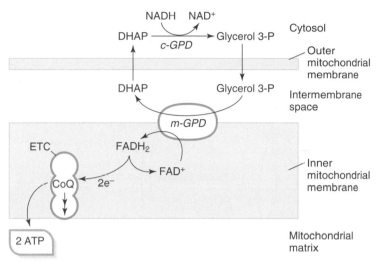

5-9: *Glycerol phosphate shuttle for transporting electrons from NADH in the cytosol across the inner mitochondrial membrane. The glycerol phosphate shuttle operates in one direction only, to import electrons from the cytosol to the mitochondrial matrix. Each NADH produces 2 ATP. CoQ, coenzyme Q in the electron transport chain (ETC); DHAP, dihydroxyacetone phosphate; GPD, glycerol 3-phosphate dehydrogenase in both cytosolic (c) and mitochondrial (m) forms.*

1. NADH produced during catabolism of glucose to pyruvate (glycolysis) in the cytosol cannot cross the inner mitochondrial membrane.
2. Shuttle mechanisms permit regeneration of cytosolic NAD^+, which is necessary for glycolysis to continue.
3. Glycerol phosphate shuttle uses cytosolic NADH to reduce dihydroxyacetone phosphate to glycerol 3-phosphate, which transfers electrons to FAD^+ in the inner mitochondrial membrane (Fig. 5-9).
   - Two cytosolic NADH produce 4 ATP, whereas two mitochondria-generated NADH (e.g., β-oxidation of fatty acids) produce 6 ATP.
4. Malate-aspartate shuttle uses cytosolic NADH to reduce oxaloacetate to malate, which enters the mitochondria via an antiporter (Fig. 5-10).
   - Two cytosolic NADH via this shuttle produce 6 ATP.
C. Movement of numerous other metabolites (e.g., PO_4^{3-}, Ca^{2+}, succinate, glutamate) in or out of mitochondria depends on specific transporters in the inner membrane.

VI. Inhibitors of Mitochondrial ATP Synthesis (Table 5-1)
   A. Most inhibitors of mitochondrial ATP synthesis act to block electron flow or to uncouple electron flow from ATP synthesis.
   B. Electron transport blockers: Carriers upstream of the block become highly reduced and carriers downstream become oxidized.
      1. Electron transport blockers prevent maintenance of the proton gradient so that ATP synthesis stops.
      2. Electron transport blockers include cyanide, carbon monoxide, amobarbital (Amytal), rotenone, and antimycin A (see Fig. 5-8).

Glycerol phosphate shuttle: 2 NADH produce 4 ATP

Malate-aspartate shuttle: 2 NADH produce 6 ATP

Uncouplers of ETC: pentachlorophenol, dinitrophenol, thermogenin (brown fat); destroy proton gradient

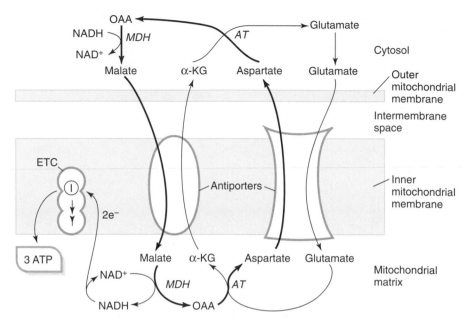

5-10: *Malate-aspartate shuttle for transporting electrons from NADH in the cytosol across the inner mitochondrial membrane. The malate-aspartate shuttle is fully reversible and operates to import electrons into the mitochondrial matrix (shown) or to export electrons to the cytosol. Each NADH produces 3 ATP. The thick arrows trace the path of malate and aspartate. AT, aminotransferase; I, complex I in the electron transport chain (ETC); α-KG, α-ketoglutarate; MDH, malate dehydrogenase; OAA, oxaloacetate.*

TABLE 5-1:

Inhibition of Mitochondrial ATP Synthesis

Inhibitor	Mode of Action	Site of Inhibition
Amobarbital (Amytal), rotenone	Blocks electron transport	Complex I (NADH dehydrogenase)
Antimycin A	Blocks electron transport	Complex III (cytochrome reductase)
CO, CN$^-$	Blocks electron transport	Complex IV (cytochrome oxidase)
Dinitrophenol, thermogenin	Acts as proton channel to reduce proton gradient, thus uncoupling ATP synthesis from electron transport	Throughout inner mitochondrial membrane
Oligomycin	Prevents ATP synthesis directly	Complex V (ATP synthase)

    C. Uncouplers: electron flow proceeds in the absence of ATP synthesis, thus eliminating respiratory control.
       1. Uncouplers carry protons through the inner mitochondrial membrane without generating ATP.
       2. Uncouplers short-circuit the proton gradient by transporting H$^+$ ions from the intermembrane space to the matrix, thereby abolishing the gradient.
       3. Uncouplers dissipate energy from electron flow as heat (risk of hyperthermia).

4. Uncouplers increase O_2 consumption.
5. Uncouplers include pentachlorophenol, dinitrophenol, and thermogenin, a natural uncoupling protein present in brown fat.
    • Unlike adults, newborns have a considerable amount of brown fat. The heat generated by electron flow in the mitochondria of brown fat is important in maintaining neonatal body temperature.
D. Nucleoside analogues (e.g., cytosine arabinoside, AZT): Inhibition of mitochondrial DNA synthesis leads to a decrease in total number of mitochondria and reduced NADH oxidation in cells.
    • Results in increased cytosolic NADH, shunting of pyruvate to lactate (lactic acidosis), hyperglycemia due to increased gluconeogenesis, and fatty liver due to inability to oxidize fatty acids.

Carbohydrate Metabolism

TARGET TOPICS

- Glycolysis: hexokinase versus glucokinase, regulated enzymes, interfaces with other pathways, effect of insulin and glucagon, energy yield under aerobic and anaerobic conditions
- Pyruvate dehydrogenase and the fate of pyruvate during fed state and fasting state
- Gluconeogenesis: reactions that bypass irreversible steps in glycolysis, allosteric regulators, relation to glycolysis, carbon sources
- Glycogen synthesis and degradation: key enzymes, reciprocal effect of hormones (glucagon, epinephrine, insulin), functions in liver and muscle
- Metabolism of galactose and fructose

- Pentose phosphate pathway: role in supplying NADPH, ribose 5-phosphate, and intermediates for glycolysis and gluconeogenesis; antioxidant function of reduced glutathione
- Glycosaminoglycans, glycoproteins, proteoglycans, and lysosomal storage diseases
- Clinical correlations: glucose-6-phosphate dehydrogenase (G6PD) deficiency, pyruvate kinase deficiency, pyruvate dehydrogenase deficiency, galactokinase deficiency, galactosemia, essential fructosuria, hereditary fructose intolerance, glycogen storage diseases, I cell disease, Hurler's and Hunter's diseases

I. Glycolysis and the Fate of Pyruvate
  A. Aerobic glycolysis (the oxidation of glucose to pyruvate) and anaerobic glycolysis (the oxidation of glucose to lactate) occur in the cytosol of all body cells.
  B. Steps of glycolysis (Fig. 6-1)
    1. Step 1: Phosphorylation of glucose to glucose 6-phosphate, the first regulated step in glycolysis, is irreversible and traps glucose inside the cell.
       a. The reaction utilizes 1 ATP.

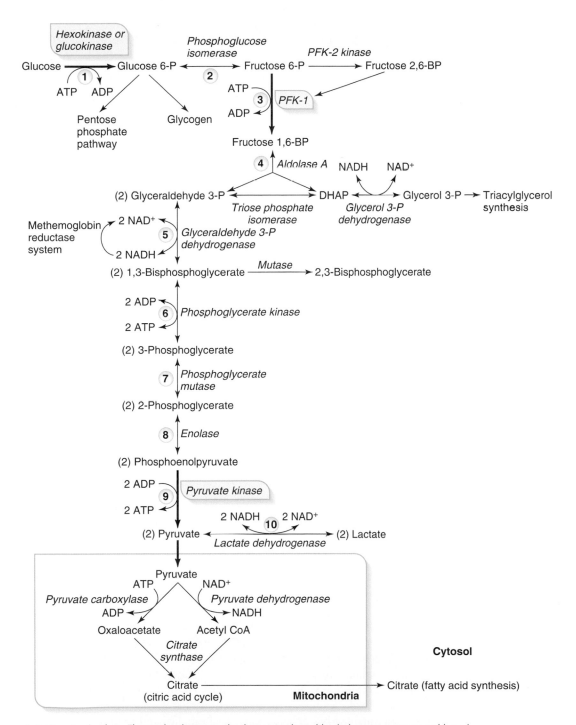

6-1: Steps in glycolysis. The regulated steps in glycolysis are indicated by thick one-way arrows and boxed enzymes. Reversible reactions are identified by two-way arrows. Interfaces with other pathways are also identified. BP, bisphosphate; MetHb, methemoglobin; P, phosphate; PFK, phosphofructokinase.

TABLE 6-1:

Comparison of Hexokinase and Glucokinase

Characteristic	Hexokinase	Glucokinase
Tissue location	All	Liver and pancreatic β cells
K_m	Low (high substrate affinity)	High (low substrate affinity)
V_{max}	Low	High
Inhibited by glucose 6-phosphate	Yes	No
Inducible by insulin	No	Yes
Substrate specificity	Glucose, fructose, galactose	Glucose only
Physiologic role	Provides cells with basal level of glucose 6-phosphate needed for energy production	Permits accumulation of intracellular glucose for conversion to glycogen or triacylglycerols

Hexokinase: phosphorylates glucose; low K_m, low V_{max}; inhibited by glucose 6-phosphate

Glucokinase: phosphorylates glucose; high K_m, high V_{max}; not inhibited by glucose 6-phosphate

   b. The two enzymes that catalyze this step, hexokinase and glucokinase, are specialized to function under different conditions (Table 6-1).
- All the kinase reactions are irreversible and serve a regulatory role in glycolysis.

   c. Hexokinase is present in all tissues.
    (1) Hexokinase is active at low glucose concentrations (low K_m) and cannot rapidly phosphorylate large amounts of glucose (low V_{max}).
    (2) Hexokinase is inhibited by glucose 6-phosphate, the reaction product.

   d. Glucokinase is present in the liver and pancreatic β cells.
    (1) Glucokinase is highly active only at high glucose concentrations (high K_m) and rapidly phosphorylates large amounts of glucose (high V_{max}).
    (2) Induction by insulin and lack of inhibition by glucose 6-phosphate promote clearance of blood glucose by the liver in the fed state.

2. Step 2: Reversible reaction involving the conversion of glucose 6-phosphate to fructose 6-phosphate by phosphoglucose isomerase

3. Step 3: Irreversible reaction involving the conversion of fructose 6-phosphate to fructose 1,6-bisphosphate by phosphofructokinase-1 (PFK-1), which is the rate-limiting enzyme of glycolysis
   a. The reaction utilizes 1 ATP.
   b. Inhibitors of PFK-1 include ATP (indicates that energy stores are high) and citrate (indicates that the cell is actively making ATP).
   c. Activators of PFK-1 include AMP (indicates that energy stores are depleted) and fructose 2,6-bisphosphate, which is formed by phosphofructokinase-2 (PFK-2).
   d. The fructose 2,6-bisphosphate level is controlled by the insulin:glucagon ratio via its effect on PFK-2, which is a bifunctional enzyme that has different activities in the fed and fasting states (Fig. 6-2).
    (1) In the fed state (i.e., high insulin, low glucagon), insulin dephosphorylates PFK-2, giving it kinase activity, which converts

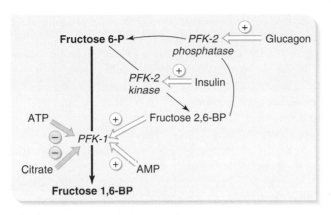

6-2: *Regulation of phosphofructokinase-1 (PFK-1). Fructose 2,6-bisphosphate (fructose 2,6-BP), the most potent activator of PFK-1, is formed by a separate enzyme, phosphofructokinase-2 (PFK-2). PFK-2 is a bifunctional enzyme that acts as a kinase at high insulin levels (fed state) and converts fructose 6-phosphate (fructose 6-P) into fructose 2,6-BP. In the fasting state, when glucagon levels are high, PFK-2 acts as a phosphatase, causing fructose 2,6-BP to convert back to fructose 6-P.*

fructose 6-phosphate to fructose 2,6-bisphosphate, leading to activation of PFK-1 and enhanced glycolysis.

High insulin:low glucagon ratio: favors glycolysis

   (2) In the fasting state (i.e., low insulin, high glucagon), protein kinase A (activated by glucagon) phosphorylates PFK-2, giving it phosphatase activity, resulting in conversion of fructose 2,6-bisphosphate back to fructose 6-phosphate, hence favoring gluconeogenesis.

4. Step 4: Reversible conversion of fructose 1,6-bisphosphate to two 3-carbon intermediates by aldolase A.
   a. Triose phosphate isomerase reversibly converts glyceraldehyde 3-phosphate to dihydroxyacetone phosphate (DHAP).
   b. DHAP is reversibly converted to glycerol 3-phosphate by glycerol 3-phosphate dehydrogenase, which utilizes NADH as a cofactor.
     (1) Glycerol 3-phosphate is the primary substrate for synthesis of triacylglycerol in the liver in the fed state (see Chapter 7).
     (2) Glycerol 3-phosphate is used to shuttle NADH to the electron transport chain in the inner mitochondrial membrane (see Chapter 5).
     (3) In the fasting state, glycerol 3-phosphate is converted to DHAP, which is used as a substrate for gluconeogenesis.
5. Step 5: Reversible conversion of glyceraldehyde 3-phosphate to 1,3-bisphosphoglycerate (1,3-BPG) by glyceraldehyde 3-phosphate dehydrogenase using NAD^+ as a cofactor.
   a. NAD^+ must be replenished for glycolysis to continue.
   b. NADH is shuttled into the electron transport chain by the glycerol phosphate shuttle or the malate-aspartate shuttle (see Chapter 5).
   c. The methemoglobin reductase system and the pathway for synthesizing 2,3-BPG are ancillary pathways that emanate from this reaction.

6. Step 6: Reversible conversion of 1,3-BPG to 3-phosphoglycerate by phosphoglycerate kinase
   - This reaction generates 2 ATP per glucose molecule, which replace the 1 ATP used in step 1 and the 1 ATP used in step 3.
7. Step 7: Reversible conversion of 3-phosphoglycerate to 2-phosphoglycerate by phosphoglycerate mutase
8. Step 8: Reversible conversion of 2-phosphoglycerate to phosphoenolpyruvate (PEP) by enolase
9. Step 9: Regulated, irreversible reaction involving the conversion of PEP to pyruvate by pyruvate kinase
   a. During glycolysis, pyruvate kinase is stimulated by fructose 1,6-bisphosphate, the product of the PFK-1 reaction.
   b. During gluconeogenesis, pyruvate kinase is inhibited by high levels of ATP, alanine, and active protein kinase A, thereby driving glucose formation.
      - During the fasting state, inactivation of liver pyruvate kinase via phosphorylation by active protein kinase further ensures enhancement of gluconeogenesis.
   c. There is a net gain of 2 ATP per glucose molecule in this reaction.
10. Step 10: Reversible conversion of pyruvate to lactate by lactate dehydrogenase using NADH as a cofactor
    a. This reaction primarily occurs in anaerobic glycolysis associated with shock and extreme exercise.
    b. This reaction also occurs in alcoholics due to an increase in NADH from alcohol metabolism (see Chapter 9).
       - Lactic acidosis is often present in alcoholics.
C. Comparison of aerobic and anaerobic glycolysis
   1. NADH produced in the glycolytic pathway must be oxidized to regenerate NAD^+ for glycolysis to continue.
   2. In aerobic glycolysis, electrons from NADH are transferred to the electron transfer chain via the glycerol phosphate shuttle or the malate-aspartate shuttle, and NAD^+ is returned to the cytosol (see Figs. 5-9 and 5-10).

Aerobic glycolysis: net gain 2 ATP and 2 NADH

   a. There is a net gain of 2 ATP and 2 NADH per glucose molecule in aerobic glycolysis.
   b. If the glycerol phosphate shuttle is used, 2 NADH produce a total of 4 ATP, whereas the malate-aspartate shuttle allows 2 NADH to produce a total of 6 ATP per glucose molecule.
   3. In anaerobic glycolysis, reduction of pyruvate to lactate by lactate dehydrogenase regenerates NAD^+ (see Fig. 6-1).

Anaerobic glycolysis: net gain 2 ATP; NAD^+ replenished

   a. There is a net gain of 2 ATP and no NADH per glucose molecule in anaerobic glycolysis.
   b. Lactate is either converted back to pyruvate in the liver or excreted in the urine.
   c. Mature red blood cells (RBCs) lack mitochondria and rely completely on anaerobic metabolism for generation of ATP.

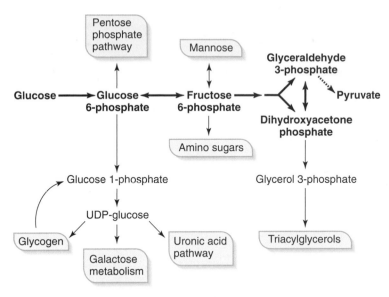

6-3: *Interface of glycolytic intermediates (boldface type) with other pathways. Note that the key glycolytic intermediates that branch off into other pathways are glucose 6-phosphate, fructose 6-phosphate, and dihydroxyacetone phosphate.*

D. Interface of glycolysis with other pathways (Fig. 6-3)
   1. Glucose 6-phosphate, the first product formed in glycolysis, connects the glycolytic pathway to the pentose phosphate pathway and to glycogen synthesis, galactose metabolism, and the uronic acid pathway.
      • Glucose 1-phosphate, a by-product of glucose 6-phosphate, is used to synthesize UDP-glucose, which is involved in glycogen synthesis, metabolism of galactose, and the synthesis of glucuronic and iduronic acid (components of glycosaminoglycans) via the uronic acid pathway.
   2. Fructose 6-phosphate is the precursor for synthesis of amino sugars (e.g., glucosamine, galactosamine), which ultimately are incorporated into glycoproteins and glycosaminoglycans (e.g., chondroitin sulfate, hyaluronic acid).
      • Fructose 6-phosphate is also used to synthesize mannose, which is involved in the synthesis of glycoproteins and lysosomal enzymes.
   3. Glycerol 3-phosphate, derived from DHAP, is used in the synthesis of triacylglycerols in the liver.
   4. 1,3-BPG is converted by a mutase to 2,3-BPG in RBCs, which is the key substrate for shifting the O_2 binding curve to the right (decreasing O_2 affinity) (see Fig. 6-1).
   5. In the reaction that converts glyceraldehyde 3-phosphate to 1,3-BPG, NADH is used by the methemoglobin reductase pathway to reduce methemoglobin (Fe^{3+}), which cannot bind O_2, to hemoglobin (Fe^{2+}), which binds O_2 to its heme iron (see step 5 in Fig. 6-1).
   6. Pyruvate, the end-product of aerobic glycolysis, is a key metabolic intermediate whose fate differs in the fed and fasting states (Fig. 6-4).

Methemoglobin reductase pathway: methemoglobin (Fe^{3+}) reduced to hemoglobin (Fe^{2+}), which can bind O_2

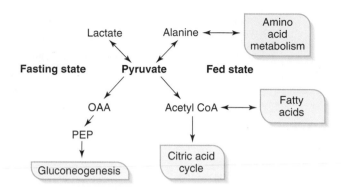

6-4: *Fate of pyruvate in the fed and fasting states. Note the importance of pyruvate in carbohydrate, protein, and fat metabolism.*

    a. In the fed state, when glucose is plentiful, pyruvate is oxidized to acetyl coenzyme A (CoA) by pyruvate dehydrogenase. Acetyl CoA enters the citric acid cycle (see Chapter 5) or is used for fatty acid synthesis (see Chapter 7).

      (1) In the fed state, pyruvate, an α-keto acid, can be converted by alanine aminotransferase to the amino acid alanine, which is used for protein synthesis.

      (2) Excessive carbohydrate intake increases the amount of acetyl CoA available for fatty acid synthesis, which in turn increases the amount available for storage in fat.

    b. In the fasting state, when glucose is in short supply, pyruvate is carboxylated to oxaloacetate, providing carbon skeletons for gluconeogenesis (see Fig. 6-1).

E. Regulation of pyruvate dehydrogenase

    1. Pyruvate dehydrogenase, a large multienzyme complex located in the mitochondrial matrix, oxidatively decarboxylates pyruvate to produce acetyl CoA.

    2. Five coenzymes are required for the previously discussed reaction.

      a. Coenzymes that are all derived from vitamins include thiamine pyrophosphate, FAD, NAD^+, and CoA.

      b. Lipoic acid is a coenzyme produced from octanoic acid.

    3. α-Ketoglutarate dehydrogenase, which carries out an analogous reaction to form succinyl CoA in the citric acid cycle, is also a multienzyme complex and requires the same coenzymes (see Chapter 5).

    4. In both dehydrogenase reactions, 2 NADH are produced for conversion to 6 ATP in the electron transport chain.

    5. Regulation of pyruvate dehydrogenase occurs by two mechanisms.

      a. There is direct inhibition of pyruvate dehydrogenase by NADH and acetyl CoA, which are the products of β-oxidation of fatty acids.

      (1) In the fasting state, inhibition of the enzyme prevents pyruvate from producing acetyl CoA and ensures its presence as a substrate for gluconeogenesis.

Pyruvate dehydrogenase: inhibited by acetyl CoA in fasting state

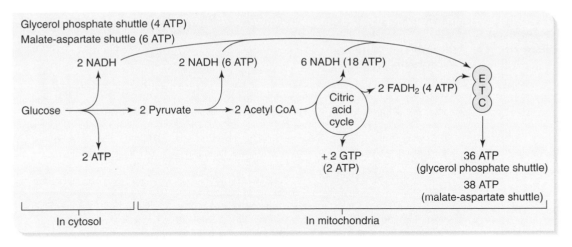

6-5: *Overview of ATP yield from complete oxidation of glucose. Substrate-level phosphorylation generates 2 ATP per glucose molecule in the cytosol; however, the bulk of the energy output is derived from electron flow through the electron transport chain (ETC) and coupled oxidative phosphorylation. Electrons from cytosolic NADH move into mitochondria via the malate-aspartate shuttle to produce 38 ATP or via the glycerol phosphate shuttle, which results in a slightly lower ATP yield (36 ATP).*

      (2) Acetyl CoA is a positive effector for pyruvate carboxylase, which favors generation of oxaloacetate as a substrate for gluconeogenesis.

  b. Cycling between inactive and active forms of pyruvate dehydrogenase is catalyzed by a specific kinase (phosphorylates the enzyme) and phosphatase (dephosphorylates the enzyme).

      (1) Active pyruvate dehydrogenase (nonphosphorylated state) is favored by high insulin (fed state) and by high ADP (indicates the need for energy).

      (2) Inactive pyruvate dehydrogenase (phosphorylated state) is favored by increased acetyl CoA and NADH from fatty acid oxidation (fasting state).

F. Maximal ATP yield from oxidation of glucose (Fig. 6-5)

  1. The maximum yield of ATP per glucose molecule depends on coupling of glycolysis with the citric acid cycle (see Chapter 5) via pyruvate dehydrogenase.

  2. The ATP count from glucose to pyruvate via aerobic glycolysis is a net gain of 2 ATP plus conversion of 2 NADH in the electron transport chain to either 4 ATP using the glycerol phosphate shuttle or 6 ATP using the malate-aspartate shuttle for a total of 6 to 8 ATP.

  3. The ATP count from conversion of pyruvate to acetyl CoA by pyruvate dehydrogenase is 6 ATP.

  4. The ATP count from the citric acid cycle is 24 ATP.

  5. The total ATP count for complete oxidation of glucose to carbon dioxide and water is 36 to 38 ATP.

G. Glycolytic enzyme defects (e.g., pyruvate kinase deficiency, pyruvate dehydrogenase deficiency) are summarized in Table 6-2.

Pyruvate dehydrogenase deficiency: lactic acidosis, decreased acetyl CoA, early death

TABLE 6-2:
Hereditary Defects in Catabolism of Sugars

Disease	Metabolic Effect	Clinical Features
Glucose and Pyruvate Metabolism		
Pyruvate kinase deficiency (autosomal recessive [AR]) most common enzyme deficiency in the glycolytic pathway	Inadequate ATP for maintaining ion pumps in RBC membrane results in loss of H_2O Damaged RBCs, subject to macrophage destruction in the spleen, lead to ↑ in unconjugated bilirubin ↑ in RBC 2,3-BPG proximal to the enzyme block	Hemolytic anemia and jaundice begin at birth; mild anemia due to ↑ in 2,3-BPG, which shifts the O_2 binding curve to the right (↓ O_2 affinity)
Pyruvate dehydrogenase deficiency (AR)	↑ in pyruvate with concomitant ↑ in lactic acid and alanine (via transamination); ↓ in production of acetyl CoA; severe reduction in ATP production	Lactic acidosis, neurologic defects, myopathy; usually fatal at early age
Galactose Metabolism		
Galactokinase deficiency (AR)	↑ in galactose and galactitol (sugar alcohol)	Cataracts
Galactosemia (AR)	Deficiency of GALT; ↑ in galactose (blood, urine), galactose 1-phosphate (very toxic), and galactitol (sugar alcohol) Galactitol osmotically active and damages tissues	Cirrhosis, mental retardation, cataracts, galactosuria Women with disorder can synthesize lactose in breast milk due to epimerase reaction
Fructose Metabolism		
Essential fructosuria (AR)	Deficiency of fructokinase; ↑ in fructose in blood and urine	Benign condition marked by fructosuria
Hereditary fructose intolerance (AR)	Deficiency of aldolase B; ↑ in fructose and fructose 1-phosphate (toxic) Excess fructose traps phosphorus in cells, leading to hypophosphatemia, ↓ in ATP, and ↑ in AMP	Toxic liver damage, renal disease Severe fasting hypoglycemia, ↑ uric acid (metabolism of AMP)
Pentose Phosphate Pathway		
Glucose-6-phosphate dehydrogenase (G6PD) deficiency (sex-linked recessive)	Inadequate NADPH production; results in reduction in antioxidant activity of glutathione in mature RBCs	Hemolytic anemia often induced by infections, oxidant drugs (e.g., dapsone, primaquine), and fava beans

II. Gluconeogenesis
   A. Precursors for gluconeogenesis
      1. Major precursors: lactate, amino acids that are convertible to pyruvate or citric acid cycle intermediates (e.g., alanine, aspartate), and glycerol
      2. Other fuels: fructose, galactose, mannose, and odd-chain fatty acids
   B. Site and function of gluconeogenesis
      1. The liver is the most important site for gluconeogenesis, whereas the kidneys and the epithelium of the small intestine assume a less important role.
         • In prolonged starvation, the kidneys assume a key role in gluconeogenesis.
      2. Gluconeogenesis is important in maintaining blood glucose levels in the fasting state for energy requirements in the brain, RBCs, exercising muscle, and the renal medulla.
      3. Gluconeogenesis occurs, in part, in the mitochondria (pyruvate carboxylase reaction) and, in part, in the cytosol.
   C. Reactions of gluconeogenesis (Fig. 6-6)
      1. Enzymes that are required to bypass the three irreversible steps in glycolysis are discussed in Box 6-1.
         a. Pyruvate carboxylase
         b. PEP carboxykinase
         c. Fructose 1,6-bisphosphatase (rate-limiting reaction)
         d. Glucose 6-phosphatase
      2. Conversion of pyruvate to PEP, which bypasses the irreversible pyruvate kinase reaction, occurs in several steps.
         a. Pyruvate carboxylase, a biotin-containing mitochondrial enzyme, converts pyruvate to oxaloacetate (OAA) in an irreversible reaction that consumes ATP (see step 1 in Fig. 6-6).
            • Biotin deficiency leads to a buildup of pyruvate, which is converted to lactic acid and leads to lactic acidosis.
         b. OAA is reduced to malate (malate shuttle), which is transported to the cytosol and then reoxidized to OAA.
            • OAA cannot exit the mitochondria and must be converted into malate, which moves freely between the mitochondria and cytosol.
         c. PEP carboxykinase decarboxylates OAA to produce PEP in a reversible reaction that consumes GTP (step 2).
      3. Conversion of PEP to fructose 1,6-bisphosphate occurs by simple reversal of six reactions in the glycolytic pathway.
      4. Fructose 1,6-bisphosphatase (rate-limiting enzyme), which dephosphorylates fructose 1,6-bisphosphate to produce fructose 6-phosphate (step 3), bypasses the irreversible PFK-1 reaction.
      5. Simple reversal of the phosphoglucose isomerase reaction converts fructose 6-phosphate to glucose 6-phosphate.
      6. Glucose 6-phosphatase dephosphorylates glucose 6-phosphate to produce glucose (step 4), thus bypassing the irreversible hexokinase or glucokinase reaction.
      7. A total of 6 ATP are consumed in gluconeogenesis.

Gluconeogenesis sites: liver (major site), kidneys (starvation), epithelium of small intestine

Fructose-1,6-bisphosphatase: rate-limiting enzyme of gluconeogenesis

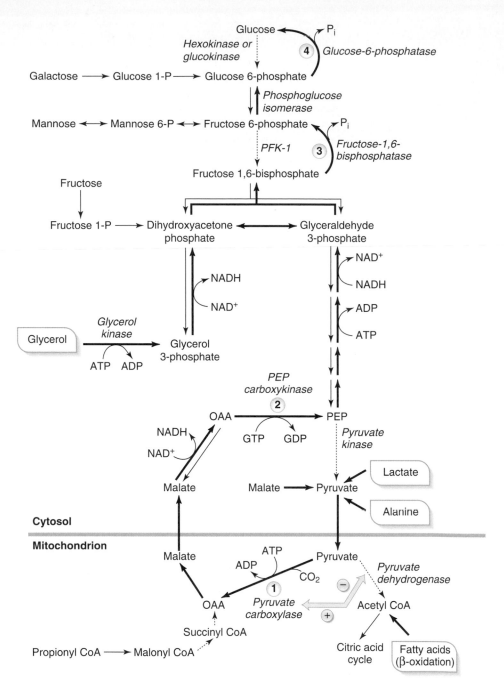

6-6: Overview of gluconeogenesis and its regulation, reading from the bottom of the figure to the top. Key enzymatic reactions that occur in the gluconeogenic pathway are numbered and labeled. Thick arrows indicate reactions leading to glucose synthesis. Dashed arrows indicate irreversible glycolytic reactions, which are blocked under conditions favoring gluconeogenesis in the fasting state. Lactate, alanine, and glycerol (boxes) are the primary sources of carbon skeletons for gluconeogenesis. Other fuels for gluconeogenesis that are also depicted include malate (malate → pyruvate in fatty acid metabolism), succinyl CoA (propionyl metabolism), dihydroxyacetone phosphate + glyceraldehyde 3-phosphate (fructose metabolism), glucose 6-phosphate (galactose metabolism), and fructose 6-phosphate (mannose metabolism). OAA, oxaloacetate; PEP, phosphoenolpyruvate.

BOX 6-1

COMPARISON OF GLYCOLYSIS AND GLUCONEOGENESIS

Of the 10 reactions in the glycolytic pathway, 7 are reversible (see Fig. 6-1). During gluconeogenesis, when these reactions proceed in the reverse direction, the gluconeogenic reactions are catalyzed by the same enzymes that are used in glycolysis.

For the three irreversible reactions in glycolysis, however, four other enzymes are required for gluconeogenesis to occur (see Fig. 6-6). Note that a pathway involving two enzymes, pyruvate carboxylase and PEP carboxylase, is required in gluconeogenesis to reverse the effect of pyruvate kinase in glycolysis. In the following list, (–) indicates inhibition, and (+) indicates activation.

Glycolysis

Hexokinase (or glucokinase)
Glucose → glucose 6-phosphate
 (step 1 in Fig. 6-1)
(–) Glucose 6-phosphate
 (hexokinase)

Phosphofructokinase 1
Fructose 6-phosphate → fructose
 1,6-bisphosphate (step 3)
(+) AMP, fructose 2,6-bisphosphate
(–) ATP, citrate
Rate-limiting reaction

Pyruvate kinase
PEP → pyruvate (step 9)
(+) Fructose 1,6-bisphosphate
(–) ATP, alanine, glucagon

Gluconeogenesis

Glucose-6-phosphatase
Glucose 6-phosphate → glucose
 (step 4 in Fig. 6-6)

Fructose 1,6-bisphosphatase
Fructose 1,6-bisphosphate → fructose
 6-phosphate (step 3)
(–) AMP, fructose 2,6-bisphosphate
(+) Citrate
Rate-limiting reaction

Pyruvate carboxylase (in mitochondria)
Pyruvate → OAA (step 1)
(+) Acetyl CoA
Requires biotin; OAA is converted to
 malate in the mitochondria, and
 malate is converted back to OAA in
 the cytosol.

PEP carboxykinase (in cytosol)
OAA → PEP (step 2)
Only reversible reaction in
 gluconeogenesis

D. Regulated steps in gluconeogenesis (see Fig. 6-6)
1. Reciprocal regulation ensures that either gluconeogenesis or glycolysis predominates, preventing futile cycling of glucose to pyruvate to glucose.
2. Acetyl CoA is a positive allosteric effector of pyruvate carboxylase, which diverts pyruvate into the gluconeogenic pathway rather than the citric acid cycle.
3. The ratio of insulin:glucagon regulates pyruvate kinase (PEP conversion to pyruvate) and fructose 2,6-bisphosphate (see Fig. 6-2), which in turn activates PFK-1.
   a. High insulin:low glucagon (fed state) leads to increased pyruvate kinase activity and increased fructose 2,6-bisphosphate levels.
      • Result: increased glycolysis (particularly in the liver) and decreased gluconeogenesis
   b. Low insulin:high glucagon (fasting state) leads to decreased pyruvate kinase activity and decreased fructose 2,6-bisphosphate levels.
      • Result: decreased glycolysis (particularly in the liver) and increased gluconeogenesis (maintains blood glucose)

Low insulin:high glucagon ratio favors gluconeogenesis.

4. Three allosteric effectors have opposite effects on fructose 1,6-bisphosphate and PFK-1.
   a. Fructose 2,6-bisphosphate and AMP
      (1) Stimulate PFK-1, which results in increased glycolysis
      (2) Inhibit fructose 1,6-bisphosphatase, which results in decreased gluconeogenesis
   b. Citrate
      (1) Inhibits PFK-1, which leads to decreased glycolysis
      (2) Stimulates fructose 1,6-bisphosphatase, which leads to increased gluconeogenesis
E. Pathways that supply carbon skeletons for gluconeogenesis
1. Lactate provides approximately one-third of the carbon skeletons used in gluconeogenesis.
   • In the Cori cycle, lactate produced in exercising muscle and RBCs travels in the bloodstream to the liver for conversion to glucose, which then travels back to muscle and RBCs.

Cori cycle: liver conversion of lactate (muscle, RBCs) to glucose via gluconeogenesis

2. Glucogenic amino acids, derived from degradation of muscle protein, supply carbon atoms for gluconeogenesis by transamination to pyruvate (alanine), α-ketoglutarate (glutamate), and OAA (aspartate) (see Chapter 8).
3. Glycerol is an important source of carbon atoms for gluconeogenesis in fasting or starvation conditions, when triacylglycerols in adipose tissue are mobilized.
   • Glycerol kinase, present only in the liver, converts glycerol to glycerol 3-phosphate, which is further converted to DHAP and used as a substrate for gluconeogenesis.
F. Gluconeogenic enzyme deficiencies result in fasting hypoglycemia.
   • Example: In von Gierke's disease, a glycogen storage disease, the absence of glucose 6-phosphatase leads to a decrease in glucose synthesis.

Gluconeogenic enzyme deficiencies: fasting hypoglycemia

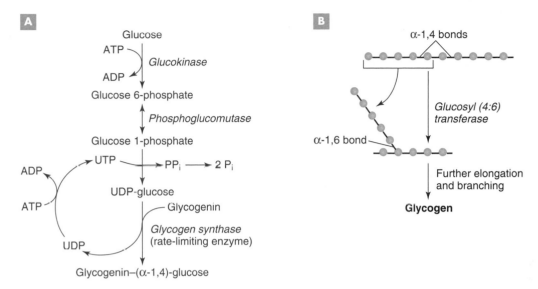

6-7: *Glycogenesis.* **A,** *Formation of UDP-glucose and α-1,4 linkages in glycogen. Phosphoglucomutase isomerizes glucose 6-phosphate to glucose 1-phosphate in a reversible reaction. Glucose 1-phosphate is converted to UDP-glucose, which is the activated form of glucose required for glycogen synthesis. Glycogen synthase, the rate-limiting enzyme, adds one glucose unit at a time, in a 1,4 linkage, to the nonreducing end of glycogenin.* **B,** *Branch formation. After the main glycogen chain reaches a certain length, a block of α-1,4-linked residues is split from the end and reattached in an α-1,6 linkage by the branching enzyme, glucosyl 4:6 transferase.*

III. Glycogen Metabolism
   A. Glycogen is a highly branched glucose polymer found primarily in liver and skeletal muscle.
      • Glycogen constitutes a reserve supply of glucose that is rapidly mobilized in the fasting state.
   B. Reactions of glycogen synthesis (fed state) and degradation (fasting state)
      1. Glycogenesis, the synthesis of glycogen, requires a preexisting fragment of glycogen or a primer glycoprotein (glycogenin) plus the activated glucose donor UDP-glucose (Fig. 6-7A).
         a. Phosphoglucomutase isomerizes glucose 6-phosphate to glucose 1-phosphate by a reversible reaction.
         b. Glucose 1-phosphate plus uridine triphosphate (UTP) produces uridine diphosphate-glucose (UDP-glucose), which is the activated form of glucose that is necessary for glycogen synthesis.
         c. Glycogen synthase (rate-limiting enzyme) forms an α-1,4 glycosidic bond between a glucose unit from UDP-glucose at the nonreducing end of an existing glycogen fragment or glycoprotein (glycogenin).
         d. The branching enzyme, glucosyl (4:6) transferase, removes a block of glucose units from the nonreducing end of a growing glycogen chain and reattaches glucose units in an α-1,6 linkage at a different site, creating a branch point (Fig. 6-7B).

Glycogen synthase: rate-limiting enzyme of glycogen synthesis

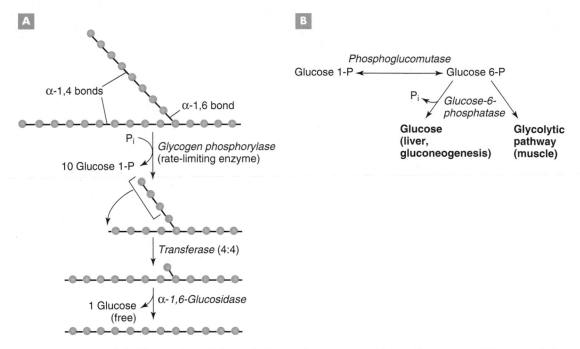

6-8: *Glycogenolysis. **A**, Action of glycogen phosphorylase and debranching enzyme, which catalyzes both transferase (4:4) and glucosidase (1:6) reactions. The ratio of glucose 1-phosphate to free glucose released depends on the number of branch points and length of the branches. **B**, Fate of glucose 1-phosphate in liver and muscle. Both tissues contain phosphoglucomutase, which catalyzes the reversible reaction between glucose 1-phosphate and glucose 6-phosphate. The liver contains glucose-6-phosphatase (gluconeogenic enzyme), so glucose 6-phosphate is primarily converted to glucose. Muscle oxidizes glucose 6-phosphate into ATP, which is used to power muscle contraction.*

- Branching increases the rate of glycogen synthesis and degradation by increasing the number of ends at which glucose units are added or removed.

2. Glycogenolysis entails the initial breakdown of glycogen to glucose 1-phosphate and free glucose in a ratio of approximately 10:1 (Fig. 6-8A).

   a. Shortening of chains is catalyzed by glycogen phosphorylase (rate-limiting enzyme), which cleaves α-1,4 bonds with inorganic phosphate (P_i) to produce glucose 1-phosphate.

   - Glycogen phosphorylase sequentially removes glucose units from the ends of all chains but stops four glucose units from each branch point.

   b. Branch removal of the four remaining glucose units is accomplished by a single debranching enzyme, which carries out two reactions.

   (1) Three glucose units remaining at one branch point are transferred to the nonreducing end of the linear glycogen chain by 4:4 transferase activity.

   (2) The last glucose unit at a branch point is split off by α-1,6 glucosidase activity, releasing a free glucose.

      c. Phosphoglucomutase reversibly converts glucose 1-phosphate to glucose 6-phosphate and is therefore functional in both glycogenesis and glycogenolysis (Fig. 6-8B).

      d. The fate of glucose 6-phosphate derived from glycogenolysis differs in muscle and liver.

         (1) Liver contains glucose 6-phosphatase, a gluconeogenic enzyme that converts glucose 6-phosphate to free glucose, which helps maintain the blood glucose level in the fasting state.

         (2) Muscle glycogen is converted to glucose 6-phosphate, which is oxidized in the muscle to produce ATP.

      e. A small amount of glycogen is degraded in lysosomes by α-1,4 glucosidase (acid maltase).

C. Regulated steps in glycogen synthesis and degradation

    1. Reciprocal regulation ensures that either synthesis or degradation predominates, preventing the wasteful operation of both pathways simultaneously.

    2. Hormonal regulation involves cAMP-mediated signaling that controls cycling of glycogen synthase and glycogen phosphorylase between phosphorylated and nonphosphorylated forms, which differ in their activity (Fig. 6-9).

      a. High insulin (low glucagon), typical of the fed state, promotes glycogen synthase activity leading to glycogen synthesis.

        • Insulin activates hepatic protein phosphatase, which then removes phosphate groups from glycogen synthase (activating the enzyme), phosphorylase kinase (inactivating the enzyme), and glycogen phosphorylase (inactivating the enzyme).

      b. High glucagon (low insulin), typical of the fasting state, activates adenylate cyclase, leading to sequential activation of protein kinase A, phosphorylase kinase, and phosphorylase in the liver, and it inactivates glycogen synthase (phosphorylation inhibits the enzyme), leading to glycogen degradation in the liver.

      c. Epinephrine (β-adrenergic), unlike glucagon, enhances glycogenolysis in both muscle and liver.

    3. Allosteric regulation of enzymes increases glycogen synthesis or degradation more rapidly than hormone-induced activation of enzymes.

      a. Glucose 6-phosphate, which is elevated in the liver in the fed state, directly stimulates glycogen synthase b (the less active phosphorylated form), which leads to an immediate increase in glycogen synthesis.

      b. Calcium, which is released from sarcoplasmic reticulum in contracting muscle, directly activates phosphorylase kinase, which leads to an immediate increase in glucose 6-phosphate from glycogen degradation and a concomitant increase in ATP production to power muscle contraction.

D. Interface of glycogen metabolism with other pathways

    1. Glucose 1-phosphate is the key metabolite linking glycogen synthesis to the glycolytic pathway (see Fig. 6-3).

Insulin (fed state) activates glycogen synthase; glucagon (fasting state) activates glycogen phosphorylase.

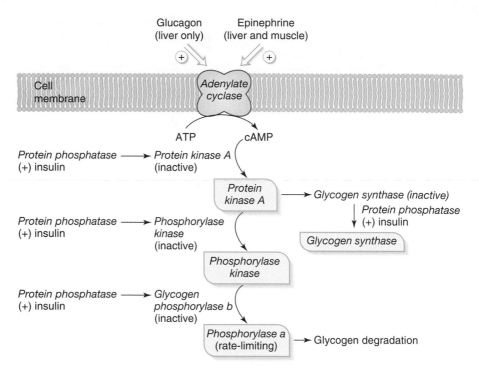

6-9: *Hormonal regulation of glycogen synthesis and degradation involves cAMP signaling. Shading indicates activated forms of the enzymes. Active protein kinase A phosphorylates glycogen synthase, which inactivates the enzyme and prevents glycogenesis. Active protein kinase A activates phosphorylase kinase, which in turn activates phosphorylase a, the rate-limiting reaction of glycogenolysis. Insulin activates hepatic protein phosphatase, which activates glycogen synthase and inactivates protein kinase A, phosphorylase kinase, and phosphorylase a.*

Pompe's disease: deficiency of α-1,4-glucosidase (lysosomal enzyme)

Von Gierke's disease: deficiency of glucose-6-phosphatase (gluconeogenic enzyme)

2. Excess glucose is shunted to glycogen synthesis in liver and muscle when the ATP supply is adequate.
3. Mobilization of glucose from glycogen occurs in muscle when ATP is needed for contraction and in liver when blood glucose levels fall.

E. Overview of glycogen storage diseases

1. The glycogenoses are autosomal recessive disorders that increase glycogen synthesis (e.g., von Gierke's disease) or prevent glycogenolysis (e.g., Pompe's disease, debranching enzyme deficiencies) and lead to an accumulation of either structurally normal or abnormal glycogen within cells (Table 6-3).
2. Branching and debranching enzyme disorders produce structurally abnormal glycogen, whereas the other types accumulate normal glycogen.
3. Clinical manifestations depend on which tissues (e.g., muscle and/or liver, kidney) are affected by glycogen accumulation.
4. Hypoglycemia occurs only in glycogenoses that interfere with gluconeogenesis (e.g., von Gierke's disease) or liver glycogenolysis (e.g., deficiency of liver phosphorylase).

TABLE 6-3:
Glycogen Storage Diseases

Disease	Deficient Enzyme	Glycogen Structure	Clinical Features
Von Gierke's (autosomal recessive [AR])	Glucose-6-phosphatase (liver and kidney)	Normal	Severe fasting hypoglycemia, ketosis, hyperlipidemia, lactic acidosis, enlarged liver and kidneys
Pompe's (AR)	α-1,4-Glucosidase (lysosomes)	Normal	Infant form: mental retardation, hypotonia, cardiomegaly leading to death by age 2 years. Adult form: gradual skeletal myopathy
Cori's (AR)	Debranching enzyme (muscle and liver), amylo-α-1,6-glucosidase	Abnormal: many short-branched chains (α-limit dextrins)	Mild hypoglycemia, hepatomegaly ↓ in free glucose after epinephrine challenge
Andersen's (AR)	Branching enzyme (liver and spleen), glucosyl-4,6-transferase	Few long chains with very few branches	Hepatosplenomegaly, cirrhosis, liver failure leading to death by age 2 years
McArdle's (AR)	Muscle glycogen phosphorylase	Normal	Muscle cramping, fatigue, and myoglobinuria with strenuous exercise; no increase in lactic acid after exercise
Hers' (AR)	Liver glycogen phosphorylase	Normal	Similar to von Gierke's disease but less severe

5. Muscle glycogenoses (e.g., McArdle's disease) do not result in hypoglycemia since muscle utilizes its glycogen to supply glucose for generation of ATP.

IV. Metabolism of Galactose and Fructose
   A. Galactose metabolism (Fig. 6-10)
      1. The major dietary source of galactose is the disaccharide lactose, which is present in milk and milk products.
         • Lactase, a brush border disaccharidase enzyme located in the epithelium of the small intestine, converts lactose to glucose and galactose.
      2. Galactose undergoes an exchange reaction with UDP-glucose to produce glucose 1-phosphate and UDP-galactose, utilizing the rate-limiting enzyme galactose 1-phosphate uridyltransferase (GALT).
         a. Glucose 1-phosphate is converted to glucose 6-phosphate by phosphoglucomutase.
         b. In the fed state, glucose 6-phosphate is used as a substrate in glycolysis; in the fasting state, it is used as a substrate for gluconeogenesis.

McArdle's disease: deficiency of muscle glycogen phosphorylase

Lactase in epithelium of small intestine converts lactose to glucose + galactose.

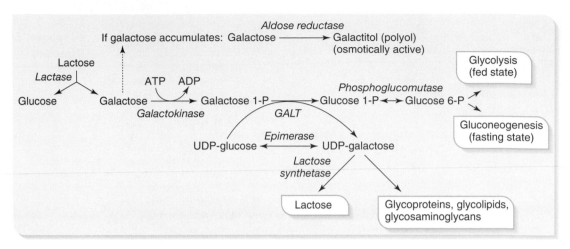

6-10: *Galactose metabolism. Lactose is the primary source of galactose. Galactose 1-phosphate uridyltransferase (GALT) is the rate-limiting reaction. Glucose 1-phosphate is converted to glucose 6-phosphate, which is used as a substrate for glycolysis (fed state) or gluconeogenesis (fasting state). UDP-galactose is used in the synthesis of lactose and other compounds. Aldolase reductase converts excess galactose (e.g., galactokinase deficiency) into a sugar alcohol (galactitol), which is osmotically active.*

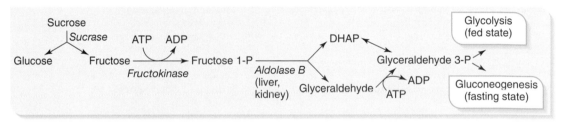

6-11: *Fructose metabolism. Sucrose is the primary source of fructose. Aldolase B, the rate-limiting enzyme, converts fructose 1-phosphate to dihydroxyacetone phosphate (DHAP) and glyceraldehyde, which is further converted to glyceraldehyde 3-phosphate. DHAP and glyceraldehyde 3-phosphate are used as substrates for glycolysis (fed state) or gluconeogenesis (fasting state).*

GALT: rate-limiting enzyme of galactose metabolism; deficient in galactosemia

    c. UDP-galactose provides galactose units for lactose synthesis in breast tissue (epimerase reaction) and synthesis of glycoproteins, glycolipids, and glycosaminoglycans in other tissues.

    d. If galactose accumulates in tissues containing aldose reductase (e.g., lens, neural tissue), it is converted into a sugar alcohol (polyol) called galactitol, which is osmotically active.

    e. Galactokinase deficiency and galactosemia, which are caused by a deficiency of GALT, are summarized in Table 6-2.

B. Fructose metabolism (Fig. 6-11)

    1. The major dietary source of fructose is the disaccharide sucrose, which is present in table sugar, fruits, and honey.

      • Sucrase, a brush border disaccharidase enzyme located in the epithelium of the small intestine, converts sucrose into glucose and fructose.

2. Aldolase B, the rate-limiting enzyme in fructose metabolism, is primarily located in the liver and, to a lesser extent, the small intestine and proximal renal tubules.
   a. Aldolase B converts fructose 1-phosphate into the 3-carbon intermediates (trioses) DHAP and glyceraldehyde.
   b. Glyceraldehyde is further converted into glyceraldehyde 3-phosphate by a kinase.
   c. In the fed state, glyceraldehyde 3-phosphate and DHAP are used as intermediates in the glycolytic pathway; in the fasting state, they are converted to glucose 6-phosphate and used for glucose synthesis.
3. Essential fructosuria and hereditary fructose intolerance, which is caused by a deficiency of aldolase B, are summarized in Table 6-2.

V. Pentose Phosphate Pathway
   A. The pentose phosphate pathway is both the major source of NADPH for reductive biosynthesis and a source of ribose 5-phosphate for nucleotide synthesis in all cells.
      • The pentose phosphate pathway, also known as the hexose monophosphate pathway, occurs in the cytosol.
   B. Reactions of the pentose phosphate pathway
      1. The oxidative branch consists of three irreversible reactions that convert glucose 6-phosphate to ribulose 5-phosphate with release of CO_2 and formation of NADPH (Fig. 6-12).
         a. Glucose 6-phosphate dehydrogenase (G6PD) is the rate-limiting enzyme that converts glucose 6-phosphate to 6-phosphogluconolactone, which is then converted via a series of intermediate reactions to ribulose 5-phosphate.
            • G6PD is competitively inhibited by NADPH.
         b. The 2 NADPH formed are used for reductive biosynthesis and for maintaining glutathione (GSH) in the reduced state.
            • GSH is an antioxidant that neutralizes the oxidant activity of hydrogen peroxide (H_2O_2) by converting it to H_2O utilizing the enzyme glutathione peroxidase.
      2. The nonoxidative branch consists of a series of reversible reactions that interconvert various sugars that produce ribose 5-phosphate and intermediates used in glycolysis or gluconeogenesis.
         a. Transketolase reactions (thiamine dependent) are responsible for 2-carbon transfer reactions, whereas transaldolase reactions are involved in 3-carbon transfer reactions.
         b. In the fed state, fructose 6-phosphate and glyceraldehyde 3-phosphate are used as substrates in the glycolytic pathway; in the fasting state, they are used as intermediates in gluconeogenesis.
   C. Pentose pathway function
      1. Function of the pathway is tailored to different cellular needs according to the relative needs of the cell for NADPH (e.g., reductive biosynthesis) and ribose 5-phosphate (e.g., RNA and DNA synthesis).

Aldolase B: rate-limiting enzyme of fructose metabolism; deficient in hereditary fructose intolerance

Pentose phosphate pathway: major source of NADPH (reductive biosynthesis); source of ribose 5-phosphate (RNA, DNA synthesis)

Glucose 6-phosphate dehydrogenase: rate-limiting enzyme of pentose phosphate pathway

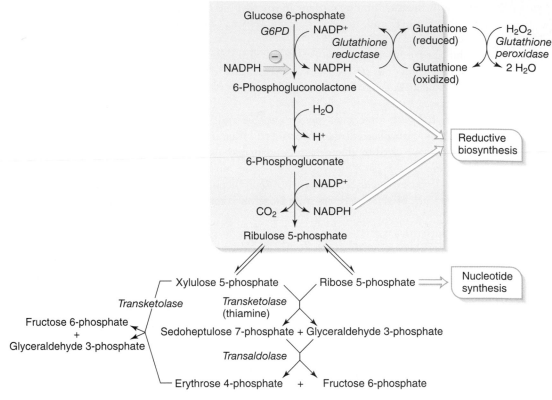

6-12: *Pentose phosphate pathway. The oxidative branch (shaded) consists of three irreversible reactions. Glucose-6-phosphate dehydrogenase (G6PD), the rate-limiting enzyme, converts glucose 6-phosphate to 6-phosphogluconolactone, which is further converted in a series of reactions to ribulose 5-phosphate. The 2 NADPH formed are used for reductive biosynthesis and for maintaining the antioxidant glutathione in its reduced form. All of the reactions of the nonoxidative branch (unshaded) are reversible and produce ribose 5-phosphate for RNA and DNA synthesis. Also produced are the intermediates fructose 6-phosphate and glyceraldehyde 3-phosphate for glycolysis (fed state) or gluconeogenesis (fasting state).*

G6PD deficiency: decreased reduced glutathione; hemolytic anemia from oxidizing drugs (e.g., primaquine, dapsone)

2. Increased pathway activity occurs in tissues that consume NADPH in reductive biosynthetic pathways.
   a. Adipose tissue for fatty acid synthesis
   b. Gonads and adrenal cortex for steroid hormone synthesis
   c. Liver for fatty acid and cholesterol synthesis
3. G6PD deficiency is summarized in Table 6-2.

VI. Glycosaminoglycans, Glycoproteins, and Proteoglycans
   A. Glycosaminoglycans (GAGs)
      1. GAGs are complexes of branched, negatively charged polysaccharide chains containing amino sugars (e.g., glucosamine or galactosamine) and acid sugars (e.g., iduronic acid or glucuronic acid).
         a. Carbohydrates are the primary component of GAGs.
         b. Most GAGs attach to a linear core of protein.

2. GAGs are the major components of ground substance in the interstitial tissue.
3. Clinically important GAGs
   a. Chondroitin sulfate, the most abundant GAG, is an important component in cartilage.
      • Chondroitin sulfate is destroyed in osteoarthritis, where there is a wearing down of articular cartilage.
   b. Heparan sulfate is primarily responsible for the strong negative charge of the glomerular basement membrane.
   c. Heparin is an anticoagulant that enhances antithrombin III activity, leading to inactivation of serine protease coagulation factors (e.g., XII, XI, X).
   d. Keratan sulfate is found in cartilage and is associated with chondroitin sulfate.
   e. Hyaluronic acid is the major component of synovial fluid (joint lubricant).
   f. Dermatan sulfate is primarily found in skin and valvular tissue in the heart.
4. GAGs are degraded in lysosomes.
5. Lysosomal enzyme synthesis, I cell disease, and lysosomal storage diseases, such as Hurler's disease and Hunter's disease, are discussed in Box 6-2.

B. Glycoproteins are proteins with attached short, branch-chained oligosaccharides whose glycosidic linkages may be N- (contain dolichol phosphate) or O-linked.
   1. Important functions of glycoproteins
      a. Glycoproteins are components of blood group antigens on RBCs (Box 6-3) and other circulating blood proteins (e.g., coagulation factors, tumor markers such as prostate-specific antigen).
      b. Glycoproteins serve as integrins, which are cell surface receptors that mediate cellular attachment (e.g., neutrophils to endothelial cells) and bind to different extracellular matrix components, such as fibronectin (an adhesive glycoprotein), laminin (a glycoprotein in basement membranes), and collagen.
      c. Glycoproteins are components of lysosomal enzymes (e.g., mannose oligosaccharides; see Box 6-2).
   2. The protein portion of glycoproteins is synthesized in rough endoplasmic reticulum (RER), and the carbohydrate portion (oligosaccharide) is attached to the protein in the lumen of the RER and in the Golgi apparatus.
      • Carbohydrate precursors for glycoproteins are sugar nucleotides (e.g., UDP-galactose, UDP-glucose).

C. Proteoglycans consist of a core protein to which is attached numerous long, linear chains of GAGs.
   • Proteoglycans are an important component of the extracellular matrix, where they interact with collagen and elastin, fibronectin, and laminin.

Chondroitin sulfate: most abundant GAG, destroyed in osteoarthritis

I cell disease: inability to phosphorylate mannose residues of Golgi lysosomal enzymes; inclusion bodies in lysosomes; psychomotor retardation, early death

Lysosomal storage diseases: deficiencies of lysosomal enzymes; complex substrates accumulate in lysosomes

SYNTHESIS OF LYSOSOMAL ENZYMES AND LYSOSOMAL DISEASES

Lysosomes, located in the cytosol of a cell, contain hydrolytic enzymes. These enzymes are glycoproteins that are initially synthesized in the rough endoplasmic reticulum. From there, the enzymes are transported to the Golgi apparatus, where mannose residues on their side chains are phosphorylated to become mannose 6-phosphate. Receptors located on the inner surface of the Golgi apparatus membranes bind to the mannose 6-phosphate residues, and then transport vesicles containing the receptor-bound enzymes pinch off from the Golgi membrane. In the cytosol, the vesicles fuse with lysosomes, releasing their enzymes into the lysosomes. The receptors from the vesicles return to the Golgi apparatus and repeat the process.

Clinical Disorders Involving Lysosomes

I cell disease is characterized by an inability to phosphorylate the mannose residues of the lysosomal enzymes in the Golgi apparatus. The lysosomes therefore lack lysosomal enzymes and are unable to degrade complex substrates, which accumulate in the lysosomes as inclusion bodies. Patients have psychomotor retardation and an early death.

Deficiencies of degrading enzymes in lysosomes lead to the accumulation of complex substrates in lysosomes, hence the term lysosomal storage disease. Lysosomal storage diseases include genetic disorders with defects in degradation of sphingolipids (e.g., Tay-Sachs disease; see Chapter 7), defects in degradation of glycosaminoglycans (mucopolysaccharidoses, such as Hurler's and Hunter's diseases), and a single disorder with a defect in the degradation of glycogen by α-1,4-glucosidase in lysosomes called Pompe's disease.

Hurler's disease is an autosomal recessive disease associated with a deficiency of α-L-iduronidase, which leads to lysosomal accumulation of dermatan sulfate and heparan sulfate. Clinical findings include severe mental retardation, coarse facial features, hepatosplenomegaly, corneal clouding, coronary artery disease (lipid accumulates in coronary vessels), and vacuoles in the lysosomes of peripheral blood leukocytes.

Hunter's disease is an X-linked recessive disease associated with a deficiency of iduronate sulfatase, leading to lysosomal accumulation of dermatan and heparan sulfate. It is milder than Hurler's disease.

BOX 6-3

ABO BLOOD GROUP ANTIGENS

ABO blood group antigens are genetically determined and are present on RBCs as well as on epithelial cells located throughout the body. Individuals are identified as having O, A, B, or AB antigens on their RBCs. These antigens are produced by the H gene, which occurs in most individuals and codes for a glycosyltransferase that attaches fucose to a glycolipid to produce H antigen on RBCs. Individuals with the A gene, which codes for an *N*-acetylgalactosamine transferase that attaches *N*-acetylgalactosamine to the H antigen, produce A antigen. People with the B gene, which codes for a galactosyltransferase that attaches galactose to the H antigen, produce B antigen. In blood group AB individuals, A and B genes code for both transferases, so their RBCs contain both A and B antigens. Individuals with the O gene cannot synthesize transferases, so the surfaces of their RBCs contain only H antigens.

After birth, individuals develop IgM antibodies (isohemagglutinins) against antigens they do not have on the surface of their RBCs (e.g., blood group A individuals develop anti-B IgM antibodies). Blood group O individuals develop anti-A IgM and anti-B IgM antibodies, as well as anti-A,B IgG antibodies, which can cross the placenta and potentially attack and destroy fetal RBCs containing either A or B antigen. This is called ABO hemolytic disease of the newborn. The elderly often lose their isohemagglutinins.

ABO Blood Group Summary

Type	Antibodies	Comments
O	Anti-A IgM; anti-B IgM; anti-A,B IgG	Individuals with blood group O are universal donors; their RBCs can be transfused into all blood groups since there are no antigens on the surface of the RBCs to react with recipient isohemagglutinins. Blood group O individuals can only receive O blood. Most common blood group.
A	Anti-B IgM	Individuals have a predisposition for gastric carcinoma.
B	Anti-A IgM	
AB	None present	Individuals with blood group AB are universal recipients; they can be transfused with any blood group since they do not have isohemagglutinins to react against A or B antigens. Least common blood group.

Lipid Metabolism

I. Fatty Acid and Triacylglycerol Synthesis
  A. Introduction
    1. Fatty acids are the major energy source (9 kcal/g) in human metabolism.
    2. Sources of fatty acids include their synthesis in the liver and the hydrolysis of chylomicrons and very low-density lipoproteins (VLDLs) by capillary lipoprotein lipase in peripheral tissues.

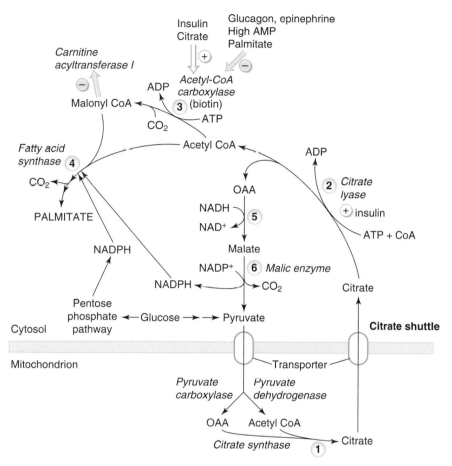

7-1: *Overview of fatty acid synthesis. Fatty acid synthesis primarily occurs in the fed state and is enhanced by insulin. Palmitate, a 16-carbon saturated fat, is the end-product of fatty acid synthesis. NADPH is required for synthesis of palmitate and elongation of the chain.*

B. Reactions involving fatty acid synthesis (Fig. 7-1)
  • Excess dietary carbohydrate is the major carbon source for fatty acid synthesis, which occurs primarily in the liver during the fed state.
  1. Step 1: The citrate shuttle transports acetyl coenzyme A (CoA) generated in the mitochondrion to the cytosol (see Fig. 7-1).
    a. Acetyl CoA *cannot* move across the mitochondrial membrane and must be converted into citrate.
    b. Acetyl CoA and oxaloacetate (OAA) undergo an irreversible condensation by citrate synthase to form citrate, which is transported across the mitochondrial membrane into the cytosol.
    c. Citrate remaining in the mitochondrion is used in the citric acid cycle.
  2. Step 2: Citrate is converted back to acetyl CoA and OAA by citrate lyase, an insulin-enhanced enzyme, in a reaction that requires ATP.

Fatty acid synthesis: acetyl CoA carboxylase is rate-limiting enzyme; occurs in cytosol in fed state

3. Step 3: Acetyl CoA is converted to malonyl CoA, an important intermediate in fatty acid synthesis, by acetyl CoA carboxylase in an irreversible rate-limiting reaction that consumes ATP and requires biotin as a cofactor.

Malonyl CoA: inhibits carnitine acyltransferase I

- Malonyl CoA inhibits carnitine acyltransferase I, preventing movement of newly synthesized fatty acids across the inner mitochondrial membrane into the matrix, where fatty acids undergo β-oxidation (futile cycling is thereby avoided).

4. Step 4: Fatty acid synthase, a large multifunctional enzyme complex, initiates and elongates the fatty acid chain in a cyclical reaction sequence.
   a. Palmitate, a 16-carbon saturated fatty acid, is the final product of fatty acid synthesis.
      - Saturated fatty acids lack double bonds.
   b. One glucose produces 2 acetyl CoA, and each acetyl CoA contains 2 carbons; therefore, four glucose molecules are required to produce the 16 carbons of palmitic acid.

5. Step 5: OAA is converted to malate.

6. Step 6: Malate is converted to pyruvate by malic enzyme, producing 1 NADPH.
   a. NADPH is required for synthesis of palmitate and elongation of fatty acids.
   b. NADPH is produced in the cytosol by both malic enzyme and the pentose phosphate pathway, which is the primary source.

C. Regulation of acetyl CoA carboxylase (see Fig. 7-1, step 3)
   1. Formation of malonyl CoA from acetyl CoA, the irreversible regulated step in fatty acid synthesis, is controlled by two mechanisms.
      a. Allosteric regulation of acetyl CoA carboxylase
         (1) Stimulation by citrate ensures that fatty acid synthesis proceeds in the fed state.
         (2) End-product inhibition by palmitate downregulates synthesis when there is an excess of free fatty acids.
      b. Cycling between active and inactive forms of acetyl CoA carboxylase
         (1) High AMP level (low energy charge) inhibits fatty acid synthesis by phosphorylation of acetyl CoA carboxylase, which inactivates the enzyme.
         (2) Glucagon and epinephrine (fasting state) inhibit acetyl CoA carboxylase by phosphorylation (via protein kinase); insulin (fed state) activates the enzyme by dephosphorylation (via phosphatase).
   2. Inhibition of acetyl CoA carboxylase enhances the oxidation of fatty acids because malonyl CoA is no longer present to inhibit carnitine acyltransferase I.

D. Synthesis of longer chain fatty acids and unsaturated fatty acids
   1. Chain-lengthening systems in the smooth endoplasmic reticulum (SER) and mitochondria convert palmitate (16 carbons) to stearate (18 carbons) and other longer saturated fatty acids.
      a. NADPH provides the reducing equivalents for elongation.
      b. Malonyl CoA donates the two-carbon units for elongation in the SER.

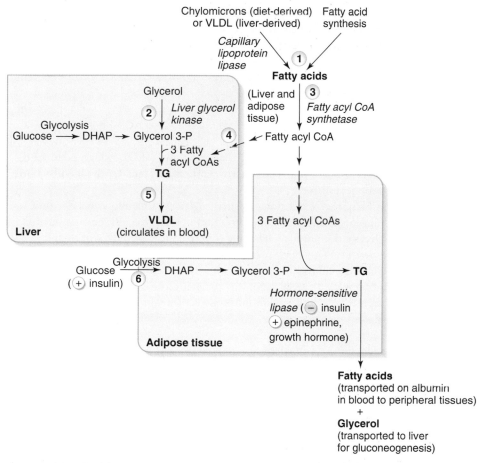

7-2: *Triacylglycerol synthesis in liver and adipose tissue. Sources of fatty acids range from synthesis in the liver to hydrolysis of diet-derived chylomicrons and liver-derived VLDL (step 1). In the liver, glycerol 3-phosphate is derived from either glycolysis or conversion of glycerol to glycerol 3-phosphate by liver glycerol kinase (step 2). In adipose tissue, glycerol 3-phosphate is derived only from glycolysis (step 6). DHAP, dihydroxyacetone phosphate; TG, triacylglycerol.*

   c. Acetyl CoA donates the two-carbon units for elongation in the
      mitochondria.
   2. Desaturation of fatty acids to produce unsaturated fatty acids occurs in the
      SER in a complex process that requires oxygen and NADPH.
      • Unsaturated fatty acids contain one or more double bonds.
E. Conversion of fatty acids to triacylglycerols in liver and adipose tissue
   (Fig. 7-2)
   1. Step 1: In the fed state, fatty acids synthesized in the liver or released from
      chylomicrons and VLDL by capillary lipoprotein lipase are used to
      synthesize triacylglycerol in liver and adipose tissue (see Fig. 7-2).
   2. Step 2: Glycerol 3-phosphate is derived from dihydroxyacetone phosphate
      during glycolysis or from the conversion of glycerol into glycerol
      3-phosphate by liver glycerol kinase.

a. Glycerol 3-phosphate is the carbohydrate intermediate that is used to synthesize triacylglycerol.

b. Decreasing the intake of carbohydrates is the most effective way of decreasing the serum concentration of triacylglycerol.

> Glycerol kinase: present only in liver, converts glycerol to glycerol 3-phosphate (precursor for triacylglycerol synthesis)

3. Step 3: Newly synthesized fatty acids or those derived from hydrolysis of chylomicrons and VLDL are converted into fatty acyl CoAs by fatty acyl CoA synthetase.

4. Step 4: Addition of three fatty acyl CoAs to glycerol 3-phosphate produces triacylglycerol in the liver.

5. Step 5: Liver triacylglycerols are packaged into VLDL, which is stored in the liver and also transports newly synthesized lipids via the bloodstream to peripheral tissues.

6. Step 6: Synthesis and storage of triacylglycerol in adipose tissue requires insulin-mediated uptake of glucose, leading to glycolysis and production of glycerol 3-phosphate, which is converted to triacylglycerol by the addition of 3 fatty acyl CoAs.

> Hormone-sensitive lipase: inhibited by insulin, prevents lipolysis

a. Insulin inhibits hormone-sensitive lipase, which allows adipose cells to accumulate triacylglycerol for storage during the fed state.

b. Epinephrine and growth hormone activate hormone-sensitive lipase during the fasting state.

II. Lipolysis and Fatty Acid Oxidation (Fig. 7-3)

A. Mobilization of stored fatty acids from adipose tissue (lipolysis)

- Lipolysis occurs in the fasting state when fat is required for energy.

> Hormone-sensitive lipase: activated by epinephrine and growth hormone, promotes lipolysis

1. Step 1: Hormone-sensitive lipases in adipose tissue hydrolyze free fatty acids and glycerol from triacylglycerols stored in adipose tissue (see Fig. 7-3).

a. Epinephrine and growth hormone activate lipolysis by converting hormone-sensitive lipase to an active phosphorylated form via their activation of protein kinase.

b. Insulin (fed state) activates phosphatase, which inhibits lipolysis by converting hormone-sensitive lipase into an inactive dephosphorylated form.

c. Glycerol released during lipolysis is transported to the liver, phosphorylated into glycerol 3-phosphate by glycerol kinase, and used as a substrate for gluconeogenesis.

- Note the difference between the fate of glycerol in fatty acid synthesis (synthesis of triacylglycerol) and the fate of glycerol in lipolysis (substrate for gluconeogenesis).

2. Step 2: Free fatty acids released from adipose tissue are carried in the bloodstream bound to serum albumin.

3. Step 3: Bound to serum albumin, the fatty acids are delivered to peripheral tissues (e.g., liver, skeletal muscle, heart, kidney).

a. The fatty acids dissociate from the albumin and are transported into cells, where they are acetylated by fatty acyl CoA synthetase in the cytosol, forming fatty acyl CoAs.

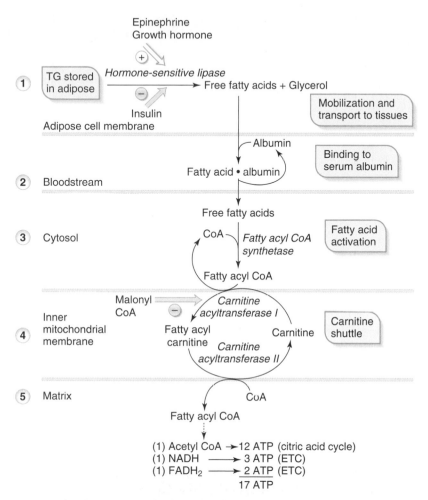

Epinephrine
Growth hormone

7-3: *Overview of lipolysis and oxidation of long-chain fatty acids. Lipolysis occurs in the fasting state. Carnitine acyltransferase I is the rate-limiting reaction and is inhibited by malonyl CoA during the fed state. Oxidation of fatty acids yields the greatest amount of energy of all nutrients. ETC, electron transport chain; TG, triacylglycerol.*

  b. Fatty acyl CoAs are shuttled into the mitochondrial matrix and
     oxidized to supply energy.
B. Characteristics of fatty acid oxidation reactions
  • Saturated fatty acyl CoA derivatives are catabolized by the sequential
    removal of two-carbon units, termed β-oxidation, in the mitochondrial
    matrix.
  1. Step 4: The carnitine shuttle transports long-chain (≥12-carbon) acetylated
     fatty acids across the inner mitochondrial membrane (see Fig. 7-3).
    • Fatty acids with less than 12 carbons enter the mitochondrion directly
      and are activated by mitochondrial synthetases.
    a. Carnitine acyltransferase I (rate-limiting reaction) on the outer surface
       of the inner mitochondrial membrane removes the fatty acyl group

β-Oxidation of fatty acids: occurs in mitochondrial matrix in fasting state

TABLE 7-1:
Comparison of Fatty Acid Synthesis and Oxidation

Property	Synthesis	Oxidation
Primary tissues	Liver	Muscle, liver
Subcellular site	Cytosol	Mitochondrial matrix
Carriers of acetyl and acyl groups	Citrate (mitochondria → cytosol)	Carnitine (cytosol → mitochondria)
Redox coenzyme	NADPH	NAD^+, FAD
Insulin effect	Stimulates	Inhibits
Epinephrine/growth hormone effect	Inhibits	Stimulates
Allosterically regulated enzyme	Acetyl CoA carboxylase (citrate stimulates; excess fatty acids inhibit)	Carnitine acyltransferase I (malonyl CoA inhibits)
Product of pathway	Palmitate	Acetyl CoA

Carnitine acyltransferase I: rate-limiting enzyme of fatty acid oxidation, shuttle for fatty acyl CoA

from fatty acyl CoA and transfers it to carnitine to form fatty acyl carnitine.
  • Malonyl CoA inhibits the above enzyme, thereby preventing transport of newly synthesized fatty acids into the mitochondrion.
  b. Carnitine acyltransferase II on the inner surface of the inner mitochondrial membrane removes the fatty acyl group from fatty acyl carnitine and transfers it to CoA to form fatty acyl CoA in the mitochondrial matrix.
2. Step 5: The oxidation system consists of four enzymes that act sequentially to yield a fatty acyl CoA that is two carbons shorter than the original and 1 acetyl CoA, 1 NADH, and 1 $FADH_2$.

Acetyl CoA: end-product of even-chain saturated fatty acids

  a. Repetition of four reactions eventually degrades even-numbered carbon chains entirely to acetyl CoA.
  b. Acetyl CoA enters the citric acid cycle and produces 12 ATP.
  c. In the electron transport chain, NADH yields 3 ATP and $FADH_2$ yields 2 ATP.
C. Reciprocal regulation of fatty acid oxidation and synthesis
  • Several features distinguish fatty acid synthesis and degradation, which are regulated so that one process predominates (Table 7-1).
  1. Fed state (↑ insulin, ↓ glucagon) leads to increased synthesis of fatty acids and decreased oxidation of fatty acids.
    a. Insulin promotes the active form of acetyl CoA carboxylase and the inactive form of hormone-sensitive lipase, thereby stimulating fatty acid synthesis over degradation.
    b. Malonyl CoA inhibition of the carnitine shuttle also prevents fatty acid degradation while synthesis is progressing.

High insulin:glucagon ratio (fed state) leads to fatty acid synthesis; low insulin:glucagon ratio (fasting state) leads to fatty acid degradation

  2. Fasting and starvation (↑ insulin; ↓ glucagons, epinephrine, and growth hormone) lead to decreased synthesis and increased oxidation of fatty acids.
    a. Epinephrine and growth hormone promote the active form of the hormone-sensitive lipase and the inactive form of acetyl CoA

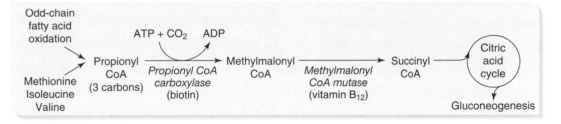

7-4: *Sources of propionyl CoA (odd-chain fatty acid) and its conversion to succinyl CoA. Vitamin B_{12} is a cofactor in odd-chain fatty acid metabolism, and succinyl CoA is used as a substrate for gluconeogenesis.*

carboxylase, thereby stimulating release of fatty acids from adipose tissue and inhibiting fatty acid synthesis.

    b. Glucagon has a weak effect on adipose tissue but promotes gluconeogenesis in the liver, which in turn is supported by the energy from mobilized free fatty acids.

D. Energy yield from fatty acid oxidation

    1. Each cycle of oxidation yields products that are used to generate ATP via the citric acid cycle and the electron transport chain (see Fig. 7-3).

       • *Example:* Oxidation of palmityl CoA yields 131 ATP (8 acetyl CoA yields 96 ATP from the citric acid cycle; 7 NADH yields 21 ATP; and 7 FADH yields 14 ATP).

    2. Total energy yield from oxidation of long-chain fatty acids (e.g., palmitate, stearate) is more than 100 ATP per molecule.

E. Other pathways of fatty acid oxidation

    1. Odd-numbered fatty acids undergo oxidation by the same pathway as saturated fatty acids, except that propionyl CoA (3 carbons) remains after the final cycle (Fig. 7-4).

      a. Propionyl CoA is converted first to methylmalonyl CoA and then to succinyl CoA, a citric acid cycle intermediate that enters the gluconeogenic pathway.

        (1) Vitamin B_{12} is a cofactor for one of the enzymes (methylmalonyl CoA mutase) in this pathway.

        (2) A major difference between odd-chain fatty acid metabolism and even-chain fatty acid metabolism is that succinyl CoA is used as a substrate for gluconeogenesis, and acetyl CoA is not.

      b. Catabolism of methionine, isoleucine, and valine also produces propionyl CoA.

    2. Unsaturated fatty acids are degraded by oxidation enzymes, but double bonds undergo reduction or rearrangement by other enzymes to produce intermediates recognized by the same enzymes involved in β-oxidation.

    3. Peroxisomal oxidation of very long-chain fatty acids (20-26 carbons) is similar to mitochondrial oxidation but generates no ATP.

F. Disorders resulting from defective fatty acid catabolism

    1. Carnitine deficiency or carnitine acyltransferase deficiency impairs the use of long-chain fatty acids via the carnitine shuttle for energy production.

Defective fatty acid
catabolism: carnitine and
MCAD deficiencies,
adrenoleukodystrophy,
Refsum's disease

a. Clinical findings include muscle aches and fatigue following exercise, elevated free fatty acids in blood, and reduced ketone production in the liver during fasting (acetyl CoA is necessary for ketone production).

b. Hypoglycemia occurs because all tissues are competing for glucose for energy.

2. Deficiency of medium-chain acyl CoA dehydrogenase (MCAD), the first enzyme in the oxidation sequence, is an autosomal recessive disorder.

   • Clinical findings include recurring episodes of hypoglycemia (all tissues are competing for glucose), vomiting, lethargy, and minimal ketone production in the liver.

3. Adrenoleukodystrophy is an X-linked recessive disorder associated with defective peroxisomal oxidation of very long-chain fatty acids.

   • Clinical findings include adrenocortical insufficiency and diffuse abnormalities in the cerebral white matter, leading to neurologic disturbances such as progressive mental deterioration and spastic paralysis.

4. Refsum's disease is an autosomal recessive disease that is marked by an inability to degrade phytanic acid, a branched-chain fatty acid that is present in dairy products.

   a. Clinical findings include retinitis pigmentosa; dry, scaly skin; chronic polyneuritis; cerebellar ataxia; and elevated protein in the cerebrospinal fluid.

   b. Accumulation of phytanic acid in plasma and tissues is caused by a defect in omega oxidation, a minor fat oxidation pathway.

III. Ketone Body Synthesis and Degradation for Fuel

Ketone bodies (acetone,
acetoacetic acid, β-
hydroxybutyric acid): fuel
for muscle (fasting), brain
(starvation), kidneys

   • In the fasting and starvation states, ketone bodies (acetone, acetoacetate, and β-hydroxybutyrate) are utilized for fuel by muscle (skeletal and cardiac), the brain (starvation), and the kidneys.

   A. Ketone body synthesis (Fig. 7-5)

      1. Ketone body synthesis occurs in the mitochondrial matrix during the fasting state when excessive β-oxidation of fatty acids results in excess amounts of acetyl CoA.

      2. The liver is the primary site for ketone body synthesis.

         • HMG CoA synthase is the rate-limiting enzyme.

Ketone body synthesis:
mitochondrial matrix of
liver in fasting state;
HMG CoA synthase is
rate-limiting enzyme

      3. The sequence of biochemical reactions leading up to HMG CoA (3-hydroxy-3-methylglutaryl CoA) is similar to those in cholesterol synthesis; however, in ketone body synthesis, HMG CoA lyase (rather than HMG CoA reductase) is used (see Fig. 7-5).

      4. Conditions associated with an excess production of ketone bodies include diabetic ketoacidosis, starvation, and pregnancy.

         a. An increase in acetoacetate and/or β-hydroxybutyrate produces an increased anion gap metabolic acidosis.

         b. The usual test for measuring ketone bodies in serum or urine (nitroprusside reaction) only detects acetoacetate and acetone, a spontaneous decomposition product of acetoacetate (see Fig. 7-5).

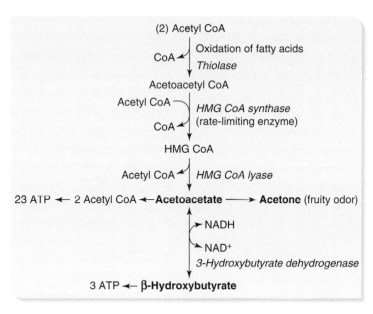

7-5: *Ketone body synthesis. Synthesis of ketone bodies occurs primarily in the liver from leftover acetyl CoA. Ketone bodies are acetone, acetoacetate, and β-hydroxybutyrate, and they are used as fuel by muscle (fasting), brain (starvation), and kidneys.*

- Acetone is a ketone with a fruity odor that can be detected in a patient undergoing a physical examination.

   c. Due to increased production of NADH in alcohol metabolism, the primary ketoacid that develops in alcoholics is β-hydroxybutyrate (NADH forces the reaction in the direction of β-hydroxybutyrate), which is not detected by standard laboratory tests.

B. Degradation of ketone bodies in peripheral tissue (see Fig. 7-5)

   1. Acetoacetate is oxidized into 2 acetyl CoA, which enter the citric acid cycle.

     - Activation of acetoacetate consumes 1 ATP, and the total amount of ATP from metabolism of 2 acetyl CoA is 24 − 1 = 23 ATP.

   2. Conversion of β-hydroxybutyrate back into acetoacetate generates 1 NADH, which produces an additional 3 ATP (total of 26 ATP) after entering the electron transport chain.

   3. The liver cannot use ketones for fuel because it lacks the enzyme succinyl CoA:acetoacetate CoA transferase, which is necessary to convert acetoacetate into 2 acetyl CoA.

Liver lacks transferase; cannot use ketones for fuel.

IV. Cholesterol and Steroid Metabolism

  A. Introduction

    1. Cholesterol, the most abundant steroid in human tissue, is important in cell membranes and is the precursor for bile acids and all the steroid hormones including vitamin D, which is synthesized in the skin from 7-dehydrocholesterol.

Cholesterol functions: cell membrane, bile acid synthesis, steroid hormone synthesis

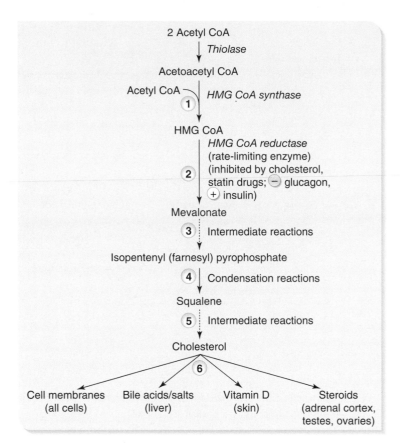

2 Acetyl CoA

↓ *Thiolase*

Acetoacetyl CoA

Acetyl CoA ⤵ | *HMG CoA synthase*

(1)

HMG CoA

HMG CoA reductase
(rate-limiting enzyme)
(inhibited by cholesterol,
(2) statin drugs; ⊖ glucagon,
⊕ insulin)

Mevalonate

(3) Intermediate reactions

Isopentenyl (farnesyl) pyrophosphate

(4) Condensation reactions

Squalene

(5) Intermediate reactions

Cholesterol

(6)

Cell membranes (all cells) — Bile acids/salts (liver) — Vitamin D (skin) — Steroids (adrenal cortex, testes, ovaries)

7-6: *Overview of cholesterol synthesis. HMG CoA reductase is the rate-limiting enzyme, and it is inhibited by statin drugs as well as by cholesterol. Glucagon favors the inactive form of the enzyme; insulin favors the active form.*

    2. Although almost all tissues synthesize cholesterol, the liver, intestinal mucosa, adrenal cortex, testes, and ovaries are the major contributors to the body's cholesterol pool.

B. Cholesterol synthesis and regulation (Fig. 7-6)

    • Enzymes in both the cytosol and SER participate in cholesterol synthesis.

    1. Step 1: HMG CoA is formed by condensation of three molecules of acetyl CoA.

        • In the liver, HMG CoA is also produced in the mitochondria matrix, where it serves as an intermediate in the synthesis of ketone bodies.

    2. Step 2: HMG CoA reductase conversion of HMG CoA to mevalonate is the rate-limiting step in cholesterol synthesis.

        a. Cholesterol, an allosteric inhibitor of gene expression of HMG CoA reductase, provides rapid feedback control of cholesterol synthesis within cells.

- Statin drugs, such as atorvastatin, simvastatin, and pravastatin, act as competitive inhibitors with mevalonate for binding to HMG CoA reductase.

HMG CoA reductase: rate-limiting enzyme in cholesterol synthesis, blocked by statin drugs

  b. Hormones control cycling between the inactive and active forms of HMG CoA reductase via phosphorylation and dephosphorylation, respectively.

   (1) Glucagon favors the inactive form and leads to decreased cholesterol synthesis.

   (2) Insulin favors the active form and leads to increased cholesterol synthesis.

  c. Sterol-mediated decrease in expression of HMG CoA reductase provides long-term regulation.

   - Delivery of cholesterol to liver and other tissues via plasma lipoproteins, such as low-density lipoproteins (LDLs) and high-density lipoproteins (HDLs), leads to a reduction in *de novo* cholesterol synthesis and a decrease in the synthesis of LDL receptors.

3. Step 3: Isopentenyl (farnesyl) pyrophosphate is formed in several reactions from mevalonate and is the key five-carbon isoprenoid intermediate in cholesterol synthesis.

   - Isopentenyl pyrophosphate is also a precursor in the synthesis of coenzyme Q (ubiquinone) and dolichol, which functions in the synthesis of carbohydrate side chains in glycoproteins.

4. Step 4: Squalene, a 30-carbon molecule, is formed by several condensation reactions involving isopentenyl pyrophosphate.

5. Step 5: Conversion of squalene to cholesterol requires several reactions and involves NADPH reduction.

6. Step 6: Cholesterol is excreted in bile or used to synthesize bile acids and salts.

   - Excess cholesterol in bile and/or a deficiency of bile acids and salts may lead to gallstones.

7. Treatment of hypercholesterolemia

  a. Reduce cholesterol intake: 50% reduction in intake lowers serum cholesterol by only approximately 5%.

  b. Decrease cholesterol synthesis by inhibiting HMG CoA reductase with statin drugs

  c. Increase cholesterol excretion with bile-acid binding drugs (e.g., cholestyramine): leads to bile salt and acid deficiency and subsequent upregulation of LDL receptor synthesis in hepatocytes for synthesis of bile salts and acids by using cholesterol

Treating hypercholesterolemia: ↓ cholesterol intake, ↓ cholesterol synthesis, ↑ cholesterol excretion

C. Bile salts and bile acids

1. Bile salts are primarily used to emulsify fatty acids and monoacylglycerols and package them into micelles, along with fat-soluble vitamins, phospholipids, and cholesteryl esters, for reabsorption by villi in the small bowel (see Chapter 4).

2. Primary bile acids (e.g., cholic acid, chenodeoxycholic acid) are synthesized in the liver from cholesterol.

3. Secondary bile salts, formed by conjugation of bile acids with either taurine (taurochenodeoxycholic acid) or glycine (glycocholic acid), are secreted into the bile and eventually released into the duodenum.
   a. Some secondary bile salts are converted into secondary bile acids (glycine and taurine are removed) by anaerobic intestinal bacteria.
   b. Secondary bile acids are deoxycholic and lithocholic acid.
4. The enterohepatic circulation in the terminal ileum recycles approximately 95% of bile salts and acids back to the liver.
5. Bile salt deficiency leads to malabsorption of fat and fat-soluble vitamins (see Box 4-2).

D. Steroid hormones in the adrenal cortex (Fig. 7-7)
1. Synthesis of steroid hormones begins with cleavage of the cholesterol side chain to yield pregnenolone, the C_{21} precursor of all the steroid hormones.
   a. ACTH stimulates conversion of cholesterol to pregnenolone in the adrenal cortex.
   b. Cytochrome P450 hydroxylases (mixed function oxidases) catalyze the addition of hydroxyl groups in reactions that utilize O_2 and NADPH.
      • Similar enzymes also function in detoxification of many drugs in the liver.
2. Steroid hormones in the adrenal cortex contain 21, 19, or 18 carbon atoms (see Fig. 7-7).
   a. Progestins (C_{21}) are synthesized in the zona fasciculata.
      • 17-Hydroxyprogesterone prepares the uterine lining during the secretory phase of the menstrual cycle for implantation of the ovum on day 21; it also contributes to the maintenance of pregnancy.

> Zona fasciculata: synthesis of glucocorticoids (e.g., cortisol)

   b. Glucocorticoids (C_{21}) are synthesized in the zona fasciculata.
      (1) Cortisol promotes glycogenolysis and gluconeogenesis in the fasting state and has a negative feedback relationship with ACTH.
      (2) The 17-hydroxycorticoids are 11-deoxycortisol, cortisol, and their metabolic end-products.

> Zona glomerulosa: synthesis of mineralocorticoids (e.g., aldosterone)

   c. Mineralocorticoids (C_{21}) are synthesized in the zona glomerulosa.
      (1) Aldosterone acts on the distal and the collecting tubules of the kidneys to promote sodium reabsorption and potassium and proton excretion.
      (2) Angiotensin II activates 18-hydroxylase, which converts corticosterone into aldosterone.
      (3) 11-Deoxycorticosterone and corticosterone are weak mineralocorticoids.

> Zona reticularis: synthesis of sex hormones (e.g., androstenedione, testosterone, estrogen)

   d. Androgens (C_{19}) are synthesized in the zona reticularis.
      (1) The 17-ketosteroids, dehydroepiandrosterone and androstenedione, are weak androgens.
      (2) Testosterone is responsible for the development of secondary sex characteristics in males.
      (3) Testosterone is converted to dihydrotestosterone by 5-α-reductase and to estradiol by aromatase.
   e. Estrogens (C_{18}) are synthesized in the zona reticularis.

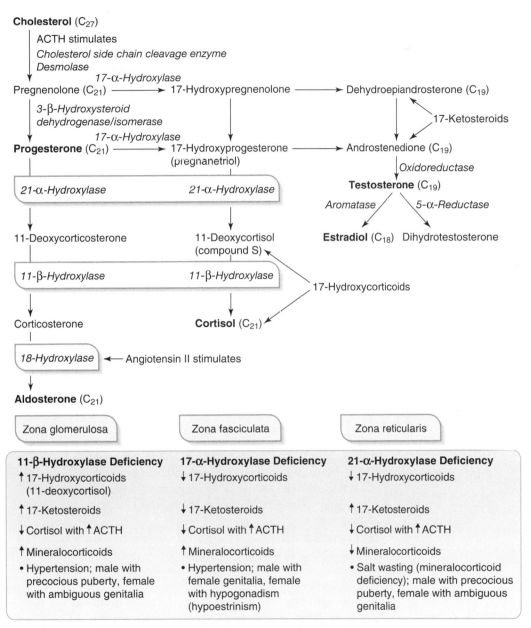

Cholesterol (C_{27})

| ACTH stimulates
| *Cholesterol side chain cleavage enzyme*
| *Desmolase*
| *17-α-Hydroxylase*
↓
Pregnenolone (C_{21}) ⟶ 17-Hydroxypregnenolone ⟶ Dehydroepiandrosterone (C_{19})

| *3-β-Hydroxysteroid*
| *dehydrogenase/isomerase*   17-Ketosteroids
| *17-α-Hydroxylase*
↓
Progesterone (C_{21}) ⟶ 17-Hydroxyprogesterone ⟶ Androstenedione (C_{19})
                              (pregnanetriol)
                                                        | *Oxidoreductase*
| ⎡ *21-α-Hydroxylase*   *21-α-Hydroxylase* ⎤   ↓
| ⎣   ⎦   **Testosterone** (C_{19})
| *Aromatase*   *5-α-Reductase*
↓   ↙   ↘
11-Deoxycorticosterone   11-Deoxycortisol   **Estradiol** (C_{18})   Dihydrotestosterone
                              (compound S)

⎡ *11-β-Hydroxylase*   *11-β-Hydroxylase* ⎤
⎣   ⎦ ← 17-Hydroxycorticoids
↓   ↓
Corticosterone   **Cortisol** (C_{21})

⎡ *18-Hydroxylase* ⎤ ← Angiotensin II stimulates

↓
Aldosterone (C_{21})

| Zona glomerulosa | | Zona fasciculata | | Zona reticularis |

11-β-Hydroxylase Deficiency	**17-α-Hydroxylase Deficiency**	**21-α-Hydroxylase Deficiency**
↑17-Hydroxycorticoids (11-deoxycortisol)	↓17-Hydroxycorticoids	↓17-Hydroxycorticoids
↑17-Ketosteroids	↓17-Ketosteroids	↑17-Ketosteroids
↓Cortisol with ↑ACTH	↓Cortisol with ↑ACTH	↓Cortisol with ↑ACTH
↑Mineralocorticoids	↑Mineralocorticoids	↓Mineralocorticoids
• Hypertension; male with precocious puberty, female with ambiguous genitalia	• Hypertension; male with female genitalia, female with hypogonadism (hypoestrinism)	• Salt wasting (mineralocorticoid deficiency); male with precocious puberty, female with ambiguous genitalia

7-7: *Overview of steroid hormone synthesis from cholesterol in the adrenal cortex. The outer layer of the cortex, the zona glomerulosa, synthesizes mineralocorticoids (e.g., aldosterone); the middle zona fasciculata synthesizes glucocorticoids (e.g., cortisol); and the inner zona reticularis synthesizes sex hormones (e.g., androstenedione, testosterone).*

- Estradiol is responsible for development of female secondary sex characteristics and the proliferative phase of the menstrual cycle.

f. 17-α-Hydroxylase converts pregnenolone and progesterone to the 17-ketosteroids.

g. 21-α-Hydroxylase converts progesterone to 11-deoxycorticosterone in the mineralocorticoid pathway and 17-hydroxyprogesterone to 11-deoxycortisol in the glucocorticoid pathway.

h. 11-β-Hydroxylase converts 11-deoxycorticosterone to corticosterone in the mineralocorticoid pathway and 11-deoxycortisol to cortisol in the glucocorticoid pathway.

i. The ovaries and testes contain only the 17-α-hydroxylase enzyme, which enables them to synthesize 17-ketosteroids, testosterone, 17-hydroxyprogesterone, and estrogen (via aromatization).

E. Adrenogenital syndrome (congenital adrenal hyperplasia)

1. The adrenogenital syndrome is a group of autosomal recessive disorders associated with deficiencies of enzymes involved in the synthesis of adrenal steroid hormones from cholesterol (see Fig. 7-7).

2. Decreased cortisol production in all types of adrenogenital syndrome causes compensatory secretion of ACTH and subsequent bilateral adrenal hyperplasia.

   - Enzyme deficiencies result in an increase in compounds proximal to the enzyme block; compounds distal to the block are decreased.

3. 21-α-Hydroxylase deficiency, the most common type of adrenogenital syndrome, exhibits variable clinical features depending on the extent of the enzyme deficiency.

   a. Less severe cases are marked only by masculinization due to increased androgen production (17-ketosteroids and testosterone).

   b. More severe cases are also associated with deficiency of the mineralocorticoids, leading to sodium wasting and, if untreated, life-threatening volume depletion and shock. The 17-hydroxysteroids are also decreased.

4. 11-β-Hydroxylase deficiency is marked by salt retention (increase in 11-deoxycorticosterone), leading to hypertension, masculinization (increase in 17-ketosteroids and testosterone), and an increase in 11-deoxycortisol (a 17-hydroxycorticoid).

5. 17-α-Hydroxylase deficiency is marked by increased production of the mineralocorticoids (hypertension) and decreased production of 17-ketosteroids and 17-hydroxycorticoids.

V. Plasma Lipoproteins

A. Structure and composition of lipoproteins

1. Spherical lipoprotein particles have a hydrophobic core of triacylglycerols and cholesteryl esters surrounded by a phospholipid layer associated with cholesterol and protein.

2. Four classes of plasma lipoproteins differ in the relative amounts of lipid and the protein they contain (Table 7-2).

21-α-Hydroxylase deficiency: salt wasting, most common cause of adrenogenital syndrome

11-β-Hydroxylase deficiency: salt retention, leads to hypertension

TABLE 7-2:
**Plasma
Lipoproteins**

Type	Components	Function and Metabolism
Chylomicron	Triacylglycerols: highest Cholesterol: lowest Protein: lowest Apolipoproteins: B-48, C-II, E	Transports dietary triacylglycerol to peripheral tissues (e.g., muscle and adipose tissue) and dietary cholesterol to liver Formed and secreted by intestinal mucosa; triacylglycerol-depleted remnants endocytosed by liver
VLDL	Triacylglycerols: moderate Cholesterol: moderate Protein: low Apolipoproteins: B-100, C-II, E	Transports liver-derived triacylglycerol to extrahepatic tissues (e.g., adipose tissue and muscle) Formed and secreted by liver; converted to LDL by hydrolysis of fatty acids by capillary lipoprotein lipase
LDL	Triacylglycerols: low Cholesterol: highest Protein: moderate Apolipoprotein: B-100	Delivers cholesterol from liver to extrahepatic tissues Derived from VLDL; endocytosed by target cells with LDL receptors and degraded, releasing cholesterol, which decreases further uptake of cholesterol
HDL	Triacylglycerols: low Cholesterol: moderate Protein: high Apolipoproteins: A-I, C-II, E	Takes up cholesterol from cell membranes in periphery and returns it to liver (reverse cholesterol transport) Secreted by liver and intestine; activates LCAT to form cholesteryl esters; transfers apoC-II and apoE to nascent chylomicrons and VLDL "Good cholesterol"; the higher the concentration, the lower the risk for coronary artery disease

- As the lipid:protein ratio decreases, particles become smaller and more dense in the following order: chylomicron > VLDL > LDL > HDL.
3. Functions of apolipoproteins
    a. Apolipoprotein A-I (apoA-I) activates lecithin cholesterol acyltransferase (LCAT), which esterifies tissue cholesterol picked up by HDL.
    b. Apolipoprotein C-II (apoC-II) activates capillary lipoprotein lipase, which releases fatty acids and glycerol from chylomicrons, VLDL, and intermediate-density lipoproteins (IDLs).
    c. Apolipoprotein B-48 (apoB-48) is required for secretion of chylomicrons from intestinal mucosa into the lymphatics and from there into the peripheral circulation.
    d. Apolipoprotein B-100 (apoB-100) contains the B-48 domain plus the LDL receptor recognition domain; therefore, it binds to cell surface LDL receptors, mediating delivery of LDL cholesterol to tissues.
    e. Apolipoprotein E (apoE) mediates uptake of chylomicron remnants and IDLs by the liver.

ApoB-48: transport of chylomicrons

ApoB-100: transport of LDL

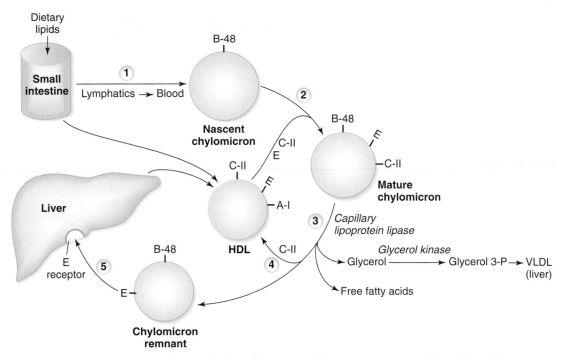

7-8: *Transport of dietary lipids via chylomicrons. Chylomicrons represent triacylglycerol derived from the diet and are a source of fatty acids and glycerol for the synthesis of triacylglycerol in the liver.*

B. Functions and metabolism of lipoproteins
  1. Chylomicrons transport dietary lipids (long-chain fatty acids) from the intestine to the peripheral tissues (Fig. 7-8).
      a. Step 1: Nascent chylomicrons formed in the intestinal mucosa are secreted into the lymph and eventually enter the subclavian vein through the thoracic duct.
          (1) Nascent chylomicrons are rich in dietary triacylglycerols (85%) and contain apoB-48, which is necessary for assembly of the chylomicron.
          (2) They contain only a minimal amount (<3%) of dietary cholesterol.
      b. Step 2: Addition of apoC-II and apoE from HDL leads to the formation of mature chylomicrons.
      c. Step 3: Capillary lipoprotein lipase is activated by apoC-II and hydrolyzes triacylglycerols in chylomicrons, releasing glycerol and free fatty acids into the blood.
          (1) Glycerol is phosphorylated in the liver by glycerol kinase into glycerol 3-phosphate, which is used to synthesize more VLDL.
          (2) Free fatty acids enter the adipose tissue to produce triacylglycerols for storage.
          (3) In muscle, the fatty acids are oxidized to provide energy.
      d. Step 4: ApoC-II returns to HDL.

Chylomicrons: contain diet-derived triacylglycerols

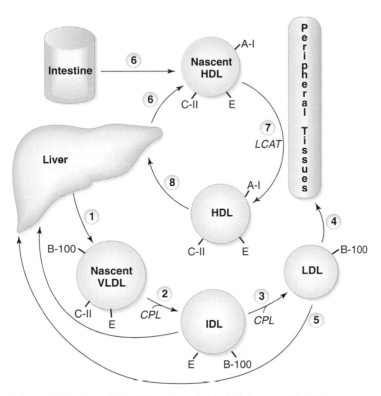

7-9: *Metabolism of VLDL, LDL, and HDL. VLDL is degraded by hydrolysis into LDL. HDL is a reservoir for apolipoproteins and transports cholesterol from tissue to the liver. CPL, capillary lipoprotein lipase; LCAT, lecithin cholesterol acyltransferase.*

 e. Step 5: Chylomicron remnants that remain after the removal of free fatty acids attach to apoE receptors in the liver and are endocytosed.

  (1) Dietary cholesterol delivered to the liver via chylomicron remnants is used for bile acid synthesis and also depresses *de novo* cholesterol synthesis.

  (2) Excess cholesterol is excreted in bile.

2. VLDL carries triacylglycerols synthesized in the liver to peripheral tissues (Fig. 7-9).

 a. Step 1: In addition to triacylglycerols, nascent VLDL particles formed in the liver also contain some cholesterol (~17%) and apoB-100; these VLDL particles obtain apoC-II and apoE from HDL.

 b. Steps 2 and 3: Conversion of circulating nascent VLDL particles into LDL particles proceeds via IDL particles.

  (1) Degradation of triacylglycerols by apoC-II-activated capillary lipoprotein lipase converts nascent VLDL particles into IDL remnants, which are then converted into LDL particles.

  (2) Fatty acids and glycerol are released into the bloodstream.

VLDL: contain liver-derived triacylglycerols and cholesterol

Capillary lipoprotein lipase: hydrolyzes triacylglycerols and VLDL into fatty acids and glycerol

3. Steps 4 and 5: LDL particles remaining after metabolism of VLDL and IDL are enriched in cholesterol (45%), which they deliver to peripheral tissues or to the liver (see Fig. 7-9).

   a. ApoB-100, the major apolipoprotein on LDL, binds to LDL receptors on the cell membrane of target cells in the liver and other tissues.

   - Following receptor-mediated endocytosis, LDL is degraded in lysosomes, releasing free cholesterol for use in membrane synthesis, bile salt synthesis (liver), or steroid hormone synthesis (endocrine tissues, ovaries, and testes).

   b. Excess cholesterol not needed by cells is esterified by acyl CoA:cholesterol acyltransferase (ACAT) and stored as cholesteryl esters.

   c. Free cholesterol in the cytosol has the following regulatory functions:

      (1) Activates ACAT

      (2) Suppresses HMG CoA reductase; decreases *de novo* synthesis of cholesterol

      (3) Suppresses further LDL receptor synthesis; decreases further uptake of LDL

4. Step 6: HDL, the "good cholesterol," is synthesized in the liver and small intestine and carries out reverse transport of cholesterol from extrahepatic tissues to the liver (see Fig. 7-9).

   a. HDL also acts as a repository of apolipoproteins (e.g., apoC-II, apoE), which are required in the metabolism of VLDL and chylomicrons.

   b. Step 7: LCAT mediates esterification of free cholesterol removed from peripheral tissues by HDL.

   - HDL is converted from a discoid shape to a spherical shape when esterified cholesterol is transferred into the center of the molecule.

   c. HDL transfers cholesteryl esters to VLDL in exchange for triacylglycerols (not shown in Fig. 7-9).

      (1) The transfer is mediated by cholesteryl ester transfer protein.

      (2) This transfer explains why an increase in VLDL leads to a decrease in HDL cholesterol levels.

   d. Step 8: Cholesteryl esters are returned to the liver via receptor-mediated endocytosis of HDL.

   e. HDL is increased by estrogen (women therefore have higher HDL levels), exercise, and red wine (increases synthesis of apoA-I).

C. Hereditary disorders related to defective lipoprotein metabolism

1. Abetalipoproteinemia is a rare autosomal recessive lipid disorder characterized by a lack of apoB lipoproteins.

   a. Without apoB, chylomicrons, VLDL, and LDL are absent and levels of triacylglycerol and cholesterol are extremely low.

   b. Clinical findings include an accumulation of triacylglycerols in intestinal mucosal cells leading to malabsorption of fat and fat-soluble vitamins.

   c. Spinocerebellar ataxia, retinitis pigmentosa, and hemolytic anemia respond to megadoses of vitamin E.

2. Genetic and acquired hyperlipoproteinemias (Table 7-3)

TABLE 7-3:
Acquired and Genetic Hyperlipoproteine-mias

Lipid Disorder and Pathogenesis	Clinical Associations	Laboratory Findings
Type I Familial lipoprotein lipase deficiency ApoC-II deficiency Pathogenesis: inability to hydrolyze chylomicrons	Rare childhood disease	↑ chylomicron and triacylglycerol, normal cholesterol and LDL Standing chylomicron test: supranate but no infranate
Type II Familial hypercholesterolemia Pathogenesis: absent or defective LDL receptors	Autosomal dominant disorder with premature coronary artery disease Achilles tendon xanthomas are pathognomonic Acquired causes: diabetes, hypothyroidism, obstructive jaundice, progesterone in birth control pills	Type IIa: ↑ LDL (often >260 mg/dL) and cholesterol, normal triacylglycerol Type IIb: ↑ LDL, cholesterol, and triacylglycerol
Type III Familial dysbetalipoproteinemia "remnant disease" Pathogenesis: deficiency of apoE; chylomicron and IDL remnants not metabolized in liver	↑ risk for coronary artery disease Hyperuricemia, obesity, diabetes	Cholesterol and triacylglycerol equally ↑ ↑ chylomicron and IDL remnants
Type IV Familial hypertriglyceridemia Pathogenesis: decreased catabolism or increased synthesis of VLDL	Autosomal dominant disorder Most common hyperlipoproteinemia ↑ triacylglycerol begins at puberty ↑ incidence of coronary artery disease and peripheral vascular disease Acquired causes: alcoholism, diuretics, β-blockers, renal failure	↑ triacylglycerol, slightly ↑ cholesterol Standing chylomicron test: turbid infranate ↑ HDL (inverse relationship with VLDL)
Type V Most commonly a familial hypertriglyceridemia with exacerbating factors Pathogenesis: combination of type I and type IV mechanisms	Particularly common in alcoholics and individuals with diabetic ketoacidosis Hyperchylomicronemia syndrome: abdominal pain, pancreatitis, dyspnea (impaired oxygen exchange), hepatosplenomegaly (fatty change), papules on skin	↑↑ triacylglycerol, normal LDL Standing chylomicron test: supranate and infranate

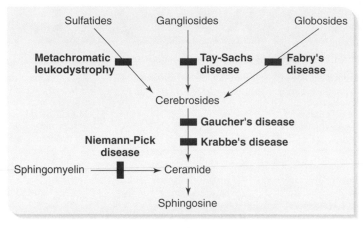

7-10: *Overview of sphingolipid degradation.*

TABLE 7-4:
Sphingolipidoses (Lysosomal Storage Diseases)

Disease	Accumulated Material (Deficient Enzyme)	Clinical Associations
Fabry's disease (X-linked recessive)	Ceramide trihexosides (α-galactosidase)	Paresthesia in extremities; reddish-purple skin rash; cataracts; death due to kidney or heart failure
Gaucher's disease, adult (autosomal recessive [AR])	Glucocerebrosides (β-glucosidase)	Hepatosplenomegaly; macrophage accumulation in liver, spleen, bone marrow; "crinkled paper"–appearing macrophages; compatible with life
Krabbe's disease (AR)	Galactocerebrosides (β-galactosidase)	Progressive psychomotor retardation; abnormal myelin; large "globoid bodies" in brain white matter; fatal early in life
Metachromatic leukodystrophy (AR)	Sulfatides (arylsulfatase A)	Mental retardation; developmental delay; abnormal myelin; peripheral neuropathy; urine arylsulfatase decreased; death within first decade
Niemann-Pick disease (AR)	Sphingomyelin (sphingomyelinase)	Hepatosplenomegaly; mental retardation; "bubbly" appearance of macrophages; fatal early in life
Tay-Sachs disease (AR)	GM_2 gangliosides (hexosaminidase A)	Muscle weakness and flaccidity; blindness, cherry-red macular spot; no hepatosplenomegaly; occurs primarily in eastern European Ashkenazi Jews; fatal at an early age

VI. Sphingolipid Degradation
- Sphingolipids are essential components of membranes throughout the body and are particularly abundant in nervous tissue.
  A. Ceramide, a derivative of sphingosine (sphingosine + fatty acids = ceramide), is the immediate precursor of all the sphingolipids.
      1. Sphingomyelin contains phosphorylcholine linked to ceramide.
      2. Cerebrosides, globosides, gangliosides, and sulfatides—the other classes of sphingolipids—all contain different types and numbers of sugars or sugar derivatives linked to ceramide.
  B. Lysosomal enzymes degrade sphingolipids to sphingosine via a series of irreversible hydrolytic reactions (Fig. 7-10).
  C. Sphingolipidoses are a group of hereditary lysosomal enzyme deficiency diseases caused by a deficiency of one of the hydrolases in the degradative pathway (Table 7-4; see also Box 6-2).
      1. A block in the degradation of sphingolipids leads to accumulation of the substrate for the defective enzyme within lysosomes.
      2. Neurologic deterioration occurs in most of these diseases, leading to early death.
      3. Autosomal recessive inheritance is shown by most of the sphingolipidoses: Gaucher's disease, Krabbe's disease, metachromatic leukodystrophy, Niemann-Pick disease, and Tay-Sachs disease.
      4. Fabry's disease is the only X-linked recessive sphingolipidosis.

> Sphingolipidoses: lysosomal enzyme deficiencies caused by deficiency of a hydrolase in degradative pathway

8

Nitrogen Metabolism and Nucleotide Synthesis and Metabolism

TARGET TOPICS

- Biosynthesis of the nonessential amino acids
- Degradation of amino acids by transamination and oxidative deamination
- Urea cycle: conversion of ammonia to urea, sources of ammonia, causes and treatment of hyperammonemia
- Catabolic pathways of amino acids: carbon skeletons of amino acids; degradation of phenylalanine, tyrosine, branched-chain amino acids, methionine; role of S-adenosylmethionine (SAM) in methyl group transfer reactions
- Amino acid derivatives: catecholamines, porphyrin synthesis, heme degradation, serotonin, melatonin, niacin, γ-aminobutyrate, histamine, creatine

- Nucleotide synthesis and metabolism: nucleotide structure, purine synthesis, pyrimidine synthesis, degradation of purines and pyrimidines, purine salvage
- Clinical correlations: hyperammonemia, phenylketonuria (PKU), dihydrobiopterin reductase deficiency, albinism, alkaptonuria, tyrosinosis, maple syrup urine disease, homocystinuria, propionic acidemia, methylmalonic acidemia, pheochromocytoma, neuroblastoma, porphyrias, lead poisoning, jaundice, carcinoid syndrome, anticancer drugs and DNA synthesis, adenosine deaminase deficiency, gout, Lesch-Nyhan syndrome

Nonessential amino acids: majority synthesized from intermediates of glycolysis and citric acid cycle

I. Biosynthesis of Nonessential Amino Acids
   A. Eleven of the 20 amino acids are synthesized in the body (nonessential amino acids), and the remaining 9 amino acids are required in the diet (essential amino acids).
      1. Ten of the nonessential amino acids are derived from glucose via intermediates derived from glycolysis and the citric acid cycle.
      2. Tyrosine is an exception in that it is derived from phenylalanine, which is an essential amino acid.

TABLE 8-1:
Synthesis of
Nonessential
Amino Acids

Amino Acid	Source of Carbon Skeleton	Comments
Alanine	Pyruvate	Transamination of precursor
Arginine	Ornithine	Reversal of arginase reaction in urea cycle
Asparagine	Oxaloacetate	Amide group from glutamine
Aspartate	Oxaloacetate	Transamination of precursor
Cysteine*	Serine	Sulfur group from methionine
Glutamate	α-Ketoglutarate	Transamination of precursor
Glutamine	α-Ketoglutarate	Amide group from free NH_4^+
Glycine	3-Phosphoglycerate	From serine via transfer of methylene group to tetrahydrofolate
Proline	Glutamate	Cyclization of glutamate semialdehyde
Serine	3-Phosphoglycerate	Oxidation to keto acid, transamination, hydrolysis of phosphate
Tyrosine*	Phenylalanine	Hydroxylation by phenylalanine hydroxylase (tetrahydrobiopterin cofactor)

*Can be synthesized only if methionine and phenylalanine are available from the diet.

3. Cysteine receives its carbon skeleton from serine (product of 3-phosphoglycerate in glycolysis); however, its sulfur comes from the essential amino acid methionine.
4. Many of the nonessential amino acids are synthesized by transamination reactions, where an amino group is added to an α-keto acid to produce an amino acid.
   - Example: Addition of an amino group from glutamate to the α-keto acids pyruvate, oxaloacetate, and α-ketoglutarate produces alanine, aspartate, and glutamate, respectively.
B. The sources of the nonessential amino acids are summarized in Table 8-1.

II. Removal and Disposal of Amino Acid Nitrogen
   A. Catabolism of amino acids
      1. Removal of the α-amino group from amino acids is the initial step in the catabolism of amino acids.
      2. Nitrogen from the amino group is either excreted as urea or incorporated into other compounds.
   B. Transamination and oxidative deamination (Fig. 8-1)
      1. Step 1: Transamination entails the transfer of the α-amino group of an α-amino acid to α-ketoglutarate, producing an α-keto acid from the amino acid and glutamate from α-ketoglutarate (see Fig. 8-1, left).
         a. Aminotransferases (transaminases) catalyze reversible transamination reactions that occur in both the synthesis and the degradation of amino acids.
         b. The two most common aminotransferases transfer nitrogen from aspartate and alanine to α-ketoglutarate, providing α-keto acids that are used as substrates for gluconeogenesis.
            (1) Aspartate aminotransferase (AST) reversibly transaminates aspartate to oxaloacetate.

Synthesized from essential amino acids: tyrosine (from phenylalanine) and cysteine (from methionine)

Transamination: reversible conversion of amino acids to their corresponding keto acids

AST, ALT: enzymes elevated in inflammatory liver diseases (e.g., viral and alcoholic hepatitis)

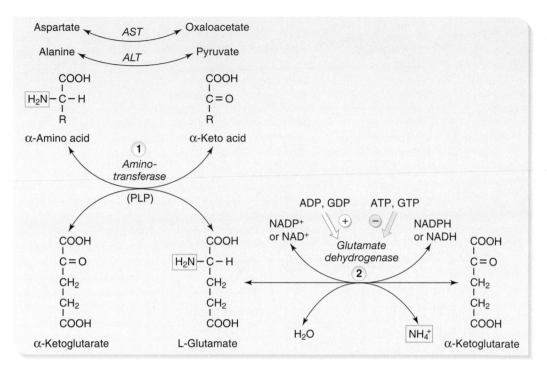

8-1: *Transamination and oxidative deamination reactions. Transamination reactions (left) are used to synthesize and degrade amino acids. Oxidative deamination of glutamate (right), the product of transamination, releases ammonia, which is disposed of in the urea cycle. ALT, alanine aminotransferase; AST, aspartate aminotransferase; PLP, pyridoxal phosphate.*

(2) Alanine aminotransferase (ALT) reversibly transaminates alanine to pyruvate.
  • Plasma AST and ALT are primarily elevated in inflammatory liver diseases such as viral hepatitis (ALT > AST) and alcoholic hepatitis (AST > ALT).
  c. Pyridoxal phosphate (PLP), derived from vitamin B_6 (pyridoxine), is a required cofactor for all aminotransferases (see Chapter 4).

Oxidative deamination: primarily in liver, kidney; releases NH_4^+ from glutamate for conversion to urea

2. Step 2: Oxidative deamination of glutamate (the product of transamination) is the major mechanism for the release of amino acid nitrogen as charged ammonia (NH_4^+), and it occurs primarily in the liver and kidneys (see Fig. 8-1, right).
  a. Glutamate dehydrogenase catalyzes this reversible reaction, using either NAD^+ or $NADP^+$.
  b. In amino acid catabolism, the enzyme reaction results in the conversion of glutamate to α-ketoglutarate and NH_4^+.
3. Allosteric regulation of glutamate dehydrogenase favors release of NH_4^+ when the energy supply is inadequate.
  a. ATP and guanosine triphosphate (GTP) are signals of high energy charge and inhibit the enzyme.

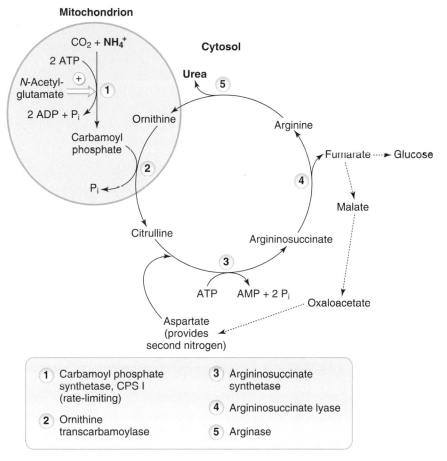

8-2: *The urea cycle. The urea cycle is located in the liver and is the primary mechanism for disposal of toxic ammonia.*

  b. ADP and guanosine diphosphate (GDP) are signals of low energy
     charge and stimulate the release of nitrogen from amino acids, freeing
     their carbon skeletons for use as fuel.
C. Urea cycle (Fig. 8-2)
  1. The urea cycle operates mainly in the liver and converts highly toxic NH_4^+
     to nontoxic urea.
  2. Glutamate is the primary source of NH_4^+ that is used in the urea cycle;
     however, much larger amounts of ammonia are produced from other
     sources that are metabolized by the cycle.
  3. Urea cycle reactions occur in the mitochondrial matrix and cytosol.
     a. Two mitochondrial reactions generate citrulline, which is transported
        to the cytosol.
       (1) Step 1: Carbamoyl phosphate synthetase I (CPS I) catalyzes the
           first, rate-limiting step in which NH_4^+ (which contains the first
           nitrogen), CO_2, and ATP react to produce carbamoyl phosphate
           (see Fig. 8-2).

Urea cycle: in liver, toxic
NH_4^+ converted to
nontoxic urea; CPS I
is rate-limiting
mitochondrial enzyme

(2) *N*-Acetylglutamate is a required activator of CPS I and is in ample supply after eating a high-protein meal.

(3) Step 2: Carbamoyl phosphate, with the addition of ornithine, is converted into citrulline by ornithine transcarbamoylase.

b. Three cytosolic reactions incorporate nitrogen from aspartate to form ornithine, which reenters mitochondria, and urea, which leaves the cell.

(1) Step 3: Citrulline reacts with aspartate (provides a nitrogen) and is converted into argininosuccinate by argininosuccinate synthetase.

(2) Step 4: Argininosuccinate is converted into arginine by argininosuccinate lyase and releases fumarate, which enters the citric acid cycle to produce glucose or aspartate via transamination.

(3) Step 5: Arginine is converted into urea and ornithine by arginase, which is an enzyme located only in the liver.

- Note that the amino acid arginine is synthesized in the urea cycle.

c. Urea enters the blood and most of it is filtered and excreted in the urine. However, a small amount diffuses into the intestine, where it is converted by bacterial ureases into ammonia for elimination in the feces as charged ammonia (NH_4^+).

- In the laboratory, urea is measured as blood urea nitrogen (BUN).

4. Regulation of the urea cycle involves both short-term and long-term mechanisms.

a. *N*-Acetylglutamate is a required allosteric activator of CPS I, providing short-term control.

b. Elevated NH_4^+ causes increased expression of the urea cycle enzymes, providing long-term control.

- This occurs during prolonged starvation when muscle proteins are metabolized to provide energy with release of high levels of NH_4^+.

D. Ammonia metabolism

1. Ammonia is primarily converted into urea, with the exception of ammonia derived from glutamine, which is used to acidify urine.

2. Sources of ammonia

a. Glutamate: ammonia is derived from oxidative deamination of glutamate by glutamate dehydrogenase (see Fig. 8-1).

- Glutamate receives amino groups from amino acids via transamination.

b. Glutamine: in the proximal tubules of the kidneys, glutamine is converted by glutaminase into ammonia and glutamate.

c. Monoamines: amine oxidases release ammonia from epinephrine, serotonin, and histamine.

d. Dietary protein: bacterial ureases release ammonia from amino acids in dietary protein, as well as from urea diffusing into the gut.

(1) Depending on the pH, ammonia released by ureases is either charged (NH_4^+) and nondiffusible through tissue or uncharged (NH_3) and diffusible through tissue.

(2) At physiologic pH, NH_4^+ is produced, which is eliminated in the stool.

Bacterial ureases: release NH_4^+ from amino acids derived from dietary protein

(3) In alkalotic conditions (respiratory and metabolic alkalosis), NH_3 is produced (fewer protons available), which is reabsorbed into the portal vein for delivery to the liver urea cycle.

 e. Purines and pyrimidines: ammonia is released from amino acids in the catabolism of these nucleotides.

3. Ammonia produced in extrahepatic tissues is toxic and is transported in the circulation primarily as urea and glutamine.
   - Glutamine is synthesized from glutamate utilizing the enzyme glutamine synthetase, which combines ammonia, ATP, and glutamate to form glutamine.

4. Ammonia carried by glutamine is important in acidifying urine.
   a. In the proximal renal tubules, glutamine is converted by glutaminase into glutamate and NH_4^+.
   b. The ammonia diffuses into the lumen of the collecting tubules as uncharged ammonia (NH_3), which combines with protons to produce ammonium chloride (acidifies the urine).

> Glutamine: carries ammonia in nontoxic state; ammonia released in kidneys for urine acidification

5. Hyperammonemia results primarily from the inability to detoxify NH_4^+ in the urea cycle, leading to elevated blood levels of ammonia.
   a. Hereditary hyperammonemia is due to defects in urea cycle enzymes.
      - Deficiencies of enzymes that are used earlier in the cycle (e.g., CPS I and ornithine transcarbamoylase) are associated with higher blood ammonia levels and more severe clinical manifestations than deficiencies of enzymes that are used later in the cycle (e.g., arginase).
   b. Acquired hyperammonemia most commonly occurs in alcoholic cirrhosis and Reye's syndrome due to disruption of the urea cycle.
      (1) In cirrhosis, the architecture of the liver is distorted, leading to shunting of portal blood into the hepatic vein or backup of blood in the portal vein (portal hypertension).
         - Serum ammonia is increased, whereas the serum BUN is decreased.

> Cirrhosis: dysfunctional urea cycle leads to hyperammonemia and decreased BUN

      (2) In Reye's syndrome, diffuse fatty change in hepatocytes and damage to the mitochondria by salicylates compromise the function of the urea cycle, resulting in high levels of ammonia.
         - Reye's syndrome occurs primarily in children with either influenza or chickenpox who are given salicylates.

> Reye's syndrome: fatty liver; salicylates compromise mitochondrial function

   c. Signs and symptoms of hyperammonemia include mental status abnormalities (e.g., coma), vomiting, lethargy, subnormal temperature, and irritability. Death may result if signs and symptoms are not treated.
      - Excess ammonia shifts the glutamate dehydrogenase reaction to formation of glutamate, reducing the concentration of α-ketoglutarate and its important role in generating ATP in the citric acid cycle (see Fig. 8-1).
   d. Nonpharmacologic treatment is a low-protein diet.
      - Decreasing protein intake reduces the release of ammonia from amino acids by bacterial ureases.

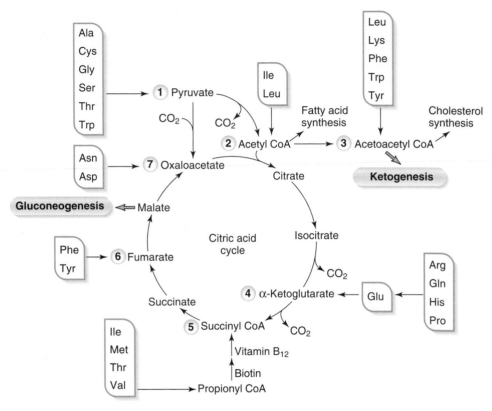

8-3: *Metabolic intermediates formed by degradation of amino acids. Acetyl CoA and acetoacetyl CoA are ketogenic; all other products are glucogenic.*

e. Pharmacologic treatment includes oral intake of lactulose (provides H^+ ions to combine with NH_3 to form NH_4^+, which is excreted) and oral neomycin (kills bacteria that release ammonia from amino acids).

III. Catabolic Pathways of Amino Acids

A. Carbon skeletons of amino acids (Fig. 8-3)

1. Amino acids are classified as glucogenic (degraded to pyruvate or intermediates in citric acid cycle), ketogenic (degraded to acetyl CoA or acetoacetyl CoA), or both glucogenic and ketogenic.

2. Carbon skeletons remaining after removal of the α-amino group from amino acids are degraded to intermediates that can be used to produce energy in the citric acid cycle or to synthesize glucose, amino acids, fatty acids, or ketone bodies.

a. Step 1: Pyruvate is formed from six amino acids that are exclusively glucogenic (except for tryptophan, which is both glucogenic and ketogenic): alanine, cysteine, glycine, serine, threonine, and tryptophan (see Fig. 8-3).

Glucogenic amino acids: degraded to pyruvate or intermediates in citric acid cycle

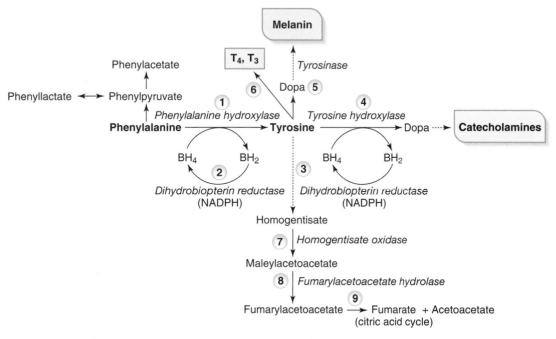

8-4: *Degradation of phenylalanine and tyrosine. Note the relationship of tyrosine to the synthesis of thyroid hormones (triiodothyronine [T$_3$] and thyroxine [T$_4$]), melanin, and catecholamines. BH$_2$, dihydrobiopterin; BH$_4$, tetrahydrobiopterin.*

   b. Step 2: Acetyl CoA is formed from two amino acids: isoleucine (ketogenic and glucogenic) and leucine (exclusively ketogenic).
   c. Step 3: Acetoacetyl CoA, which is interconvertible with acetyl CoA, is formed from five amino acids: leucine and lysine (both exclusively ketogenic), and phenylalanine, tryptophan, and tyrosine (all are ketogenic and glucogenic).
   d. Step 4: α-Ketoglutarate is formed from five amino acids that are exclusively glucogenic: glutamate, glutamine, histidine, arginine, and proline.
   e. Step 5: Succinyl CoA is formed from four amino acids via propionyl CoA, which is a substrate for gluconeogenesis: isoleucine, valine, methionine, and threonine.
   f. Step 6: Fumarate is formed from two amino acids that are both glucogenic and ketogenic: phenylalanine and tyrosine.
   g. Step 7: Oxaloacetate is formed from two amino acids that are exclusively glucogenic: aspartate and asparagine.
B. Degradation of phenylalanine and tyrosine (Fig. 8-4)
   1. Step 1: Phenylalanine is converted into tyrosine by phenylalanine hydroxylase (see Fig. 8-4).
      a. The reaction requires tetrahydrobiopterin (BH$_4$) and oxygen.
      b. Step 2: Dihydrobiopterin (BH$_2$) is converted back into BH$_4$ by dihydrobiopterin reductase using NADPH as a cofactor.

Ketogenic amino acids: degraded to acetyl CoA or acetoacetyl CoA; Leu and Lys are ketogenic

Tetrahydrobiopterin (BH$_4$): cofactor in conversion of phenylalanine to tyrosine, tyrosine to DOPA, and tryptophan to serotonin

c. Phenylpyruvate, phenylacetate, and phenyllactate normally are not produced in large quantities unless there is a deficiency of phenylalanine hydroxylase.
  • Deficiency of phenylalanine hydroxylase produces classic phenylketonuria (PKU) (Table 8-2).
  d. Deficiency of dihydrobiopterin reductase produces a variant of PKU called "malignant" PKU (see Table 8-2).
  2. Step 3: Tyrosine is converted after an intermediate reaction into homogentisate.
    a. Tyrosine is also used to synthesize catecholamines.
      (1) Step 4: Tyrosine is converted by tyrosine hydroxylase into DOPA, which is used to synthesize the catecholamines through a series of intermediate reactions (see Fig. 8-6).
      (2) The reaction requires BH_4 and oxygen.
      (3) Dihydrobiopterin BH_2 is converted back into BH_4 by dihydrobiopterin reductase using NADPH as a cofactor.
    b. Step 5: Tyrosine can also be converted by tyrosinase into DOPA and other intermediates to produce melanin.
      • Deficiency of tyrosinase produces albinism (see Table 8-2).

    c. Step 6: Triiodothyronine (T_3) and thyroxine (T_4) synthesis in the thyroid gland begins with iodination of tyrosine residues.
      • Condensation of iodinated tyrosine residues forms T_3 and T_4.
  3. Step 7: Homogentisate is converted into maleylacetoacetate by homogentisate oxidase.
    • Deficiency of homogentisate oxidase produces alkaptonuria (see Table 8-2).

  4. Step 8: Maleylacetoacetate is converted into fumarylacetoacetate by fumarylacetoacetate hydrolase.
    • Deficiency of fumarylacetoacetate hydrolase produces tyrosinosis (see Table 8-2).
  5. Step 9: Fumarylacetoacetate is converted into fumarate, which is a substrate in the citric acid cycle, and acetoacetate, which is a keto acid.
C. Degradation of leucine, isoleucine, and valine: branched-chain amino acids
  1. Branched-chain amino acids are metabolized primarily in muscle and to a lesser extent in other extrahepatic tissues.
  2. Their metabolism involves a series of reactions resulting in the conversion of leucine (ketogenic) into acetyl CoA and acetoacetate; isoleucine (ketogenic and glucogenic) into acetyl CoA and succinyl CoA; and valine (glucogenic) into succinyl CoA.
  3. One of the enzymes used in the degradative process is branched-chain α-keto acid dehydrogenase, which is deficient in maple syrup urine disease (see Table 8-2).

    • Branched-chain keto acids cause urine to have the odor of maple syrup.
D. Degradation of methionine (Fig. 8-5)
  1. The essential amino acid methionine is the precursor of S-adenosylmethionine (SAM), which is the most important methyl group (CH_3) donor in biological methylations (e.g., norepinephrine receives a methyl group from SAM to produce epinephrine).

TABLE 8-2:
**Genetic Disorders
Associated with
Degradation of
Amino Acids**

Genetic Disorder	Associated Enzyme	Clinical Associations
Classic PKU (autosomal recessive [AR])	Phenylalanine hydroxylase: Catalyzes conversion of phenylalanine to tyrosine Deficiency leads to ↑ phenylalanine and neurotoxic phenylketones and acids and ↓ tyrosine	Mental retardation; fair skin (↓ melanin synthesis from tyrosine) Mousy odor in affected individual Vomiting simulating congenital pyloric stenosis Must screen for phenylalanine after child has been exposed to phenylalanine in breast milk *Treatment*: Restrict phenylalanine, add tyrosine, and restrict aspartame (contains phenylalanine) from diet Pregnant women with PKU must restrict phenylalanine from diet or neurotoxic damage will develop in the fetus *in utero*
"Malignant" PKU (AR)	Dihydrobiopterin reductase: Cofactor for phenylalanine hydroxylase, which converts phenylalanine to tyrosine Deficiency leads to ↑ phenylalanine and neurotoxic byproducts and ↓ tyrosine and tetrahydrobiopterin (BH_4)	Similar to classic PKU Neurologic problems occur regardless of restricting phenylalanine intake Inability to metabolize tryptophan or tyrosine (require BH_4), which causes ↓ synthesis of neurotransmitters (serotonin and dopamine, respectively) *Treatment*: Restrict phenylalanine in diet; administer L-DOPA and 5-hydroxytryptophan to replace neurotransmitters and BH_4 replacement
Albinism (AR)	Tyrosinase: Catalyzes a reaction converting tyrosine to DOPA and DOPA to melanin; melanocytes are present but do not contain melanin pigment	Absence of melanin in hair (white hair), eyes (photophobia, nystagmus), and skin (pink skin with ↑ risk of UV light-related skin cancer)
Alkaptonuria (AR)	Homogentisate oxidase: Catalyzes conversion of homogentisate to maleylacetoacetate Deficiency leads to ↑ homogentisate in urine (turns black when oxidized by light) Articular cartilage and sclera darken (ochronosis) due to homogentisate deposition	Degenerative arthritis in spine, hip, and knee
Tyrosinosis (AR)	Fumarylacetoacetate hydrolase: Catalyzes conversion of maleylacetoacetate to fumarylacetoacetate Deficiency leads to ↑ tyrosine	Liver damage (hepatitis progressing to cirrhosis and hepatocellular carcinoma) and kidneys (aminoaciduria and renal tubular acidosis)

continued

TABLE 8-2:
Genetic Disorders Associated with Degradation of Amino Acids—cont'd

Genetic Disorder	Associated Enzyme	Clinical Associations
Maple syrup urine disease (AR)	Branched-chain α-keto acid dehydrogenase: Enzyme is normally present in muscle and catalyzes the second step in degradation of isoleucine, leucine, and valine Deficiency leads to ↑ branched-chain amino acids and their corresponding keto acids in blood and urine	Feeding difficulties, vomiting, seizures, hypoglycemia, fatal without treatment Urine has odor of maple syrup *Treatment*: Restrict intake of branched-chain amino acids to the amount required for protein synthesis
Homocystinuria (AR)	Cystathionine synthase: Catalyzes conversion of homocysteine + serine into cystathionine Deficiency leads to ↑ homocysteine and methionine Homocysteine damages endothelial cells causing thrombosis and thromboembolic disease	Similar to Marfan syndrome: dislocated lens, arachnodactyly ("spider fingers"), eunuchoid features (arm span > height) Distinctive features include mental retardation, vessel thrombosis (e.g., cerebral vessels), osteoporosis *Treatment*: High doses of vitamin B_6, restriction of methionine, addition of cysteine
Propionic acidemia (AR)	Propionyl carboxylase: Catalyzes conversion of propionyl CoA to methylmalonyl CoA Deficiency leads to ↑ propionic acid and odd-chain fatty acids in the liver	Neurologic and developmental complications *Treatment*: Low-protein diet; L-carnitine (improves β-oxidation of fatty acids); ↑ intake of methionine, valine, isoleucine, and odd-chain fatty acids
Methylmalonic acidemia (AR)	Methylmalonyl CoA mutase: Catalyzes conversion of methylmalonic acid to succinyl CoA, using vitamin B_{12} as a cofactor Deficiency leads to ↑ methylmalonic and propionic acids	Neurologic and developmental complications Rule out vitamin B_{12} deficiency as a cause *Treatment*: Same as for propionic acidemia

2. Step 1: SAM is formed by the transfer of the adenosyl group from ATP to methionine (see Fig. 8-5).
3. Step 2: After donation of its methyl group, SAM becomes *S*-adenosylhomocysteine.
   - The methyl group is transferred to a variety of acceptors (e.g., norepinephrine), resulting in a methylation product (e.g., epinephrine).
4. Step 3: *S*-Adenosylhomocysteine is converted into homocysteine.
   a. Step 4: Homocysteine can resynthesize methionine with the aid of vitamin B_{12} and folate (see Chapter 4).
   b. Vitamin B_{12} removes the methyl group from N^5-methyltetrahydrofolate (N^5-methyl-FH_4) and produces tetrahydrofolate (FH_4).

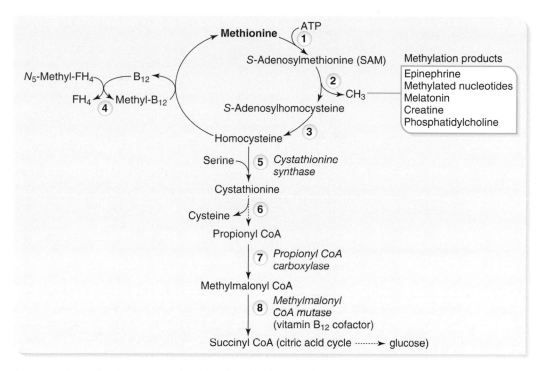

8-5: *Degradation of methionine. Note the relationship of methionine with the donation of methyl groups, resynthesis by homocysteine with the aid of vitamin B_{12} and folate, synthesis of cysteine, and production of succinyl CoA in the citric acid cycle. FH_4, tetrahydrofolate; methyl-B_{12}, methylated vitamin B_{12}.*

     c. Methylated vitamin B_{12} (methyl-B_{12}) transfers the methyl group to homocysteine, which produces methionine.

5. Step 5: Homocysteine combined with serine is converted into cystathionine by cystathionine synthase (see Fig. 8-5).
   - Deficiency of cystathionine synthase produces homocystinuria (see Table 8-2).

6. Step 6: Cystathionine, after an intermediate reaction, is converted into propionyl CoA and cysteine.
   - Propionyl CoA is also produced by the metabolism of odd-chain fatty acids (see Chapter 7) and is an intermediary product in the metabolism of the branched-chain amino acids valine and isoleucine.

7. Step 7: Propionyl CoA is converted into methylmalonyl CoA by propionyl CoA carboxylase, which uses biotin as a cofactor (see Chapter 4).
   - Deficiency of propionyl CoA carboxylase produces propionic acidemia (see Table 8-2).

8. Step 8: Methylmalonyl CoA is converted into succinyl CoA by methylmalonyl CoA mutase, which uses vitamin B_{12} as a cofactor (see Chapter 4).
   a. Succinyl CoA is a substrate in the citric acid cycle that is used to synthesize glucose (by gluconeogenesis) and heme (see Fig. 8-7).

Homocystinuria (AR): deficiency of cystathionine synthase; homocysteine produces vessel damage

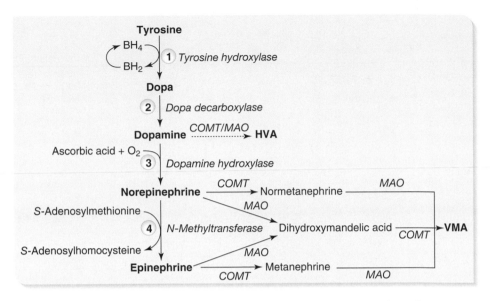

8-6: *Catecholamine synthesis and degradation. Tyrosine plays a major role in the synthesis of catecholamines, which are important neurotransmitters. BH₂, dihydrobiopterin; BH₄, tetrahydrobiopterin; COMT, catechol-O-methyltransferase; HVA, homovanillic acid; MAO, monoamine oxidase; VMA, vanillylmandelic acid.*

       b. Deficiency of methylmalonyl CoA mutase produces methylmalonic acidemia (see Table 8-2).

       c. Deficiency of vitamin B_{12} leads to an accumulation of methylmalonyl CoA and propionyl CoA, causing permanent neurologic dysfunction.

IV. Amino Acid Derivatives

   A. Catecholamines (Fig. 8-6)

     1. Catecholamines (dopamine, epinephrine, and norepinephrine) are important neurotransmitters that are derived from tyrosine and are formed by the DOPA pathway in neural tissue and the adrenal medulla.

       a. Norepinephrine is a neurotransmitter with excitatory activity in the brain (hypothalamus and brain stem) and sympathetic nervous system; dopamine (primarily located in the substantia nigra and ventral hypothalamus) is a neurotransmitter with inhibitory activity against acetylcholine.

       b. Stimulation of the sympathetic nerves to the adrenal medulla causes the release of epinephrine and norepinephrine, which affect blood vessels (vasoconstriction is greater with norepinephrine than with epinephrine), the heart (contraction is greater with epinephrine than with norepinephrine), and the gastrointestinal tract (both inhibit peristalsis).

     2. Step 1: The reaction sequence for catecholamine synthesis begins with tyrosine, which is converted into DOPA by tyrosine hydroxylase (copper-containing rate-limiting enzyme) in the cytoplasm (see Fig. 8-6).

Catecholamines (neurotransmitters derived from tyrosine): dopamine, epinephrine, norepinephrine

    a. The reaction requires BH_4.

    b. BH_2 is converted back into BH_4 by dihydrobiopterin reductase (see Fig. 8-4) using NADPH as a cofactor.

3. Step 2: DOPA is converted into dopamine by DOPA decarboxylase.

    a. This reaction occurs in storage vesicles in the adrenal medulla and synaptic vesicles in neurons.

    b. Catechol-*O*-methyltransferase (COMT) and monoamine oxidase (MAO) are involved in reactions that metabolize dopamine into homovanillic acid (HVA).

    c. Dopamine is deficient in Parkinson's disease.

> HVA: degradation product of dopamine

4. Step 3: Dopamine is converted into norepinephrine by dopamine hydroxylase (a copper-containing enzyme), which utilizes ascorbic acid as a cofactor.

    • COMT and MAO metabolize norepinephrine into vanillylmandelic acid (VMA).

5. Step 4: Norepinephrine is converted into epinephrine by *N*-methyltransferase using a methyl group donated by SAM.

> VMA: degradation product of norepinephrine and epinephrine

    a. *N*-Methyltransferase is located only in the adrenal medulla; hence, epinephrine is only synthesized in the adrenal medulla.

    b. COMT metabolizes epinephrine into metanephrine, which is converted into VMA by MAO.

> Metanephrine: degradation product of epinephrine

    c. HVA, VMA, and metanephrines are excreted in the urine, and levels are commonly measured to screen for tumors of the adrenal medulla or sympathetic nervous system.

      (1) Tumors of the adrenal medulla secrete excess catecholamines, leading to hypertension.

      (2) Pheochromocytomas are benign, unilateral tumors of the adrenal medulla that occur primarily in adults.

      (3) Neuroblastomas are malignant unilateral tumors of the adrenal medulla that occur primarily in children.

> Pheochromocytoma (benign) and neuroblastoma (malignant): adrenal medulla tumors that secrete excess catecholamines

B. Porphyrin synthesis and metabolism (Fig. 8-7)

1. Porphyrins are ring compounds that bind to iron at their center.

    a. Porphyrins are involved in oxidative or oxygen-transferring functions and are precursors for heme synthesis in the bone marrow and liver.

    b. The porphyrin heme has one iron atom (Fe^{2+}) coordinately bound in the center of the porphyrin ring and is found in hemoglobin, myoglobin, and cytochromes (e.g., cytochrome P450 system).

    c. Porphyrinogens (porphyrin precursors) are colorless and nonfluorescent in the reduced state.

      (1) When porphyrinogen compounds are oxidized in voided urine and exposed to light, they become porphyrins, which have a wine-red color and fluoresce under ultraviolet light.

      (2) Porphyrins in the peripheral circulation absorb ultraviolet light near the skin surface, becoming photosensitizing agents that damage skin and produce vesicles and bullae.

    d. Porphyrin synthesis begins in the mitochondria, moves into the cytosol, and then reenters the mitochondria.

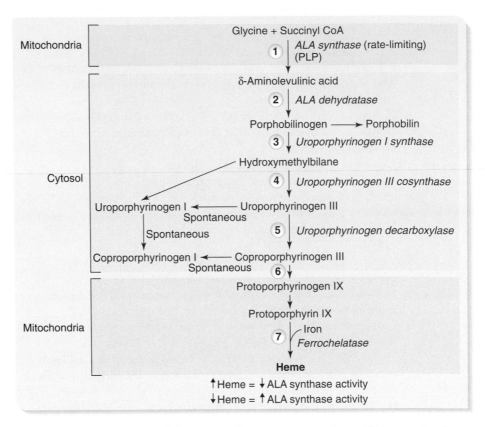

8-7: *Porphyrin synthesis and metabolism. Heme is the most important porphyrin and plays a major role in oxygen transfer reactions. Enzyme deficiencies in porphyrin synthesis result in various types of porphyria. ALA, δ-aminolevulinic acid; PLP, pyridoxal phosphate.*

2. Biochemical reactions in heme synthesis
   a. Step 1: Glycine and succinyl CoA are combined by the mitochondrial enzyme δ-aminolevulinic acid synthase (ALA synthase), which is a rate-limiting enzyme, to form δ-aminolevulinic acid (see Fig. 8-7).
      (1) The reaction requires PLP, derived from vitamin B_6, as a cofactor.
      (2) An increase in heme suppresses ALA synthase; a decrease in heme (e.g., after metabolism of a drug in the liver) increases activity of the enzyme.
      (3) Carbohydrate loading inhibits ALA synthase activity in the liver.
   b. Step 2: δ-Aminolevulinic acid is converted into porphobilinogen by the cytosolic enzyme δ-aminolevulinic acid dehydratase (ALA dehydratase).
      • Lead inhibits ALA dehydratase, leading to an increase in δ-aminolevulinic acid.
   c. Step 3: Porphobilinogen is converted into hydroxymethylbilane by the cytosolic enzyme uroporphyrinogen I synthase (Table 8-3).

Heme synthesis: ALA synthase is rate-limiting enzyme; feedback control with heme

TABLE 8-3:
Genetic Disorders Involving Porphyrin Synthesis

Genetic Disorder	Associated Enzyme	Clinical Associations
Acute intermittent porphyria (autosomal dominant [AD])	Uroporphyrinogen I synthase: Catalyzes conversion of porphobilinogen to hydroxymethylbilane Deficiency leads to ↑ porphobilinogen (PBG) and δ-aminolevulinic acid (ALA) in urine	Recurrent attacks of neurologically induced abdominal pain (mimics a surgical abdomen) Abdominal pain often leads to surgical exploration ("bellyful of scars") without finding any cause Urine exposed to light develops a wine-red color due to porphobilin ("window sill" test) Enzyme assay in RBCs is the confirming test when the patient is asymptomatic Attacks precipitated by drugs that induce the liver cytochrome P450 system (e.g., alcohol); drugs that induce ALA synthase (e.g., progesterone); and dietary restriction *Treatment*: Carbohydrate loading and infusion of heme, both of which inhibit ALA synthase activity
Congenital erythropoietic porphyria (autosomal recessive [AR])	Uroporphyrinogen III cosynthase: Catalyzes conversion of hydroxymethylbilane to uroporphyrinogen III Deficiency leads to ↑ uroporphyrinogen I and its oxidation product uroporphyrin I	Hemolytic anemia and photosensitive skin lesions with vesicles and bullae Uroporphyrin I produces a wine-red color in urine and teeth and induces a photosensitivity reaction in skin *Treatment*: Protection of skin from light; bone marrow transplantation
Porphyria cutanea tarda (PCT) (AD or acquired)	Uroporphyrinogen decarboxylase: Catalyzes conversion of uroporphyrinogen III to coproporphyrinogen III Deficiency leads to accumulation of uroporphyrinogen III, which spontaneously converts into uroporphyrinogen I and coproporphyrinogen I and their respective oxidized porphyrins	Most common porphyria in United States Predominantly associated with photosensitive skin lesions consisting of vesicles and bullae and liver disease (e.g., cirrhosis) Exacerbating factors include iron therapy, alcohol, estrogens, and hepatitis C (most common acquired cause of PCT) Uroporphyrin I produces a wine-red color in urine and predisposes to photosensitive skin lesions; PBG levels are normal *Treatment*: Phlebotomy (reduce iron levels in the liver) and chloroquine

continued

TABLE 8-3:
Genetic Disorders Involving Porphyrin Synthesis—cont'd

Genetic Disorder	Associated Enzyme	Clinical Associations
Lead poisoning (acquired)	Inhibits ALA dehydratase and ferrochelatase: ALA dehydratase catalyzes conversion of δ-ALA to PBG; inhibition leads to ↑ δ-ALA in urine Ferrochelatase combines iron with protoporphyrin IX to form heme Inhibition causes ↑ RBC protoporphyrin IX and ↓ heme Iron accumulates in mitochondria, causing a microcytic anemia with "ringed sideroblasts" (mitochondria around the RBC nucleus filled with iron) in the bone marrow Lead inhibits ribonuclease, causing persistence of ribosomes in peripheral blood RBCs (coarse basophilic stippling)	Causes include exposure to lead-based paint and working in battery factories Children develop encephalopathy with convulsions, microcytic anemia, and abdominal pain Adults develop abdominal pain and diarrhea, peripheral neuropathies, and renal disease (aminoaciduria, renal tubular acidosis) Screen for blood lead levels *Treatment*: British antilewisite, calcium disodium edetate, and D-penicillamine

Acute intermittent porphyria (AD): deficiency of uroporphyrinogen I synthase; increase in porphobilinogen and δ-ALA in urine; neurologic problems

- Uroporphyrinogen I synthase is deficient in acute intermittent porphyria.
  d. Step 4: Hydroxymethylbilane is converted into uroporphyrinogen III by the cytosolic enzyme uroporphyrinogen III cosynthase (see Table 8-3).
    (1) Some hydroxymethylbilane is nonenzymatically converted into uroporphyrinogen I, which is further converted into coproporphyrinogen I.
      - Both compounds are spontaneously oxidized into uroporphyrin I and coproporphyrin I, respectively.
    (2) Deficiency of uroporphyrinogen III cosynthase produces congenital erythropoietic porphyria.
  e. Step 5: Uroporphyrinogen III is converted into coproporphyrinogen III by the cytosolic enzyme uroporphyrinogen decarboxylase (see Table 8-3).
    (1) Both uroporphyrinogen III and coproporphyrinogen III can be spontaneously oxidized into uroporphyrinogen I and coproporphyrinogen I, respectively.
    (2) Uroporphyrinogen decarboxylase is deficient in porphyria cutanea tarda, the most common porphyria in the United States.
  f. Step 6: Coproporphyrinogen III is converted into protoporphyrinogen IX and the latter into protoporphyrin IX by oxidase reactions that occur in the mitochondria.

Porphyria cutanea tarda (AD): deficiency of uroporphyrinogen decarboxylase; skin photosensitivity

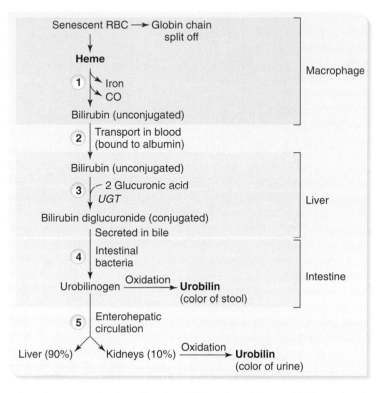

8-8: *Heme degradation. Note that the end-products of heme degradation are bilirubin and its degradative product, urobilinogen. Oxidation of urobilinogen into urobilin provides the color for both stool and urine. CO, carbon monoxide; UGT, uridine diphosphate glucuronyltransferase.*

g. Step 7: Ferrochelatase combines iron with protoporphyrin IX to form heme (see Table 8-3).

   (1) Heme has a feedback inhibition with ALA synthase.

      • Drugs metabolized by the cytochrome P450 system (e.g., alcohol and barbiturates) decrease the concentration of heme, leading to activation of ALA synthase.

   (2) Lead inhibits ferrochelatase, leading to a decrease in heme and an increase in protoporphyrin IX (see Table 8-3).

3. Heme degradation (Fig. 8-8)

  a. Most heme that is degraded comes from the hemoglobin of "old" erythrocytes, which are phagocytosed by macrophages (primarily in the spleen).

    • After globin is split off, the free heme is degraded.

  b. Step 1: Oxidases convert heme to unbound unconjugated bilirubin in macrophages located in the spleen.

   (1) Iron and carbon monoxide (CO) are released.

   (2) Unbound, unconjugated bilirubin, which is lipid soluble, is released by macrophages into the bloodstream.

Lead poisoning: inhibition of ferrochelatase and ALA dehydratase; microcytic anemia with coarse basophilic stippling

Bilirubin: end-product of heme degradation by macrophages

c. Step 2: Unconjugated bilirubin (indirect bilirubin) combines with albumin in the blood and is taken up into hepatocytes by binding proteins.
  - Unconjugated bilirubin is not filtered in urine since it is lipid-soluble and bound to albumin.
d. Step 3: In the hepatocytes, unconjugated bilirubin is conjugated by reacting with two molecules of glucuronic acid, a reaction that is catalyzed by uridine diphosphate glucuronyltransferase (UGT).
  (1) Bilirubin diglucuronide, or conjugated (direct) bilirubin, is water-soluble.
  (2) Conjugated bilirubin does not have access to the blood unless there is inflammation in the liver (e.g., hepatitis) or obstruction to bile flow (e.g., gallstone in the common bile duct).
  (3) Conjugated bilirubin is actively secreted into the bile ducts and stored in the gallbladder for eventual release into the duodenum.
e. Step 4: Intestinal bacteria hydrolyze conjugated bilirubin and reduce free bilirubin to colorless urobilinogen.
  - Oxidation of urobilinogen yields urobilin, which gives feces its characteristic brown color.
f. Step 5: Approximately 20% of urobilinogen is reabsorbed back into the blood (enterohepatic circulation) in the terminal ileum and is recycled to the liver and kidneys.
  (1) In urine, urobilinogen is oxidized into urobilin, which gives urine its yellow color.
  (2) Note that the color of both stool and urine is due to urobilin.

4. Hyperbilirubinemia results from overproduction or defective disposal of bilirubin and may lead to jaundice.

Jaundice: overproduction of bilirubin; decreased conjugation; disruption of bile ducts (hepatitis); bile duct obstruction

  a. Measuring the serum concentration of conjugated bilirubin and unconjugated bilirubin provides clues to the cause of jaundice.
    - Expressing the percentage conjugated bilirubin of the total bilirubin (conjugated bilirubin divided by total bilirubin) is most often used in classifying the types of jaundice.
  b. Predominantly unconjugated bilirubin (percentage conjugated bilirubin is less than 20% of the total) is present in hemolytic anemias associated with macrophage destruction of red blood cells (RBCs) (e.g., congenital spherocytosis) and problems with uptake and conjugation of bilirubin (e.g., Gilbert's disease and Crigler-Najjar syndrome).
    (1) Congenital spherocytosis is an autosomal dominant disorder with a defect in spectrin, the contractile protein attached to the inner surface of an RBC that helps maintain its characteristic shape.
    (2) Gilbert's disease is a benign autosomal dominant disorder with a defect in the uptake and conjugation of bilirubin and is second only to hepatitis as the most common cause of jaundice in the United States.
    (3) Crigler-Najjar syndrome is a genetic disease associated with either a partial (autosomal dominant) or a total (autosomal recessive) deficiency of UGT, the latter being incompatible with life.

    c. Viral hepatitis is associated with a mixed hyperbilirubinemia (increase in both unconjugated and conjugated bilirubin) due to problems with uptake, conjugation, and secretion of bilirubin into bile ducts.
- The percentage conjugated bilirubin is between 20% and 50% of the total bilirubin.

    d. Obstructive jaundice is primarily a conjugated type of hyperbilirubinemia (percentage conjugated bilirubin >50% of the total) and is due to obstruction of bile ducts (e.g., gallstone in the common bile duct).
- Stools are light colored and urobilinogen is not present in urine because bile containing bilirubin is prevented from reaching the small intestine.

C. Tryptophan is a precursor of serotonin, melatonin, and niacin.

  1. The first reaction in the metabolism of tryptophan is catalyzed by tryptophan hydroxylase, which converts tryptophan to 5-hydroxytryptophan.
- The reaction requires BH_4 as a cofactor.

  2. 5-Hydroxytryptophan is converted into serotonin using pyridoxine (vitamin B_6) as a cofactor.

  3. Serotonin (5-hydroxytryptamine) is synthesized primarily in the median raphe of the brain stem, pineal gland, and chromaffin cells of the gut.

    a. Serotonin is a neurotransmitter that suppresses pain and helps control mood.
- Deficiency of serotonin is associated with depression.

    b. Serotonin stimulates contraction of smooth muscle in the gastrointestinal tract, increasing peristalsis, and it increases the peripheral resistance as a vasoconstrictor of arterioles.

    c. Serotonin is converted into melatonin in the pineal gland utilizing SAM as a methyl donor.
- Melatonin is involved in regulating the sleep/wake cycle.

    d. Serotonin is excreted as 5-hydroxyindoleacetic acid (5-HIAA) in urine.

    e. The carcinoid syndrome typically occurs when a carcinoid tumor of the small intestine metastasizes to the liver.
- Serotonin produced by the metastatic nodules gains access to the systemic circulation and causes cyanotic flushing of the skin, sudden drops in blood pressure, watery diarrhea (hyperperistalsis), and an increase of 5-HIAA in urine.

  4. Tryptophan is a precursor for the synthesis of niacin (nicotinic acid).
- Deficiency of tryptophan or niacin produces pellagra (see Chapter 4).

D. Glutamate is decarboxylated to produce γ-aminobutyrate (GABA), an inhibitory neurotransmitter in the basal ganglial system.
- GABA is increased in hepatic encephalopathy.

E. Histidine is decarboxylated to produce histamine, a potent vasodilator that is released by mast cells during type I hypersensitivity reactions.

F. Arginine, glycine, and SAM are precursors of creatine.

Tryptophan: precursor of serotonin (neurotransmitter), melatonin (sleep/wake cycle), niacin (deficiency causes pellagra)

Carcinoid syndrome: carcinoid tumor leads to production of excess serotonin

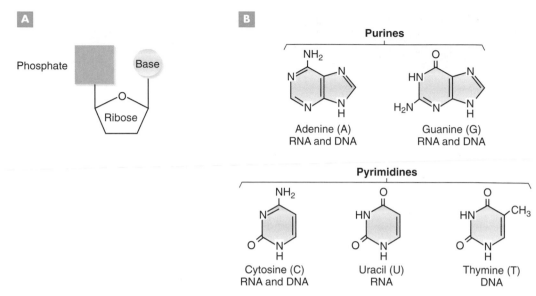

8-9: *Nucleotide structure.* **A,** *All nucleotides have three components.* **B,** *Five bases are most commonly found in nucleotides. Both RNA and DNA contain adenine (A), guanine (G), and cytosine (C); uracil (U) is present only in RNA, and thymine (T) is present only in DNA. Ribose in nucleoside diphosphates can also be reduced to deoxyribose.*

1. Creatine kinase combines creatine with ATP to produce creatine phosphate, which is a high-energy storage compound present in tissue, particularly muscle and brain.
2. Creatine phosphate provides a ready source of phosphate to regenerate ATP.
3. Creatine is spontaneously converted into creatinine, which is excreted at a constant rate in urine, hence its usefulness in measuring the glomerular filtration rate.

V. Nucleotide Synthesis and Metabolism
  A. Nucleotide structure
    1. Nucleotides consist of an organic base bound via an *N*-glycosyl linkage to a phosphorylated pentose (Fig. 8-9A).
    2. The base component has a purine (adenine, guanine) or pyrimidine (cytosine, thymine, uracil) ring structure (Fig. 8-9B).
      a. RNA and DNA contain adenine (A), guanine (G), and cytosine (C).
      b. Uracil (U) occurs only in RNA, and thymine (T) occurs only in DNA.
    3. The pentose component is the ribose in the ribonucleotides that make up RNA and the deoxyribose in the deoxyribonucleotides that make up DNA.
      a. Ribonucleotide reductase reduces nucleoside diphosphates (ADP, GDP, CDP, and UDP) to their deoxy forms (e.g., dADP) in a reaction that requires reduced thioredoxin as a cofactor.

RNA: contains ribose and A, G, C, or U

DNA: contains deoxyribose and A, G, C, or T

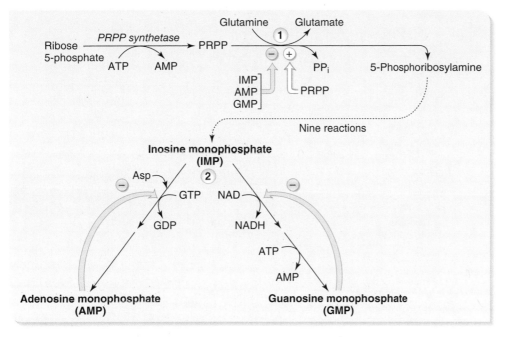

8-10: *Overview of purine synthesis. The purine ring is assembled on a ribose 5-phosphate molecule supplied by 5-phosphoribosyl 1-pyrophosphate (PRPP).*

     b. Oxidized thioredoxin must be converted back into reduced thioredoxin for continued conversion of ribonucleotides to their deoxy forms.
       (1) Thioredoxin reductase, using NADPH as a cofactor, is required for this conversion.
       (2) Note the similarity of this reaction with conversion of BH_2 back to BH_4 by dihydrobiopterin reductase.

B. Purine synthesis (Fig. 8-10)
  1. Step 1: Formation of 5-phosphoribosylamine from 5-phosphoribosyl 1-pyrophosphate (PRPP) and glutamine is a committed step in the *de novo* synthesis of purines (see Fig. 8-10).
     a. End-product feedback inhibition of this reaction by guanosine monophosphate (GMP), adenosine monophosphate (AMP), and inosine monophosphate (IMP) prevents overproduction of purines; high PRPP concentrations overcome this inhibition.
     b. Ribose phosphate pyrophosphokinase (PRPP synthetase), the rate-limiting enzyme, produces PRPP, the source of the ribose 5-phosphate on which the newly synthesized purine ring is assembled.
     c. PRPP, an activated form of ribose 5-phosphate, is also used in the purine salvage pathway and in pyrimidine synthesis.
  2. Step 2: Conversion of IMP to AMP or GMP is controlled to achieve balanced production of AMP and GMP by two mechanisms.
     a. One mechanism is cross-regulation, in which the end-product of one pathway is required for the other pathway.

Purine synthesis: PRPP synthetase is rate-limiting enzyme; purine ring assembled on ribose 5-phosphate supplied by PRPP

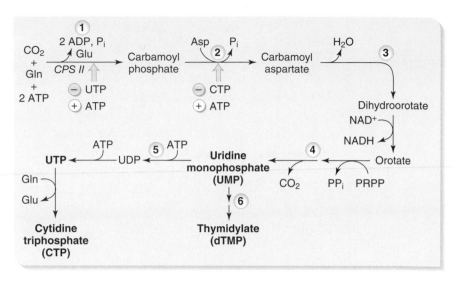

8-11: *Overview of pyrimidine synthesis. The pyrimidine ring is synthesized before the ribose 5-phosphate molecule is supplied by 5-phosphoribosyl 1-pyrophosphate (PRPP). Asp, aspartate; CPS II, carbamoyl phosphate synthetase II; Gln, glutamine; Glu, glutamate.*

- Example: the GMP pathway requires ATP; the AMP pathway requires GTP.
  b. The other mechanism is end-product inhibition of each pathway.
  3. Purine salvage pathways produce nucleotides from preformed bases by transfer of ribose 5-phosphate groups from PRPP to free bases (see Fig. 8-12).
  4. Nucleoside diphosphates and triphosphates are formed from both purine and pyrimidine nucleoside monophosphates by several kinases.
     - ATP is the usual source of high-energy phosphate groups in these reactions.
  C. Pyrimidine synthesis
  1. In contrast to the purine ring, which is assembled on a ribose 5-phosphate molecule, the pyrimidine ring is synthesized before the ribose molecule is supplied by PRPP.
  2. Chemical reaction sequence of pyrimidine synthesis (Fig. 8-11)
     a. Step 1: Carbamoyl phosphate synthetase II (CPS II) catalyzes the formation of carbamoyl phosphate from glutamine, CO_2, and 2 ATP (see Fig. 8-11).
        (1) Unlike CPS I, which is a mitochondrial enzyme in urea synthesis, CPS II is located in the cytosol and is not activated by *N*-acetylglutamate.
        (2) This reaction, the committed step in pyrimidine synthesis, is inhibited by uridine triphosphate (UTP) and activated by ATP and PRPP.
     b. Step 2: Aspartate transcarbamoylase adds aspartate to carbamoyl phosphate, producing carbamoyl aspartate.

Pyrimidine synthesis: CPS II is rate-limiting cytosolic enzyme; ring synthesized before ribose 5-phosphate molecule supplied by PRPP

TABLE 8-4:
Anticancer Drugs Inhibiting Nucleotide Synthesis

Drug	Mechanism of Action	Treatment
Methotrexate (folate analogue)	Competitively inhibits dihydrofolate reductase (DHR): DHR catalyzes reduction of dihydrofolate to tetrahydrofolate, required for synthesis of thymidine and purine nucleotides (see Chapter 4)	Molar disease (hydatidiform moles and choriocarcinoma), leukemias and lymphomas, osteogenic sarcoma, and rheumatoid arthritis
5-Fluorouracil	Converted by tumor cell enzymes to 5-fluorodeoxyuridine monophosphate, which irreversibly inhibits thymidylate synthase and prevents the synthesis of deoxythymidine monophosphate from deoxyuridine monophosphate	Breast, stomach, and colon cancers
Hydroxyurea	Inhibits ribonucleotide reductase, which converts ribonucleotides to deoxyribonucleotides ↓ deoxyribonucleotides ↓ DNA synthesis	Chronic myelogenous leukemia and sickle cell anemia, where it ↑ synthesis of hemoglobin F and ↓ sickling

   c. Step 3: Dihydroorotase converts carbamoyl aspartate into dihydroorate, which is oxidized to produce orotic acid.
   d. Step 4: Conversion of orotate to uridine monophosphate (UMP) is catalyzed by a single bifunctional enzyme (orotate phosphoribosyl transferase and orotidine phosphate decarboxylase).
      • Transfer of ribose 5-phosphate from PRPP is followed by decarboxylation to yield UMP.
   e. Step 5: UMP is the common precursor for synthesis of the remaining pyrimidines UTP and cytidine triphosphate.
   f. Step 6: UMP is converted to deoxyuridine monophosphate (dUMP), which is then converted to thymidylate (dTMP).
      • Thymidylate synthase methylates dUMP to produce dTMP, using methylene tetrahydrofolate as the carbon donor (see Fig. 4-3).
   g. Salvage of uracil and thymine (but not cytosine) and their conversion into nucleotides is catalyzed by pyrimidine phosphoribosyl transferase, which utilizes PRPP as the source of ribose 5-phosphate.
 D. Anticancer drugs that inhibit nucleotide synthesis are summarized in Table 8-4.
 E. Degradation of nucleotides and purine salvage (Fig. 8-12)
   1. Purine nucleotides are degraded to uric acid, which is excreted in urine.
   2. Chemical reactions involved in the degradation of purines to uric acid.
      a. Step 1: The first set of reactions in Figure 8-12 show the conversion of PRPP to IMP in purine synthesis (see Fig. 8-10).

Anticancer drugs inhibiting nucleotide synthesis: methotrexate, 5-fluorouracil, hydroxyurea

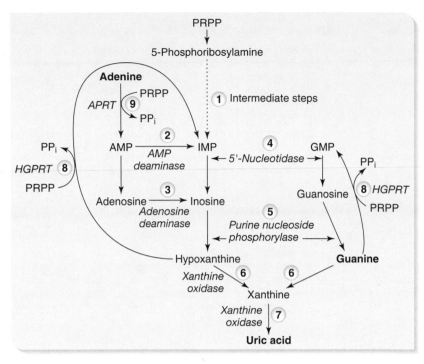

8-12: *Overview of purine degradation and purine salvage. Hypoxanthine-guanine phosphoribosyl transferase (HGPRT) and adenine phosphoribosyl transferase (APRT) are involved in salvaging purines for their conversion into nucleotides. Uric acid is the end-product of purine degradation. PP$_i$, pyrophosphate; PRPP, 5-phosphoribosyl 1-pyrophosphate.*

Adenosine deaminase deficiency (AR): combined B and T cell deficiency (SCID); first gene therapy experiment

  b. Step 2: AMP is converted to IMP by AMP deaminase; AMP is also converted to adenosine.
  c. Step 3: Adenosine is converted to inosine by adenosine deaminase.
    (1) Adenosine deaminase also catalyzes a reaction converting 2-deoxyadenosine to 2-deoxyinosine (which is not shown in Fig. 8-12).
    (2) Deficiency of adenosine deaminase is associated with severe combined immunodeficiency (Table 8-5).
  d. Step 4: IMP is converted into inosine, and GMP is converted into guanosine by 5'-nucleotidase.
  e. Step 5: Inosine is converted into hypoxanthine (purine base) and guanosine into guanine (purine base) by purine nucleoside phosphorylase.
  f. Step 6: Both guanine and hypoxanthine are converted into xanthine, the latter by xanthine oxidase.
  g. Step 7: Xanthine oxidase further converts xanthine into uric acid.
    (1) Allopurinol inhibits xanthine oxidase, resulting in reduced synthesis of uric acid and an increase in both xanthine and hypoxanthine.

TABLE 8-5:
Genetic Disorders Involving Nucleotides

Genetic Disorder	Pathogenesis	Clinical Associations
Severe combined immunodeficiency (SCID) (autosomal recessive)	Variant of SCID due to deficiency of adenosine deaminase (ADA), which catalyzes conversion of adenosine to inosine Deficiency leads to an accumulation of adenosine (toxic to B and T lymphocytes) and adenosine monophosphate (AMP), which is converted by AMP deaminase to inosine monophosphate ADA also catalyzes conversion of 2-deoxyadenosine to 2-deoxyinosine Deficiency of ADA leads to an accumulation of 2-deoxyadenosine and deoxyadenosine monophosphate (dAMP) dAMP is converted to dADP and dATP, which accumulates in the cell; dATP inhibits ribonucleotide reductase, which reduces conversion of ribonucleotides to deoxynucleotides, resulting in ↓ DNA synthesis in B and T cells	Combined B and T cell deficiency leads to recurrent infections involving bacteria, viruses, fungi, and protozoa due to loss of both humoral and cellular immunity
Gout (acquired or genetic)	Associated with either overproduction or underexcretion (most common) of uric acid, end-product of purine degradation Overproduction may be due to overactivity of ribose phosphate pyrophosphokinase (PRPP synthetase) or deficiency of hypoxanthine-guanine phosphoribosyl transferase (HGPRT), a purine salvage enzyme Underexcretion is due to defects in renal excretion of uric acid	Acute gout most often occurs in the metatarsophalangeal joint of the large toe Recurrent attacks are common hallmarks of disease: hyperuricemia with deposition of monosodium urate (MSU) crystals in synovial fluid *Treatment:* Reduce intake of red meats and alcohol Treat underexcretors with uricosuric agents (e.g., probenecid), and treat overproducers with allopurinol (blocks xanthine oxidase) Untreated, MSU accumulates in soft tissue (tophus)
Lesch-Nyhan syndrome (X-linked recessive)	Due to total deficiency of HGPRT, the salvage enzyme for hypoxanthine and guanine Loss of the enzyme results in conversion of hypoxanthine and guanine into xanthine, which is converted into uric acid, leading to hyperuricemia	Severe mental retardation, self-mutilating behavior, spasticity, gout, and urate deposition in the kidney, leading to renal failure

Gout: hyperuricemia due to overproduction or underexcretion of uric acid

Lesch-Nyhan syndrome: deficiency of HGPRT; hyperuricemia with mental retardation

Pyrimidine degradation: end product is urea

(2) Underexcretion or overproduction of uric acid may produce gout (see Table 8-5).

3. Hypoxanthine-guanine phosphoribosyl transferase (HGPRT) is involved in the salvage of the purines hypoxanthine and guanine.

  a. Step 8: Hypoxanthine and guanine are converted into IMP and GMP, respectively, utilizing PRPP as the source of ribose 5-phosphate (see Fig. 8-12).

  b. Deficiency of HGPRT is associated with Lesch-Nyhan syndrome (see Table 8-5).

4. Step 9: Adenine is salvaged with the enzyme adenine phosphoribosyl transferase (APRT), which converts adenine into AMP, utilizing PRPP as the source of ribose 5-phosphate.

F. Pyrimidine nucleotides are degraded to CO_2, NH_4^+, and β-amino acids.

  • NH_4^+ is metabolized in the urea cycle; therefore, the end-product of pyrimidine degradation is urea.

9 CHAPTER

Integration of Metabolism

TARGET TOPICS

- Summary of allosteric effectors and hormonal control of key regulatory enzymes in primary metabolic pathways
- Factors that influence release of insulin, glucagon, and epinephrine
- Metabolic adaptations and tissue interactions in well-fed, fasting, and starvation states
- Comparison of type 1 and type 2 diabetes mellitus
- Comparison of metabolic changes in untreated type 1 diabetes and starvation
- Hepatic metabolism of alcohol and its metabolic consequences; fetal alcohol syndrome

I. Hormonal Regulation of Metabolism
   A. Introduction
      1. Hormones act by triggering intracellular signaling pathways leading to coordinated activation and/or deactivation of key enzymes (usually by phosphorylation or dephosphorylation), induction and/or repression of enzyme synthesis, or both.
      2. Three hormones—insulin, glucagon, and epinephrine—play a critical role in integrating metabolism, especially energy metabolism, in different tissues (Table 9-1).
         - Allosteric effectors, molecules that bind at a site other than the active site and activate or inhibit particular enzymes, are also important in regulation of metabolic pathways (see Table 9-1).
      3. Insulin and glucagon are the key hormones in the short-term regulation of blood glucose concentration under normal physiologic conditions.
         a. Insulin acts to reduce blood glucose (hypoglycemic effect).
         b. Glucagon acts to increase blood glucose (hyperglycemic effect).
   B. Insulin is synthesized by pancreatic β cells as an inactive precursor, proinsulin.
      1. Proteolytic cleavage of proinsulin yields C-peptide and active insulin, consisting of disulfide-linked A and B chains.
      2. Secretion of insulin is regulated by circulating substrates and hormones.

> Insulin causes enzyme dephosphorylation; glucagon causes enzyme phosphorylation.

TABLE 9-1:
Allosteric and Hormonal Regulation of Metabolic Pathways

Metabolic Pathway	Major Regulatory Enzyme(s)	Allosteric Effectors*	Hormonal Effects†
Glycolysis and pyruvate oxidation	Hexokinase	Glucose 6-P (−)	—
	Glucokinase (liver)	—	Induced by insulin
	Phosphofructokinase 1	Fructose 2,6-BP, AMP (+); citrate (−)	Glucagon (↓) via decrease in fructose 2,6-BP
	Pyruvate kinase	Fructose 1,6-BP (+); ATP, alanine (−)	Glucagon (↓)
	Pyruvate dehydrogenase	ADP (+); acetyl CoA, NADH, ATP (−)	Insulin (↑)
Citric acid cycle	Isocitrate dehydrogenase	ADP (+); ATP, NADH (−)	—
Glycogenesis	Glycogen synthase	Glucose 6-P (+)	Insulin (↑); glucagons in liver, epinephrine in muscle (↓) Induced by insulin
Glycogenolysis	Glycogen phosphorylase	Ca²⁺ (+) in muscle	Glucagon in liver, epinephrine in muscle (↑)
Gluconeogenesis	Fructose-1,6-bisphosphatase	Citrate (+); fructose 2,6-BP, AMP (−)	Glucagon (↑) via decrease in fructose 2,6-BP
	PEP carboxykinase	—	
	Pyruvate carboxylase	Acetyl CoA (+)	All three enzymes induced by glucagon and cortisol; repressed by insulin
Pentose phosphate pathway	Glucose-6-phosphate dehydrogenase (G6PD)	NADPH (−)	
Fatty acid synthesis	Acetyl CoA carboxylase	Citrate (+); palmitate (−)	Insulin (↑); glucagons (↓) Induced by insulin
Lipolysis	Hormone-sensitive lipase	—	Epinephrine (↑); insulin (↓)
β-Oxidation of fatty acids	Carnitine acyltransferase	Malonyl CoA (−)	—
Cholesterol synthesis	HMG CoA reductase	Cholesterol (−)	Insulin (↑); glucagons (↓)
Urea cycle	Carbamoyl phosphate synthetase I (CPS I)	N-Acetylglutamate (+)	—
Pyrimidine synthesis	Carbamoyl phosphate synthetase II (CPS II)	PRPP, ATP (+); UTP (−)	—
Purine synthesis	PRPP amidotransferase	PRPP (+); IMP, AMP, GMP (−)	—
Heme synthesis	ALA synthase	Enzyme synthesis repressed by heme	—

*Stimulates (+) or inhibits (−) enzyme activity.
†Promotes formation of active form (↑) or inactive form (↓) of enzyme via phosphorylation/dephosphorylation.

    a. Stimulated by increased blood glucose (most important), increased individual amino acids (e.g., arginine and leucine), and gastrointestinal hormones (e.g., gastric inhibitory peptide), which are released after ingestion of food

    b. Inhibited by somatostatin and low glucose

3. Metabolic actions of insulin are most pronounced in liver, muscle, and adipose tissue.
   - Overall effect is to promote storage of excess glucose as glycogen in liver and muscle and as triacylglycerols in adipose tissue.

4. Insulin receptor is a tetramer whose cytosolic domain has tyrosine kinase activity for generating second messengers (see Chapter 3).

    a. Insulin binding triggers signaling pathways that produce several cellular responses (post-receptor functions).

    b. Increased adipose tissue downregulates insulin receptor synthesis, whereas weight loss upregulates receptor synthesis.

    c. Increased glucose uptake by muscle and adipose tissue is due to translocation of GLUT4 receptors to cell surface.

    d. Activation of energy-storage enzymes (e.g., glycogen synthase) and inactivation of energy-mobilizing enzymes (e.g., glycogen phosphorylase) are due to dephosphorylation of these enzymes.

    e. Increased enzyme synthesis (e.g., glucokinase and phosphofructokinase) is due to activation of gene transcription.

C. Glucagon and epinephrine function to prevent fasting hypoglycemia.

1. Secretion of glucagon from pancreatic α cells is regulated by circulating substrates and hormones.

    a. Stimulated by decreased blood glucose, increased amino acids, and increased epinephrine

    b. Inhibited by insulin

2. Secretion of epinephrine from the adrenal medulla is triggered by release of acetylcholine from preganglionic sympathetic nerves in response to stress, prolonged exercise, or trauma.

3. Metabolic actions of glucagon and epinephrine reinforce each other and counteract insulin action.

    a. Glucagon acts primarily on the liver to promote glycogenolysis and gluconeogenesis.

    b. Epinephrine stimulates glycogenolysis in muscle and the liver and the release of free fatty acids (lipolysis) in adipose tissue.

4. Glucagon and epinephrine receptors are both coupled to stimulatory G protein (see Chapter 3).

    a. Hormone binding activates adenylate cyclase, leading to an increase in cAMP, which activates protein kinase A.

    b. Subsequent phosphorylation by protein kinase A results in activation of energy-mobilizing enzymes (e.g., glycogen phosphorylase and hormone-sensitive lipase) and inactivation of energy-storage enzymes (e.g., glycogen synthase and acetyl CoA carboxylase in fatty acid synthesis).

> Epinephrine inhibits insulin release, promotes glucagon release, and supplements the hyperglycemic effect of glucagon.

TABLE 9-2:
Comparison of the Well-Fed, Fasting, and Starvation States

Process	Well-Fed State	Fasting State	Starvation State
Glycogenesis	Increased	None	None
Glycogenolysis	Decreased; none in the liver, some in muscle	Increased; early supply of glucose derived from liver, not muscle	None; glycogen depleted
Gluconeogenesis	None	Increased; primary source of glucose after glycogenolysis	Decreased; just enough to supply RBCs
Triacylglycerol synthesis in liver, adipose tissue	Increased	None	None
Lipolysis	None	Increased	Increased
Fate of glycerol	Synthesize more triacylglycerol in liver	Substrate for gluconeogenesis	Substrate for gluconeogenesis
β-Oxidation of fatty acids	None	Increased	Markedly increased; primary fuel for muscle
Muscle catabolism	None; increased protein synthesis and uptake of amino acids	Increased; supply amino acids for gluconeogenesis	Decreased; conserve muscle for important body functions
Urea synthesis, excretion	Remains constant; handles NH_4^+ load from protein degradation in gut by bacteria	Increased; deamination of amino acids used for gluconeogenesis increases urea synthesis	Decreased; less muscle breakdown of protein with fewer amino acids to degrade
Ketone body synthesis	None	Increased	Markedly increased; by-product of acetyl CoA from increased β-oxidation of fatty acids
Muscle use of glucose for fuel	Primary fuel	Decreased	None; mainly uses fatty acids
Muscle use of fatty acids for fuel	None	Increased; primary fuel	Markedly increased; primary fuel
Muscle use of ketones for fuel	None	Some; alternative fuel	None; allows the brain to use ketones for fuel
Brain use of glucose for fuel	Remains constant	Remains constant	Decreased; allows RBCs to primarily use glucose for fuel
Brain use of ketones for fuel	None	None	Increased; primary fuel
RBC use of glucose for fuel	Remains constant	Remains constant	Remains constant

II. The Well-Fed State
   A. Introduction
      1. The metabolic activity of various tissues interacts in order to store energy
         when ingested fuel is plentiful (well-fed state) and to draw on energy
         stores to maintain blood glucose during fasting or starvation.
      2. The period from approximately 1 to 3 hours after ingestion of a normal
         meal is marked by a high insulin:glucagon ratio and elevated blood
         glucose due to circulating absorbed dietary glucose (Table 9-2).
   B. Liver metabolism in the well-fed state (Fig. 9-1)
      1. Following a meal, the hepatic portal vein delivers venous blood containing
         absorbed nutrients (with the exception of long-chain fatty acids) and
         elevated levels of insulin directly to the liver.

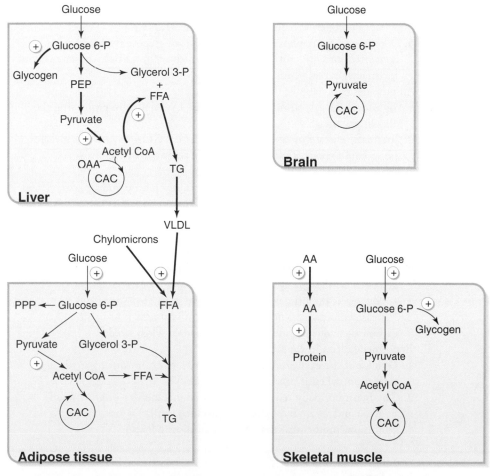

9-1: Overview of metabolism in the well-fed state. Thick arrows indicate pathways that are prominent; +
indicates steps that insulin directly or indirectly promotes. AA, amino acid; CAC, citric acid cycle; FFA, free
fatty acid; OAA, oxaloacetic acid; PEP, phosphoenolpyruvate; PPP, pentose phosphate pathway; TG,
triacylglycerol; VLDL, very low-density lipoprotein.

2. Glucokinase traps most of the large glucose influx from the portal vein as glucose 6-phosphate.
   a. In contrast to hexokinase, which is present in most tissues, liver glucokinase is active only at high glucose concentrations but is not inhibited by glucose 6-phosphate (see Table 6-1).
   b. Elevated glucose 6-phosphate immediately stimulates the less active phosphorylated form of glycogen synthase, which in turn increases glycogen synthesis.
3. Active (dephosphorylated) forms of glycogen synthase and pyruvate dehydrogenase are favored by a high insulin:glucagon ratio.
   • Increased pyruvate dehydrogenase activity provides abundant acetyl CoA for synthesis of free fatty acids, which are esterified as triacylglycerols in hepatocytes and transported to adipose tissue (as VLDLs) for synthesis of triacylglycerol for storage.
4. The oxidative branch of the pentose phosphate pathway provides NADPH, which is required for fatty acid synthesis.
5. Dihydroxyacetone phosphate produced from glucose 6-phosphate is converted into glycerol 3-phosphate, which is the carbohydrate backbone for triacylglycerol synthesis.

C. Adipose tissue metabolism in the well-fed state
   • High insulin levels stimulate triacylglycerol synthesis by promoting the following actions.
   1. Increased glucose uptake by insulin-sensitive GLUT4 provides glycerol 3-phosphate for esterification of free fatty acids and synthesis of triacylglycerol.
   2. Increased lipoprotein lipase activity promotes release and uptake of free fatty acids from chylomicrons and VLDL.
   3. Inhibition of hormone-sensitive lipase by insulin prevents fat mobilization.

D. Muscle metabolism in the well-fed state
   • High insulin:glucagon ratio promotes the following actions.
   1. Increased glucose uptake by insulin-sensitive GLUT4 and activation of glycogen synthase lead to the formation of glycogen.
      • Glucose is the primary fuel for muscle in the fed state.
   2. Increased amino acid uptake and protein synthesis lead to storage of carbon skeletons for use as an energy source when needed.

E. Brain metabolism in the well-fed state
   1. Glucose is the exclusive fuel for brain tissue, except during extreme starvation, when it can use ketone bodies.
   2. The brain normally relies on the aerobic metabolism of glucose, so hypoxia and severe hypoglycemia produce similar symptoms (e.g., confusion, motor weakness, and visual disturbances).

III. The Fasting State
   A. Introduction
      1. The period extending from 3 or 4 hours to 32 to 36 hours after a meal is marked by decreasing levels of absorbed nutrients in the bloodstream and a declining insulin:glucagon ratio.

High insulin levels (fed): ingested fuels stored as glycogen (liver, muscle), triacylglycerols (adipose, liver), and protein (muscle)

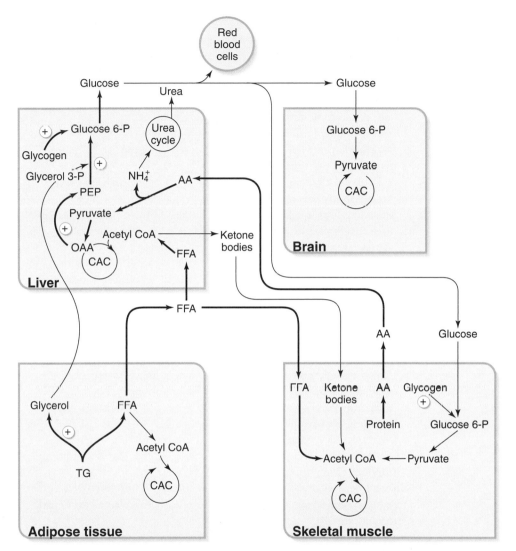

9-2: *Overview of metabolism in the fasting state. Thick arrows indicate pathways that are prominent; +
indicates steps that are promoted directly or indirectly by glucagon in the liver and epinephrine in adipose
tissue and muscle. Some glucogenic amino acids (AA) are converted to citric acid cycle (CAC) intermediates
in the liver. FFA, free fatty acid; PEP, phosphoenolpyruvate; TG, triacylglycerol.*

2. Metabolism initially shifts to increasing reliance on glycogenolysis and
   then to gluconeogenesis to maintain blood glucose in the absence of
   nutrient absorption from the gut (see Table 9-2).

B. Liver metabolism in the fasting state (Fig. 9-2)

1. Glucose 6-phosphatase, a gluconeogenic enzyme that is present in liver but
   not in muscle, allows glucose from glycogenolysis and gluconeogenesis to
   be released in blood.
   • Glucose 6-phosphatase converts glucose 6-phosphate to glucose.

Glucose-6-phosphatase:
located in liver, a blood
sugar-regulating organ,
not in muscle, a glucose-
consuming tissue

2. Glycogen degradation (glycogenolysis) is stimulated by glucagon-induced activation of glycogen phosphorylase and inhibition of glycogen synthase, which prevents futile recycling of glucose 1-phosphate.

3. Gluconeogenesis is stimulated by glucagon via several mechanisms.
   a. Reduction in fructose 2,6-bisphosphate concentration relieves inhibition of fructose 1,6-bisphosphatase (rate-limiting enzyme) and reduces activation of phosphofructokinase 1.
      - Net result = ↑ gluconeogenesis, ↓ glycolysis
   b. Inactivation of pyruvate kinase (via protein kinase A) reduces futile recycling of phosphoenolpyruvate.
      - Pyruvate kinase is also allosterically inhibited by high ATP and alanine.
   c. Increased liver uptake of amino acids (derived from protein catabolism in skeletal muscle) provides carbon skeletons for gluconeogenesis (e.g., alanine is transaminated into pyruvate).
   d. Increased synthesis of urea cycle enzymes removes NH_4^+ resulting from deamination of amino acids and increases the excretion of urea in the urine.

4. Hepatic oxidation of free fatty acids (derived from lipolysis in adipose tissue) elevates the concentration of ATP, acetyl CoA, and citrate.
   a. Citrate allosterically stimulates fructose 1,6-bisphosphatase (↑ gluconeogenesis) and inhibits phosphofructokinase 1 (↓ glycolysis).
   b. Acetyl CoA activates pyruvate carboxylase, which converts pyruvate to oxaloacetate for use in the gluconeogenic pathway.
   c. Inhibition of pyruvate dehydrogenase by acetyl CoA also increases shunting of pyruvate toward oxaloacetate.
   d. Increased ATP concentration resulting from oxidation of fatty acid-derived acetyl CoA in the citric acid cycle inhibits glycolysis and supplies energy for gluconeogenesis.

5. Glycerol derived from lipolysis in adipose tissue is phosphorylated in the liver by glycerol kinase and also contributes carbon skeletons for hepatic gluconeogenesis.

6. Some ketogenesis occurs in the liver, with ketone bodies primarily transported to muscle as an alternative fuel.

C. Adipose tissue metabolism in the fasting state
   1. Low insulin levels and epinephrine promote the active form of hormone-sensitive lipase, which splits triacylglycerols into glycerol and free fatty acids.
   2. Free fatty acids are transported in blood bound to serum albumin.
      - Liver and muscle use the free fatty acids released via β-oxidation in the mitochondria as the primary energy source during fasting.
   3. Glycerol is converted into glycerol 3-phosphate in the liver and is used as a substrate for gluconeogenesis.

D. Muscle metabolism in the fasting state
   1. Degradation of muscle protein provides carbon skeletons for hepatic gluconeogenesis.
      a. Most amino acids released from muscle protein are transported directly to the liver, where they are transaminated and converted to glucose.

Low insulin levels (fasting): stored fuels mobilized from glycogen (liver, muscle), fat (adipose), and protein (muscle); adequate blood glucose maintained for brain

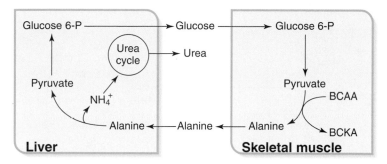

9-3: *Alanine cycle for disposing of nitrogen from branched-chain amino acids (BCAA). In contrast to other amino acids, the three BCAA (isoleucine, leucine, and valine) are metabolized to alanine and branched-chain keto acids (BCKA) in skeletal muscle (not the liver, which lacks the necessary enzymes). Glucose produced in the liver is returned to muscle to regenerate the pyruvate supply for transamination of more BCAA, resulting in no net production of glucose for use by other tissues.*

      b. Branched-chain amino acids (isoleucine, leucine, and valine), however, are converted to their α-keto acids in muscle by transamination of pyruvate, yielding alanine, which is transported to the liver.
- The alanine cycle, which disposes of nitrogen from branched-chain amino acids, results in no net production of glucose for use by other tissues (Fig. 9-3).

  2. Free fatty acids are the primary fuel source for muscle during fasting.

  3. Glycogen degradation can provide glucose as fuel for muscle for short periods of exertion.
- Skeletal muscle lacks glucose 6-phosphatase; therefore, degradation of muscle glycogen cannot contribute to blood glucose.

E. Brain metabolism in the fasting state
- Brain tissue continues to use glucose as an energy source during periods of fasting, depending on hepatic glycogenolysis and gluconeogenesis to maintain blood glucose.

IV. The Starvation State

A. Introduction

  1. After 3 to 5 days of fasting, increasing reliance on fatty acids and ketone bodies for fuel enables the body to maintain blood glucose at 60 to 65 mg/dL and to spare muscle protein for prolonged periods without food (see Table 9-2).

  2. Less NH_4^+ is produced; therefore, less urea is excreted in the urine.

B. Liver metabolism in the starvation state (Fig. 9-4)

  1. The rate of gluconeogenesis decreases as the supply of amino acid carbon skeletons from muscle protein catabolism decreases.
- Glycerol released by lipolysis in adipose tissue supports a low level of gluconeogenesis in the liver, which is the only tissue that contains glycerol kinase:

      Glycerol → Glycerol 3-P → DHAP →→→ Glucose

Fatty acids are the primary source of fuel for muscle in the fasting state.

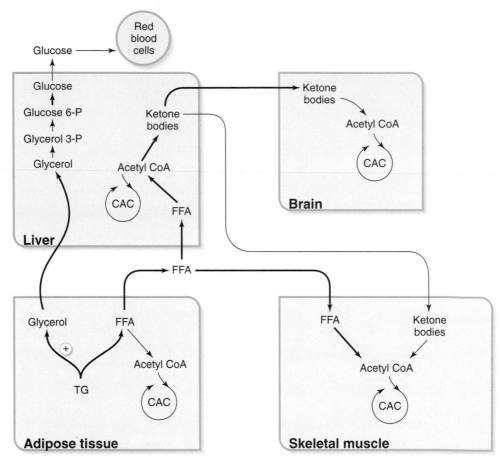

9-4: *Overview of metabolism in the starvation state. As starvation persists, the use of ketone bodies by skeletal muscle decreases, sparing this fuel source for brain tissue.*

2. Fatty acid oxidation continues at a high level.
3. Acetyl CoA accumulates as the citric acid cycle slows down.
   a. Elevated acetyl CoA is shunted to produce ketone bodies, which consist of acetoacetate, β-hydroxybutyrate, and acetone.
   b. Ketoacidosis resulting from increased hepatic production of ketone bodies is the hallmark of starvation.
      (1) Acetoacetate and β-hydroxybutyrate are metabolized to acetyl CoA and used for energy production by many tissues (e.g., muscle, brain, and kidney) but not by the red blood cells (RBCs) or the liver.
      (2) Acetone, which is not metabolized, gives a fruity odor to the breath.
C. Adipose tissue metabolism in the starvation state
   • The elevated epinephrine level caused by the stress of starvation coupled with very reduced levels of insulin increases the activity of hormone-

Starvation: fatty acids and ketone bodies supply the energy needs of all tissues except RBCs and liver

TABLE 9-3:

Comparison of Type 1 and Type 2 Diabetes Mellitus

Characteristic	Type 1	Type 2
Proportion of diagnosed diabetics	5–10%	90–95%
Usual time of onset (exceptions are common)	Childhood, adolescence, early adulthood	Older than age 40 (frequently associated with obesity)
Cause	Gradual elimination of insulin production due to autoimmune destruction of β cells; HLA relationship	Relative insulin deficiency; insulin resistance of target tissues due to decreased insulin receptors, postreceptor defects (e.g., tyrosine kinase defects); no HLA relationship
Plasma insulin (basal)	Absent	Normal to high
Metabolic disorders	Hyperglycemia, ketoacidosis, hypertriglyceridemia, muscle wasting	Hyperglycemia, hyperosmolarity; no ketosis
Symptoms	Rapid onset of polydipsia, polyuria, polyphagia	Insidious onset
Insulin therapy	Always necessary	May be necessary; diet, exercise, and oral glucose-lowering agents used primarily
Long-term complications	Atherosclerosis, microvascular disease, peripheral neuropathy, retinopathy, nephropathy	Similar to type 1, but slower onset

sensitive lipase, which further stimulates the mobilization of fatty acids from stored fat.

D. Muscle metabolism in the starvation state

1. Degradation of muscle protein decreases as the demand for blood glucose is reduced due to a reduction in gluconeogenesis.
2. Both free fatty acids and ketone bodies are used as energy sources in early starvation.
3. As starvation persists, muscle relies increasingly on free fatty acids, sparing ketone bodies for use by the brain.

E. Brain metabolism in the starvation state

1. Increasing ketone body use by the brain spares blood glucose for use by RBCs, which rely solely on glucose for energy production.
2. Decreasing glucose use by the brain reduces the need for hepatic gluconeogenesis and thus indirectly spares muscle protein.

Key metabolic adaptations to starvation: sparing of muscle protein, shift to fat as primary fuel source

V. Diabetes Mellitus

• Hyperglycemia and similar long-term complications occur in both type 1 and type 2 diabetes mellitus (DM), but the two conditions differ in their underlying cause, acute manifestations, and treatment (Table 9-3).

A. Type 1 DM (formerly called insulin-dependent diabetes mellitus)

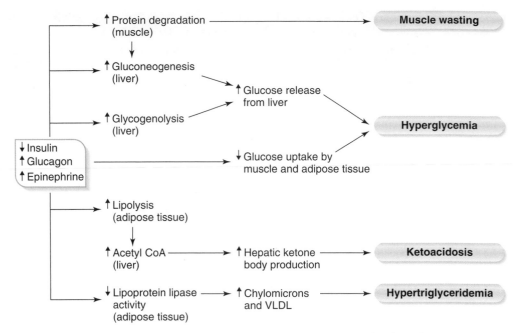

9-5: *Mechanisms of metabolic changes in untreated type 1 DM. VLDL, very low-density lipoprotein.*

1. Type 1 DM is caused by autoimmune destruction of pancreatic β cells.
   a. Total absence of endogenous insulin production eventually results, accompanied by onset of clinical symptoms.
   b. Human leukocyte antigen (HLA) genes are involved in the autoimmune destruction of β cells.
2. Polydipsia, polyuria, and polyphagia—the classic triad of presenting symptoms—are usually accompanied by weight loss, fatigue, and weakness.
3. Metabolic changes in untreated type 1 DM resemble, but are distinct from, those in starvation and lead to four characteristic metabolic abnormalities (Fig. 9-5).
   a. Muscle wasting results from exaggerated degradation of muscle protein.
      (1) Lack of insulin reduces uptake of amino acids and protein synthesis by muscle but promotes protein degradation.
         • Released amino acids are used for muscle energy production (along with free fatty acids from adipose tissue) and also are transported to the liver for gluconeogenesis.
      (2) During starvation, muscle protein is spared.
   b. Hyperglycemia is caused by increased hepatic glucose production and reduced glucose uptake by insulin-sensitive GLUT4 in adipose tissue and muscle.
      (1) Very low insulin : glucagon ratio causes increased gluconeogenesis (most important) and increased glycogenolysis in the liver despite high blood glucose.

   (2) Osmotic diuresis from glucosuria results in hypovolemic shock due to significant losses of sodium in the urine.

   (3) During starvation, blood glucose is usually maintained near the lower end of the normal range due to decreased gluconeogenesis.

   c. Ketoacidosis results from excessive mobilization of fatty acids (lipolysis) from adipose tissue.

   (1) Elevated acetyl CoA resulting from β-oxidation of fatty acids in the liver leads to accelerated ketone body production, which is much greater than in starvation.

   (2) Because blood glucose is high, brain tissue uses glucose instead of ketone bodies (as in starvation), which contributes to ketoacidosis.

   d. Hypertriglyceridemia is caused by reduced lipoprotein lipase activity in adipose tissue and excessive fatty acid esterification in the liver.

   • Reduced lipoprotein lipase activity in adipose tissue, due to lack of insulin, leads to elevated plasma levels of both chylomicrons from ingested fats and VLDL from hepatic triacylglycerol production, which often results in a type V hyperlipoproteinemia (see Table 7-3).

4. Insulin therapy reduces clinical symptoms of type 1 DM and alleviates life-threatening ketoacidosis.

   a. Successful treatment of type 1 DM also reduces the risk of long-term complications, which are thought to result primarily from prolonged hyperglycemia.

   b. Glucose-related damage is due primarily to two mechanisms.

   (1) Intracellular nonenzymatic glycosylation (glucose covalently linked to protein) of the basement membranes of arterioles and capillaries

   (2) Osmotic damage due to glucose conversion into sorbitol by aldose reductase

   c. The most common complications of insulin therapy are hypoglycemia and subsequent insulin coma due to excess insulin.

B. Type 2 (formerly called non-insulin-dependent diabetes mellitus)

1. Type 2 DM results from dysfunctional pancreatic β cells (relative insulin deficiency) and insulin resistance (reduced responsiveness of target tissues to insulin at the receptor and post-receptor level), which is associated with obesity.

   • Obesity leads to downregulation of insulin receptor synthesis.

2. Basal insulin level is normal to high, but insulin release in response to glucose is insufficient to prevent hyperglycemia.

3. Metabolic changes in untreated type 2 DM are generally milder than in type 1 DM, partly because the imbalance in insulin and glucagon levels is not as extreme.

   • Ketoacidosis does not occur, but hyperglycemia may be greater than in type 1 DM (hyperosmolar nonketotic coma).

4. Weight loss (upregulates insulin receptor synthesis), exercise, and dietary modifications can adequately control blood glucose in some type 2 diabetics.

5. In more difficult cases, insulin therapy or an oral hypoglycemic agent is necessary to reduce hyperglycemia.

Type 1 DM: absolute insulin deficiency, autoimmune destruction of pancreatic β cells, hyperglycemia, ketoacidosis

Type 2 DM: relative insulin deficiency, insulin resistance, postreceptor defects, hyperglycemia, no ketosis, obesity

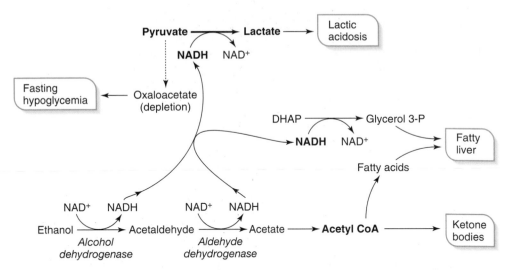

9-6: *Consequences of ethanol metabolism in the liver. Reduction in the pyruvate level as it is converted to lactate and depletion of oxaloacetate eventually lead to fasting hypoglycemia. The higher NADH : NAD$^+$ ratio also increases the conversion of dihydroxyacetone phosphate (DHAP) to glycerol 3-phosphate, leading to increased synthesis of triacylglycerol.*

VI. Alcohol Metabolism
- Metabolism of alcohol occurs primarily in the liver via two pathways, depending on the ethanol concentration.
- A. At low concentrations of ethanol, oxidation by two dehydrogenases results in an increased NADH : NAD$^+$ ratio (Fig. 9-6).
    1. Both alcohol dehydrogenase in the cytosol and aldehyde dehydrogenase in mitochondria transfer electrons to NAD$^+$ to form NADH.
        - Disulfiram, which inhibits aldehyde dehydrogenase and is used in the treatment of chronic alcoholism, causes severe perspiration, abdominal cramping, and nausea following ingestion of alcohol.
    2. Lactic acidosis results from shunting of pyruvate into lactate due to a high NADH : NAD$^+$ ratio.
    3. Fasting hypoglycemia results from depletion of pyruvate, which leads to reduced gluconeogenesis.
        - Alcohol-induced hypoglycemia most likely occurs in individuals who have not eaten recently. In this situation, liver glycogen stores are depleted and maintenance of blood glucose depends entirely on gluconeogenesis.
    4. Fatty liver in alcoholics is a consequence of prolonged imbalance in the NADH : NAD$^+$ ratio.
        a. High NADH promotes increased formation of glycerol 3-phosphate from dihydroxyacetone phosphate, which is esterified to yield triacylglycerols.
        b. Reduction in the citric acid cycle leads to shunting of acetyl CoA and to increased fatty acid synthesis.

Ethanol metabolism in liver: high NADH levels lead to lactic acidosis and hypoglycemia

    c. Impaired protein synthesis prevents assembly and secretion of VLDL, causing triacylglycerols to accumulate in the liver.

  5. Ketone bodies are produced by increased shunting of acetyl CoA from the citric acid cycle.

B. At higher concentrations of ethanol, cytochrome P450 enzymes in the smooth endoplasmic reticulum (SER), which have a relatively high K_m for ethanol, are active:

$$\text{Ethanol} + NADPH + O_2 \rightarrow \text{acetaldehyde} + NADP^+ + H_2O$$

  1. This microsomal-ethanol oxidizing system also detoxifies drugs such as barbiturates.

    • Alcohol causes the SER in liver cells to increase, which results in an increased synthesis of γ-glutamyltransferase, an enzyme located in the SER that is an excellent marker of alcohol ingestion.

  2. Ethanol oxidation by the microsomal-ethanol oxidizing system does not affect the $NADH : NAD^+$ ratio substantially and thus does not have the metabolic effects described for low concentrations of ethanol.

Gene Expression

I. Nucleic Acids: Structure and Functions
- Both DNA and RNA are polynucleotides in which the nucleotide monomers are linked by $5' \rightarrow 3'$ phosphodiester bonds between the pentose units, creating a sugar-phosphate backbone (see Chapter 8).

DNA: helix composed of two strands that are antiparallel and complementary

A. DNA, composed of deoxyribonucleotides, is a double-strand helix in which the strands are antiparallel (run in opposite directions) and complementary (adenine in one strand bonds with thymine in the other strand, and guanine bonds with cytosine) (Fig. 10-1).
1. Hydrogen bonding between bases in different strands and hydrophobic interactions between stacked, adjacent bases in the same strand stabilize the DNA double helix.
2. Chromatin is a complex of double-strand DNA associated with histone proteins and other proteins that folds and packs to form the chromosomes.
a. Histones are basic proteins (positively charged) that associate tightly with acidic DNA (negatively charged).

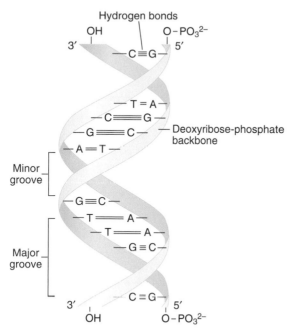

Hydrogen bonds

10-1: DNA double helix. Strands are complementary (A is always paired with T, and G with C) and antiparallel (one strand runs in the 3′ → 5′ direction and the other in the 5′ → 3′). Note that adenine-thymine (A-T) pairs have two hydrogen bonds; guanine-cytosine (G-C) pairs have three hydrogen bonds.

    b. The nucleosome, the basic structural unit of chromatin, is made up of a core containing a total of eight histones (two molecules each of histones H2A, H2B, H3, and H4), around which DNA is wrapped twice (Fig. 10-2).

    c. Linker DNA, which is associated with a fifth type of histone, histone H1, connects adjacent nucleosomes and forms the "beads on a string" form of chromatin.

    d. Supercoiling, mediated by histone H1, produces the more compact 30-nm chromatin fiber.

    e. Higher order coiling and folding of chromatin permits compaction of DNA into chromosomes.

      • Fluoroquinolone antibiotics such as ciprofloxacin, which block DNA compaction by inhibiting bacterial DNA gyrase (topoisomerase II), have little effect on the equivalent human enzyme.

  3. A gene represents a discrete region of DNA that is required for production of a functional RNA.

    • A gene contains a coding region and regulatory sequences, which may be located a substantial distance away from the coding region and contain noncoding intervening sequences.

B. RNA, composed of ribonucleotides, is a single-strand molecule that may contain internal base-paired regions, forming stem loops.

  • The three major types of RNA have specific functions in protein synthesis.

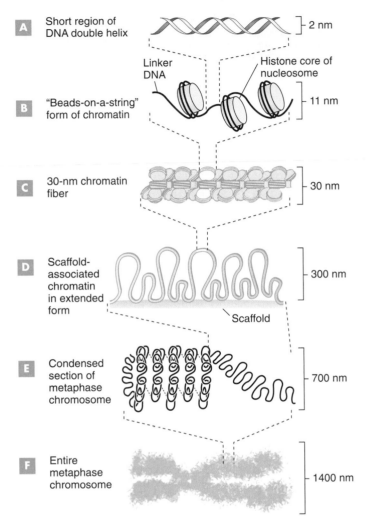

A. Short region of DNA double helix — 2 nm

B. "Beads-on-a-string" form of chromatin — 11 nm
Linker DNA
Histone core of nucleosome

C. 30-nm chromatin fiber — 30 nm

D. Scaffold-associated chromatin in extended form — 300 nm
Scaffold

E. Condensed section of metaphase chromosome — 700 nm

F. Entire metaphase chromosome — 1400 nm

10-2: *Schematic model depicting the organization of human DNA.* **A** *and* **B,** *Double-strand DNA wraps around histone cores to form nucleosomes, which are connected by intervening linker DNA to which another histone is bound.* **C,** *Supercoiling produces a more compact 30-nm chromatin fiber.* **D,** *In interphase chromosomes, long stretches of 30-nm chromatin loop out from a protein scaffold.* **E** *and* **F,** *Further folding of the scaffold yields the highly condensed structure of a metaphase chromosome.*

RNAs: mRNAs are the blueprints for protein synthesis; tRNAs transport amino acids; rRNAs form the ribosomes where proteins are synthesized

1. Messenger RNAs (mRNAs) provide the blueprint for assembly of amino acids into proteins; mRNA is approximately 5% of the total RNA.
2. Transfer RNAs (tRNAs) play an adaptor role in protein synthesis, carrying amino acids to the ribosomes for incorporation into growing protein chains; tRNA is approximately 15% of the total RNA.
3. Ribosomal RNAs (rRNAs) self-assemble with basic proteins to form ribosomes, the small ribonucleoprotein particles on which protein synthesis occurs; rRNA is approximately 80% of the total RNA.

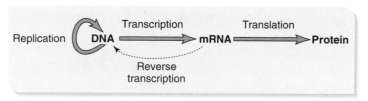

10-3: *Central dogma of the flow of information in the cell.*

C. The flow of genetic information is described by the central dogma (Fig. 10-3)
   1. Replication: DNA is replicated in dividing cells.
   2. Transcription: one strand of DNA serves as a template for synthesis of a complementary RNA strand.
      • Reverse transcription occurs in retroviruses and is the only known exception to the DNA → RNA → protein flow of information.
   3. Translation: a ribosome-mediated process in which the nucleotide sequence of mRNA is converted into the amino acid sequence of a protein according to the genetic code.
D. The genetic code is a triplet code in which sequences (codons) made up of three nucleotides specify amino acids, as well as start and stop commands. The code has the following general features:
   1. Nonoverlapping and commaless: codons are contiguous, and no nucleotide sequences represent spacers (exceptions are some viruses).
   2. Unambiguous: each codon corresponds to only one amino acid.
   3. Degenerate: some amino acids are coded by more than one codon.
      • "Wobble" at the third base of the codon allows the same aminoacyl-tRNA to pair with more than one codon.
   4. Universal: the same code is used in all protein synthesis, with minor exceptions in the mitochondria and a few microorganisms and plants.

II. DNA Replication and Repair
   A. The cell cycle is an ordered sequence of events during which proliferating cells replicate their chromosomes and separate into daughter cells (Fig. 10-4).
      1. The cell cycle consists of interphase, followed by mitosis (nuclear replication) and cytokinesis (cell division).
         a. Interphase consists of a G_1 (first gap or growth) phase, an S (synthesis) phase, and a G_2 phase.
            (1) The G_1 and G_2 phases are periods of RNA and protein synthesis for general growth of organelles and mitotic structures; no DNA synthesis occurs.
               • Resting cells in the G_0 phase reenter the cell cycle early in the G_1 phase, the most variable phase of the cell cycle.
            (2) Replication of DNA occurs during the S phase of the cycle.
         b. During mitosis and cytokinesis of the M phase, replicated chromosomes align on the mitotic spindle and then segregate evenly to the daughter cells.
      2. Cell cycle control proteins regulate progression through the cell cycle.

Cell cycle: interphase, consisting of G_1, S, and G_2 phases, followed by mitosis and cytokinesis

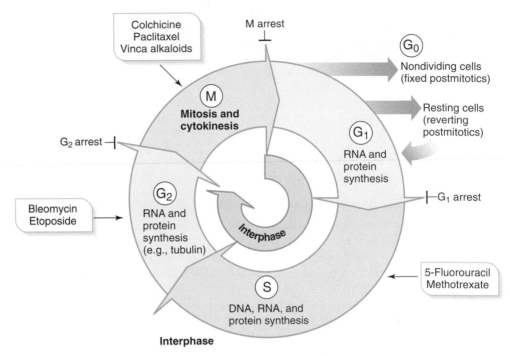

10-4: *Cell cycle in eukaryotic cells. DNA synthesis occurs only during the S (synthesis) phase; the G (gap or growth) phases are periods of growth of organelles and mitotic structures. Anticancer drugs exert their effect at different stages depending on their mode of action. Damage to DNA or improper spindle formation lead to arrest, preventing entry to the next stage.*

Cdks, activated by cyclins, regulate the progress of the cell cycle; arrests at checkpoints prevent abnormalities.

a. Cyclin-dependent protein kinases (Cdks) phosphorylate various target proteins, thereby modulating their activity at different cell cycle stages.

b. Cyclins activate Cdks by binding to them.

• Concentrations of various cyclins rise and fall throughout the cell cycle phases, leading to formation of specific cyclin-Cdk complexes that control entry into the S phase and entry into and exit from mitosis.

3. Checkpoints are points in the cell cycle where progress can be arrested to prevent formation of abnormal daughter cells (see Fig. 10-4).

a. When DNA is damaged, the G_1 checkpoint prevents entry into the S phase, and the G_2 checkpoint prevents entry into mitosis.

(1) Expression of *p53*, a tumor-suppressor gene (on chromosome 17) that is required for operation of the G_1 and G_2 checkpoints, codes for a protein product that inhibits activated Cdks.

(2) Arrest of the cell cycle allows time for DNA repair and reduces the chances for perpetuation of mutations.

(3) Inactivation of the *p53* suppressor gene is seen in most human cancers.

b. The M checkpoint prevents exit from mitosis when the spindle is abnormal, thereby preventing missegregation of chromatids and

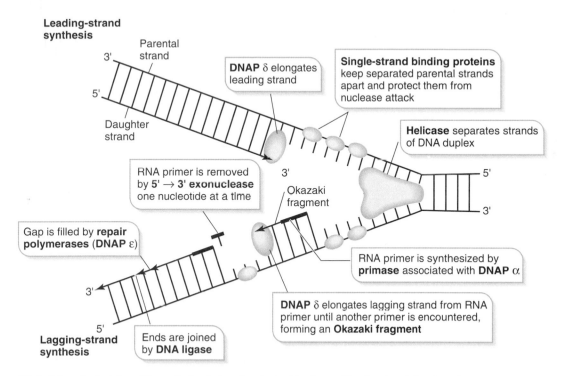

Leading-strand synthesis

Parental strand

3'

5'

Daughter strand

DNAP δ elongates leading strand

Single-strand binding proteins keep separated parental strands apart and protect them from nuclease attack

Helicase separates strands of DNA duplex

RNA primer is removed by **5' → 3' exonuclease** one nucleotide at a time

3'

Okazaki fragment

5'

3'

Gap is filled by **repair polymerases (DNAP ε)**

RNA primer is synthesized by **primase** associated with **DNAP α**

3'

DNAP δ elongates lagging strand from RNA primer until another primer is encountered, forming an **Okazaki fragment**

5'

Lagging-strand synthesis

Ends are joined by **DNA ligase**

10-5: *Schematic depiction of the replication fork and synthesis of leading and lagging strands in eukaryotic cells. Major proteins and their functions in DNA synthesis are indicated; various accessory proteins that are also required are not shown. DNAP, DNA polymerase.*

formation of daughter cells with an abnormal number of chromosomes.

B. DNA synthesis begins at specific nucleotide sequences, called replication origins, and proceeds in both directions (bidirectional).

- Replication is semiconservative; that is, each new DNA double helix contains one parental strand and one daughter strand.

1. Multiple proteins participate in initiation and elongation of daughter DNA strands at the replication fork (Fig. 10-5).

a. Helicase separates the two strands of the DNA helix, which is required for the synthesis of daughter strands; however, the unwinding causes a strain ahead of the moving fork.

b. Topoisomerase I relieves the supercoiling strain ahead of the replication fork by breaking one of the DNA strands and allowing it to rotate around the unbroken strand before rejoining the broken ends.

c. DNA polymerases catalyze the addition of deoxyribonucleoside triphosphates (dATP, dTTP, dGTP, and dCTP) to the free 3'-OH end of the growing strands with a loss of pyrophosphate (PP_i).

(1) Parental (template) strand is always read in the 3' → 5' direction.

(2) Daughter (new) strand is always synthesized in the 5' → 3' direction.

DNA polymerases always synthesize daughter strands in the 5' → 3' direction.

(3) Because of the directionality of DNA synthesis, one daughter strand is synthesized continuously (leading strand), and the other is synthesized discontinuously (lagging strand) (see Fig. 10-5).

2. Different processes are involved in the synthesis of leading and lagging strands.

 a. Leading strand synthesis, catalyzed primarily by DNA polymerase δ, proceeds continuously from a single RNA primer synthesized by DNA polymerase α.

 b. Lagging strand synthesis proceeds discontinuously from multiple RNA primers synthesized by DNA polymerase α, forming short Okazaki fragments (see Fig. 10-5).

  (1) The Okazaki fragments are extended by DNA polymerase δ, as in leading strand elongation.

  (2) Primer is removed from the fragments by a 5′→ 3′ exonuclease, and gaps are filled by DNA polymerase ε, which also functions in repair.

  (3) DNA ligase connects the ends of the adjoining fragments.

3. The proofreading activity of DNA polymerases δ and ε usually detects and corrects base-pairing errors that occur during DNA synthesis (e.g., formation of an A-C pair rather than the correct A-T pair).

 • The 3′ → 5′ exonuclease activity of the DNA polymerases removes a mismatched nucleotide, and synthesis then continues with insertion of the correct nucleotide.

C. Shortening of chromosomes during DNA replication occurs in cells that lack telomerase.

1. Dissociation of DNA polymerase from the 3′ end of the daughter strand prevents completion of the last Okazaki fragment.

 • The result is a newly synthesized DNA strand that is shortened at one end.

2. Telomerase is an enzyme that adds repeat sequences beyond the coding region to constitute the telomeric regions at the ends of chromosomes.

 a. Telomerase is a large ribonucleoprotein that has reverse transcriptase activity and contains an RNA molecule that acts as a template for synthesis of the telomeric region.

 b. Telomerase is expressed in germline cells and neoplastic cells.

Absence of telomerase in differentiated somatic cells is associated with cell aging.

3. Senescence of somatic cells, which do not express telomerase, is related to progressive shortening of chromosomes resulting from successive rounds of replication.

D. Reverse transcriptase mediates the synthesis of DNA using an RNA template.

1. HIV and other retroviruses use viral reverse transcriptase to produce a DNA copy of the viral RNA genome. Viral DNA is then integrated into the genome of the infected cell.

 a. High mutation rate in HIV and emergence of new strains are due in part to lack of proofreading activity in reverse transcriptase.

 b. Zidovudine (AZT) is a thymidine analogue that inhibits reverse transcriptase, thereby disrupting infection of cells.

       (1) AZT has a minimal effect on nuclear DNA polymerases, but the drug inhibits mitochondrial DNA replication.

       (2) Aerobic metabolism is impaired in patients treated with AZT because mitochondrial DNA encodes proteins involved in the citric acid cycle.

   2. Movement of some jumping genes, also called retrotransposons, in human cells involves reverse transcription by a cellular reverse transcriptase encoded in the genome of normal, uninfected cells.

     • Insertion of a jumping gene into an active gene causes an insertion mutation, which prevents expression of normal protein.

E. Damage to nonreplicating DNA is often repaired before initiation of the next S phase, when DNA is replicated.

   1. Exposure to radiation or certain chemicals, as well as spontaneous reactions, can damage nonreplicating DNA.

     a. Pyrimidine dimers (e.g., thymine-thymine), caused by exposure to ultraviolet (UV) light, distort the DNA helix.

       • Pyrimidine dimers are responsible for UV-induced cancers of the skin (e.g., basal cell carcinoma and squamous cell carcinoma).

     b. Deamination of cytosine to uracil (C → U) and depurination by cleavage of the bond linking A or G to deoxyribose cause base alterations.

   2. DNA repair enzymes vary depending on the specific type of damage; however, the general repair process entails the following steps:

     a. Endonucleases cleave (nick) the altered strand near the damage site.

     b. Exonucleases remove one or more nucleotides at the damage site.

     c. DNA polymerase fills in the gap using the undamaged strand as a template.

     d. DNA ligase joins the repaired segment to the remainder of the strand.

   3. Inherited defects in DNA repair enzymes increase the risk for cancer (see section VI).

F. Some antineoplastic drugs act to interrupt the cell cycle or reduce the fidelity of DNA replication, and they are most destructive to rapidly proliferating cells (see Fig. 10-4).

   1. 5-Fluorouracil (5-FU) and methotrexate are S phase-specific antimetabolites that cause reduced synthesis of dTMP and, in turn, decreased DNA replication.

   2. Bleomycin and etoposide inhibit human topoisomerase II, which normally acts in the S and G_2 phases to facilitate separation of intertwined DNA molecules during and following replication and during repair of double-strand breaks.

   3. Alkylating agents such as cyclophosphamide and nitrosoureas lead to copying errors during DNA replication and expression of abnormal proteins.

   4. Doxorubicin and dactinomycin intercalate into the DNA structure and block DNA and RNA polymerases.

   5. Vinca alkaloids (e.g., vincristine) and paclitaxel are M phase-specific agents that inhibit mitotic spindle formation and breakdown, respectively.

AZT (zidovudine) inhibits reverse transcriptase in HIV and blocks replication of mitochondrial DNA.

Pyrimidine dimers (thymine-thymine) are produced by excessive UVB light exposure and lead to skin cancer.

Certain cancer drugs block the cell cycle or reduce the accuracy of DNA replication.

III. RNA Synthesis and Processing
   A. RNA polymerase unwinds the DNA helix and transcribes the DNA template strand into RNA, beginning at the transcription start site.
      • The DNA strand complementary to the template strand is the coding, or sense, strand.
      1. The RNA chain is elongated in the $5' \rightarrow 3'$ direction by the addition of ribonucleoside triphosphates (ATP, GTP, UTP, and CTP) to the free 3'-OH end of the RNA.
      2. RNA polymerases differ in eukaryotes and prokaryotes.
         a. Eukaryotes contain three nuclear RNA polymerases, which produce different types of RNA.
            (1) RNA polymerase I produces rRNA, the most abundant type.
            (2) RNA polymerase II produces mRNA, the largest type.
            (3) RNA polymerase III produces tRNA (and other small RNAs), the smallest type.
         b. Prokaryotes (bacteria) contain a single RNA polymerase, which produces all the types of RNA.
            • Rifampin, an antibiotic used in the treatment of tuberculosis, inhibits RNA polymerase in bacteria but not in eukaryotes.
   B. mRNA synthesis in eukaryotes begins with the binding of RNA polymerase II at specific DNA sequences known as promoters.
      1. The initiation complex, containing RNA polymerase II and several basal transcription factors that bind RNA polymerase II, is assembled near the transcription start site.
         a. TATA box, a conserved promoter sequence approximately 25 bases upstream of the start site, helps orient the RNA polymerase in many eukaryotic genes.
         b. CAAT box, another conserved sequence within the promoter region, is often present approximately 70 bases upstream of the start site.
         c. CG-rich box (CG island) is the major promoter element in housekeeping genes, which encode proteins that are expressed at a low basal rate in all cells (e.g., metabolic enzymes and cytoskeleton proteins).
      2. Elongation of the RNA strand by RNA polymerase II continues until the enzyme reaches a termination signal.
      3. Primary mRNA transcript, also called hnRNA (heterogeneous nuclear RNA) or pre-mRNA, is initially produced; it contains both coding and noncoding sequences.
         a. Exons are expressed (coding) sequences within a gene, primary RNA transcript, and mRNA that code for amino acids within the protein product.
         b. Introns are intervening (noncoding) sequences within the coding region of a gene and primary transcript that do not code for amino acids in the protein product.
   C. Processing of hnRNA occurs in the nucleus, yielding functional mRNA, which is exported to the cytosol (Fig. 10-6).

Rifampin inhibits bacterial RNA polymerase but does not affect eukaryotic RNA polymerases.

Exons specify amino acids in a protein; introns carry no genetic information.

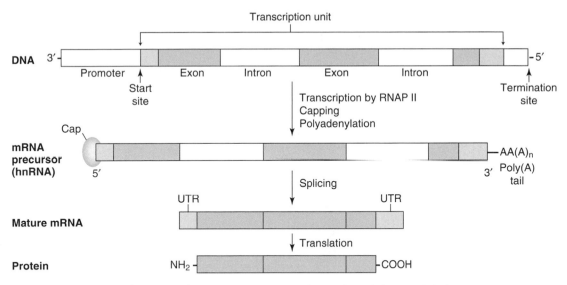

10-6: *Eukaryotic protein-coding gene and its conversion into RNA products and encoded protein. Only the template (missense) strand of DNA is depicted. Untranslated regions (UTR) at each end of a transcription unit and mRNA (gray regions) do not appear in the protein. A, adenylate; hnRNA, heterogeneous nuclear RNA; RNAP II, RNA polymerase.*

1. 7-Methylguanosine cap is added to the 5′ end of the growing mRNA before transcription is completed.
2. Cleavage and polyadenylation at the poly(A) site leads to formation of the poly(A) tail consisting of 20 to 250 adenylate residues at the 3′ end of the transcript.
3. Splicing removes introns from capped, tailed transcripts and rejoins exons in a continuous coding sequence.
   a. Splice sites, the junctions between exons and introns, usually are marked by consensus sequences: GU at the 5′ end of an intron and AG at the 3′ end.
   b. Small nuclear ribonucleoproteins (snRNPs) assemble at splice sites in hnRNA, forming a spliceosome.
      (1) Two transesterification reactions catalyzed by snRNPs result in excision of the intron as a lariat structure and joining of exons.
      (2) Systemic lupus erythematosus is an autoimmune disease in which the patient produces antibodies to snRNPs.

D. Regulation of transcription initiation is the most important mechanism for controlling gene expression.
   1. Regulatory elements in the DNA sequence, called enhancers or silencers, bind DNA regulatory proteins (specific transcription factors), which may activate or repress transcription by RNA polymerase II.
      a. Enhancers generally are located at a considerable distance upstream or downstream from the promoter region of a gene, but they also may be located within introns.

Systemic lupus erythematosus: autoimmune disease; antibodies produced to snRNPs, which function in mRNA splicing

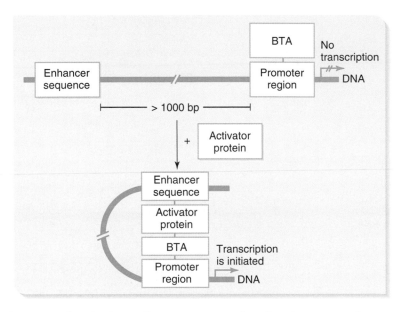

10-7: *Transcription of regulated genes. Transcription initiation depends on the interaction of an activator protein (bound to an enhancer sequence) with components of the basal transcription apparatus (BTA). Nonregulated housekeeping genes require only assembly of the BTA for transcription. bp, base pairs.*

    b. The complex made up of the enhancer and activator protein interacts with the basal transcription apparatus (BTA) at the promoter region, greatly increasing or decreasing the rate of transcription of regulated genes (Fig. 10-7).

    c. Multiple enhancers and activators often regulate a single gene.

2. Steroid hormones, when complexed to their intracellular receptors, function as transcriptional activators (see Chapter 3).

    a. Each hormone-receptor complex binds to a particular regulatory element in DNA.

    b. Tamoxifen, used in the treatment of breast cancer, is an estrogen antagonist that blocks the binding of estrogen to its intracellular receptor in estrogen-sensitive tumor cells in breast tissue.

3. Many polypeptide hormones and growth factors also regulate gene expression by triggering intracellular signaling pathways, leading to activation (or, less often, repression) of transcription (see Chapter 3).

4. Physical accessibility of DNA to transcription factors and RNA polymerase II depends on the degree of compaction of chromatin in the region of a gene.

    a. Heterochromatin is highly condensed, DNase resistant, and inactive in transcription.

    b. Euchromatin is dispersed, DNase digestible, and active in transcription.

Tamoxifen: estrogen antagonist used to treat breast cancer

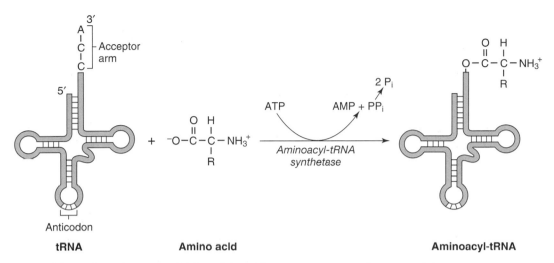

10-8: *Charging of tRNA by aminoacyl-tRNA synthetases. These enzymes recognize the amino acid that corresponds to the anticodon in a particular tRNA and link it via a high-energy bond to the 3'-adenylate residue of the acceptor arm.*

IV. Protein Synthesis
   A. Transfer RNAs are charged with an amino acid by aminoacyl-tRNA synthetases (Fig. 10-8).
      1. tRNAs have a cloverleaf shape with an acceptor arm, which receives the amino acid, and a three-base anticodon, which base pairs with the complementary codon in mRNA.
      2. Each aminoacyl-tRNA synthetase attaches one type of amino acid to all of the tRNAs specific for that amino acid.
      3. Proofreading by aminoacyl-tRNA synthetases detects and removes amino acids that are linked to the incorrect tRNA.
   B. Ribosomes are particle-like ribonucleoprotein complexes composed of small and large subunits, whose composition and function in protein synthesis differ.
      1. Small (40S) subunit (equivalent to the 30S subunit in prokaryotes)
         a. Binds mRNA and aminoacyl-tRNAs
         b. Locates AUG start codon on mRNA
      2. Large (60S) subunit (equivalent to the 50S subunit in prokaryotes)
         a. Binds to the small subunit after the start codon is located
         b. Has peptidyltransferase activity
   C. Translation of the mRNA message into a protein involves three stages: initiation, chain elongation, and termination (Fig. 10-9).
      1. Initiation of protein synthesis
         a. Start codon (AUG), at which synthesis of all proteins begins, specifies methionine (formylmethionine [f-Met] in bacteria).
         b. Initiation factors are required to bind the mRNA and beginning methionyl-tRNA (or f-Met-tRNA) to the small ribosomal subunit and then to assemble the ribosome, forming an initiation complex.

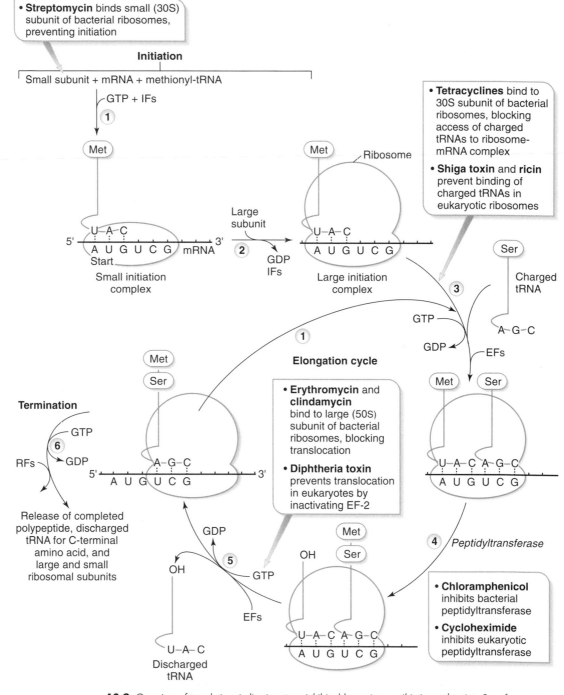

• **Streptomycin** binds small (30S) subunit of bacterial ribosomes, preventing initiation

Initiation

Small subunit + mRNA + methionyl-tRNA

GTP + IFs

1

Met

U–A–C
A U G U C G mRNA
Start

5' 3'

Small initiation complex

Large subunit

2

GDP
IFs

Met

Ribosome

U–A–C
A U G U C G

Large initiation complex

• **Tetracyclines** bind to 30S subunit of bacterial ribosomes, blocking access of charged tRNAs to ribosome-mRNA complex
• **Shiga toxin** and **ricin** prevent binding of charged tRNAs in eukaryotic ribosomes

3

Ser

Charged tRNA

A–G–C

GTP

GDP

EFs

Met   Ser

U–A–C A–G–C
A U G U C G

1

Elongation cycle

Met
Ser

• **Erythromycin** and **clindamycin** bind to large (50S) subunit of bacterial ribosomes, blocking translocation
• **Diphtheria toxin** prevents translocation in eukaryotes by inactivating EF-2

Termination

GTP

6

RFs

GDP

A–G–C
A U G U C G

5' 3'

Release of completed polypeptide, discharged tRNA for C-terminal amino acid, and large and small ribosomal subunits

GDP

5

OH

EFs

GTP

U–A–C
Discharged tRNA

Met

OH   Ser

4 *Peptidyltransferase*

U–A–C A–G–C
A U G U C G

• **Chloramphenicol** inhibits bacterial peptidyltransferase
• **Cycloheximide** inhibits eukaryotic peptidyltransferase

10-9: *Overview of translation, indicating steps inhibited by various antibiotics and toxins. Specific protein initiation factors (IFs), elongation factors (EFs), and release factors (RFs) are required in both prokaryotes and eukaryotes. During step 5 (translocation), the ribosome moves toward the 3' end of the mRNA by one codon, freeing the site for another aminoacyl-tRNA. The polypeptide chain is elongated by repetition of steps 3, 4, and 5 with different charged tRNAs. Termination occurs when the ribosome encounters a stop codon.*

2. Elongation of the protein chain
   a. Direction of synthesis of the protein chain proceeds from the amino end to the carboxyl end.
      • During translation, the ribosome shifts by one codon in the $5' \to 3'$ direction along the mRNA in a process known as translocation.
   b. Peptide bond formation is catalyzed by peptidyltransferase activity of an rRNA component with enzyme function (a ribozyme) in the large ribosomal subunit.
   c. Elongation factors facilitate the reading of the mRNA and translation into the amino acid sequence of the specified polypeptide.
3. Termination of protein synthesis
   a. Stop codons (UGA, UAG, or UAA) signal termination of chain elongation.
      • No tRNAs exist that have anticodons complementary to stop codons.
   b. Release factors bind to a stop codon and stimulate the release of the newly synthesized polypeptide chain, the final tRNA, and the dissociated ribosome.
D. Several antibiotics act by selectively inhibiting bacterial protein synthesis (see Fig. 10-9).
   1. Streptomycin binds to the small (30S) ribosomal subunits of bacteria and interferes with formation of the initiation complex.
      • Aminoglycosides, tetracycline, and spectinomycin are other inhibitors of small ribosomal subunits.
   2. Tetracyclines bind to the small ribosomal subunits of bacteria and block the binding of incoming aminoacyl-tRNAs.
   3. Chloramphenicol inhibits peptidyltransferase activity of the large (50S) ribosomal subunits of bacteria.
   4. Erythromycin and clindamycin also bind to the large ribosomal subunits, thus preventing translocation of the ribosome along the bacterial mRNA.
E. Some toxins and antibiotics disrupt eukaryotic protein synthesis.
   1. Shiga toxin (*Shigella dysenteriae*) and shiga-like toxin (enterohemorrhagic *Escherichia coli*) cleave the 28S rRNA in the large (60S) ribosomal subunits of eukaryotes, preventing binding of incoming aminoacyl-tRNAs.
   2. Diphtheria toxin (*Corynebacterium diphtheriae*) inactivates an elongation factor, EF-2, thereby preventing translocation in the eukaryotic ribosome.
   3. Ricin, a protein found in castor beans, inactivates large ribosomal subunits in the same manner as does shiga toxin.
   4. Cycloheximide, which is used as a fungicide and rat repellent, inhibits eukaryotic peptidyltransferase.
F. Polyribosomes (polysomes) are extended arrays of individual ribosomes all associated with a single strand of mRNA.
   • By carrying out synthesis of multiple copies of the same protein concurrently, polyribosomes increase the rate of protein synthesis.
G. Synthesis of secreted, lysosomal, and membrane proteins begins in the cytosol but is completed on the rough endoplasmic reticulum (RER).

Many antibiotics target differences between prokaryotic and eukaryotic ribosomes, selectively inhibiting bacterial protein synthesis.

Eukaryotic protein synthesis: targeted by certain toxins and antibiotics

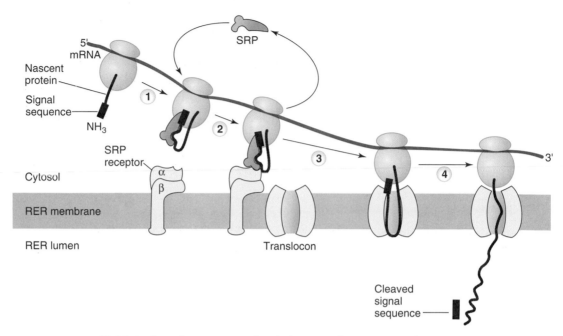

10-10: *Synthesis of proteins on rough endoplasmic reticulum (RER). A signal sequence on a nascent protein interacts with a signal recognition particle (SRP) and an SRP receptor on the RER. The growing polypeptide passes through a translocon into the RER lumen, where it may be glycosylated.*

1. A signal sequence at the amino terminus of the nascent polypeptide guides the nascent polypeptide to the RER membrane and ultimately into the RER lumen (Fig. 10-10).
   a. Steps 1 and 2: After synthesis of the signal sequence on a free ribosome in the cytosol, the ribosome attaches to the RER membrane with the aid of a signal recognition particle (SRP) and SRP receptor (see Fig. 10-10).
   b. Step 3: The SRP dissociates, the ribosome-nascent protein associates with a translocon in the RER membrane, and the polypeptide chain enters the open channel in the translocon.
   c. Step 4: As translation continues, the elongating polypeptide is translocated into the RER lumen, amino end first, and the signal sequence is cleaved and digested.
      • Once translation is completed, the new protein may be glycosylated in the RER lumen.
2. Transport vesicles that bud off from the RER carry newly formed proteins to the Golgi apparatus, where they undergo various post-translational modifications.
   • Post-translational modifications of many proteins are required for their biological activity (Table 10-1).
3. Hydrolytic enzymes destined for lysosomes are tagged with mannose 6-phosphate residues by enzymes in the lumen of the Golgi apparatus.

TABLE 10-1:
Post-translational Modifications in Proteins

Type of Modification	Example
Proteolytic cleavage	Digestive enzymes (e.g., trypsinogen → trypsin) Clotting factors (e.g., prothrombin → thrombin) Hormones (e.g., proinsulin → insulin + C-peptide)
Disulfide bond formation	Secreted proteins
Attachment of prosthetic group	Covalent linkage of biotin to carboxylases
Glycosylation (sugars attached to amino acids) (serine, threonine, and asparagines residues)	Membrane and secreted proteins (e.g., glycosylated membrane proteins, ABO blood group determinants, immunoglobulins)
Phosphorylation (serine, threonine, and tyrosine residues)	Hormonally regulated enzymes (e.g., glycogen synthase, acetyl CoA carboxylase, pyruvate kinase)
Hydroxylation (lysine and proline residues)	Collagen α-chains
γ-Carboxylation (glutamine residues)	Clotting factors II, VII, IX, X, and proteins C and S

a. The mannose 6-phosphate residues on the enzymes bind tightly to specific receptors in the Golgi membrane, and vesicles containing the bound enzymes bud off and eventually fuse with lysosomes.

b. I cell disease is a lysosomal storage disease that results from an inherited deficiency of the phosphotransferase needed to form the mannose 6-phosphate tag on lysosomal enzymes (see Box 6-2).

(1) Lysosomal enzymes are produced normally, but because they lack the mannose 6-phosphate tag, they are secreted into the blood rather than being directed to lysosomes.

(2) Other lysosomal storage diseases, such as mucopolysaccharidoses, Pompe's disease, and sphingolipidoses, are caused by inherited defects in the lysosomal enzymes (see Chapters 6 and 7).

> I cell disease: cannot form mannose 6-phosphate on enzymes targeted for lysosomes; lysosomes have no enzymes

V. Mutations and Inherited Diseases

A. A mutation is a change in the base sequence of DNA that escapes detection and correction by proofreading or repairing enzymes and is permanently "locked in" to a cell's genome at the next cell division.

- Inherited diseases originate from mutations in germ cells that are passed on to the offspring and incorporated into all of their cells (e.g., inactivation of the *Rb* suppressor gene on chromosome 13 causes retinoblastoma).

B. Different types of mutations have varying phenotypic effects.

1. Alterations in a single nucleotide base, known as point mutations, within a protein-coding gene can have three possible outcomes (Fig. 10-11):

a. Silent mutation occurs when the altered codon specifies the same amino acid; therefore, there is no phenotypic effect.

b. Missense mutation occurs when the altered codon specifies a different amino acid, causing variable phenotypic effects.

- Example: Altered hemoglobins resulting from different missense mutations cause symptoms ranging from benign (HbC, which causes a mild, chronic anemia) to moderate (HbS, sickle cell

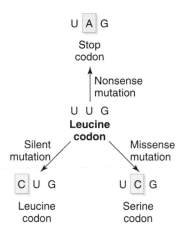

10-11: *Possible outcomes resulting from a point mutation that alters a single nucleotide base in the coding region of mRNA. As seen here for the leucine codon, a point mutation can result in no change in the amino acid (silent mutation), a change in the amino acid (missense mutation), or a premature termination of synthesis of the polypeptide (nonsense mutation).*

hemoglobin) and severe (HbM, associated with methemoglobinemia) (see Chapter 2).

Point mutations cause silent, missense, or nonsense mutations.

    c. Nonsense mutation occurs when the altered codon is a stop codon, causing premature termination during protein synthesis, which usually results in deleterious phenotypic effects.

2. Frameshift mutations are caused by insertion or deletion of any number of nucleotides not divisible by three, which shifts the reading frame during translation of mRNA (Fig. 10-12).

Tay-Sachs disease: frameshift mutation caused by four-nucleotide insertion

    a. A frameshift mutation results in a randomly incorrect amino acid sequence on the carboxyl side of the mutation and usually a truncated protein caused by the introduction of a premature stop codon.

    b. Example: Tay-Sachs disease is the result of a four-nucleotide insertion that causes a frameshift mutation and defective hexosaminidase.

3. Trinucleotide repeat mutations are caused by errors in DNA replication that lead to an abnormal number of repeated trinucleotides (e.g., CGG, CAG, and CTG) within a gene.

    a. Huntington's disease, Friedreich's ataxia, fragile X syndrome, and myotonic dystrophy are caused by this type of mutation.

    b. These disorders worsen in future generations due to the addition of trinucleotides; this is called anticipation.

4. Translocation mutations are caused by movement of all or part of a gene from its normal position to another position in the genome.

    a. Translocation mutations are generally caused by mistakes during homologous recombination, a normal process that occurs in meiosis and in repair of double-strand breaks in DNA.

    b. These mutations cause various effects ranging from no protein production to reduced expression of normal protein.

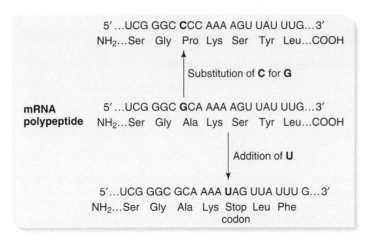

5'...UCG GGC **C**CC AAA AGU UAU UUG...3'
NH₂...Ser Gly Pro Lys Ser Tyr Leu...COOH

Substitution of **C** for **G**

mRNA   5'...UCG GGC **G**CA AAA AGU UAU UUG...3'
polypeptide NH₂...Ser Gly Ala Lys Ser Tyr Leu...COOH

Addition of **U**

5'...UCG GGC GCA AAA **U**AG UUA UUU G...3'
NH₂...Ser Gly Ala Lys Stop Leu Phe
                                codon

10-12: *Effect of mutations resulting from a base addition or base substitution of a single nucleotide in the coding region of mRNA. With the base substitution of C for G, CCC codes for Pro rather than Ala (a missense mutation). When U is added, UAG becomes a stop codon (a nonsense mutation). Had the addition of U not produced a stop codon, a frameshift mutation would have occurred resulting in changes in the amino acid sequence of the protein (e.g., UUA, leucine, UUU, and phenylalanine). The normal mRNA sequence and corresponding amino acid sequence are shown in the middle.*

    c. Examples: Burkitt's lymphoma (t8;14) and chronic myelogenous leukemia (t9;22)

5. Mutations may involve a gain or a loss of an entire chromosome.
    a. Example: trisomy 21, with three copies of chromosome 21, causes Down syndrome.
    b. Most chromosomal number disorders are due to nondisjunction, when homologous chromosomes or chromatids fail to separate properly in the first phase of meiosis, resulting in one or more extra chromosomes in some gametes and fewer chromosomes in other gametes.

6. Mutations may involve a loss of a small portion of a chromosome (microdeletion).
    a. Microdeletion on chromosome 15 may result in Prader-Willi syndrome if the abnormal chromosome is of paternal origin.
    b. Angelman syndrome may result if the particular abnormal chromosome is of maternal origin.
    c. The mechanism of Prader-Willi and Angelman syndromes is genomic imprinting, meaning that the phenotypic outcome depends on whether the chromosome is maternal or paternal in origin.

C. Mendelian inheritance is shown by inherited diseases resulting from single-gene defects in nuclear DNA (Box 10-1).

D. Mitochondrial diseases resulting from a mutation in mitochondrial DNA exhibit maternal transmission because mitochondria from sperm do not enter the fertilized egg.
    • Examples: Leber's hereditary optic neuropathy, Kearns-Sayre syndrome (see Chapter 5)

> Down syndrome: caused by extra copy of chromosome 21

BOX 10-1

MENDELIAN INHERITANCE PATTERNS

Autosomal dominant: One defective copy of the gene on an autosomal (non-sex) chromosome produces the disease. A child has a 50% chance of having the disease if one of the parents is heterozygous. Both males and females are affected. Clinical symptoms may not develop until adulthood. Some patients with the abnormal gene do not develop clinical symptoms (less than 100% penetrance), but all can transmit the disease to their children.

- *Examples:* Familial hypercholesterolemia, Huntington's disease, Marfan's syndrome, osteogenesis imperfecta, von Willebrand's disease, congenital spherocytosis, adult polycystic kidney disease, neurofibromatosis

Autosomal recessive: Two defective copies (alleles) of the gene, each on an autosomal chromosome, are needed to produce the disease. Each child of two heterozygous (asymptomatic carriers) parents has a 25% chance of having the disease (homozygous). Both males and females are affected. Clinical symptoms usually develop in infancy or childhood and commonly are more severe than in dominant disorders.

- *Examples:* Most inborn errors of metabolism (e.g., glycogen storage diseases, maple syrup urine disease, phenylketonuria, Tay-Sachs disease), sickle cell disease, cystic fibrosis, adrenogenital syndrome, Wilson's disease

X-linked recessive: Each son of a heterozygous mother, who is usually an asymptomatic carrier, has a 50% chance of being affected. Affected males transmit the abnormal X chromosome to all of their daughters (carriers) but to none of their sons. Heterozygous females may show minor effects, but males, with only one X chromosome, manifest clinical symptoms.

- *Examples:* Duchenne-type muscular dystrophy, Fabry's disease, hemophilia A and B, Hunter's syndrome, Lesch-Nyhan syndrome, glucose 6-phosphate dehydrogenase deficiency

E. Multifactorial disorders are associated with multiple gene defects and are commonly influenced by environmental factors.
   1. Although multifactorial disorders tend to occur in families, they do not exhibit simple Mendelian inheritance patterns.
   2. Examples: Coronary artery disease, epilepsy, gout, type 2 diabetes mellitus, essential hypertension
F. Hemoglobinopathies that involve altered rates of globin synthesis produce hemolytic anemias called thalassemias.
   1. Mutations cause reduced production of α-globin or β-globin.

      a. Complete deletion of globin genes

      b. Impaired RNA synthesis

      c. Impaired primary mRNA splicing (most common type)

      d. Abnormal globins due to frameshift or nonsense mutations (quickly degraded)

  2. α-Thalassemias are caused by defects in the synthesis of α-globin, which normally involves two genes on each chromosome 16, for a total of four genes.

     • The progressive loss of the four α-globin genes results in more severe microcytic anemias.

  3. β-Thalassemias are caused by defects in the synthesis of β-globin, which normally involves a single gene on each chromosome 11.

      a. Thalassemia major, caused by a mutation of both β-globin genes, is lethal by the age of 2 years unless regular transfusions are administered.

      b. Thalassemia minor, caused by a mutation of one of the β-globin genes, produces mild microcytic anemia.

α-Thalassemia: caused by defects in α-globin synthesis; β-thalassemia is caused by defects in β-globin synthesis

VI. Mutations and Cancer

  A. Introduction

    1. Most cancers are noninherited disorders resulting from the accumulation over time of multiple mutations in somatic cells.

    2. Mutations in proto-oncogenes, tumor-suppressor genes, and DNA repair genes are primarily associated with the development of cancer.

  B. Proto-oncogenes encode proteins that promote cell proliferation or inhibit apoptosis (programmed cell death) (Table 10-2).

    1. Gain-of-function mutations occur in proto-oncogenes, converting them into oncogenes, which act dominantly.

      • Oncogenes code for oncoproteins, and only one copy of an oncogene is needed to produce an effect.

    2. Oncoproteins may be constitutively active forms of normal proteins or normal proteins that are expressed in excessive amounts, in the wrong tissue, or at the wrong time during development.

Gain-of-function mutations in proto-oncogenes (e.g., ras) exhibit dominance.

  C. Tumor-suppressor genes encode proteins that inhibit cell proliferation or promote apoptosis (see Table 10-2).

    1. Loss-of-function mutations in tumor-suppressor genes act recessively.

      • Both alleles of a tumor-suppressor gene must be mutated to permit development of a cancer.

    2. Genetic predisposition to certain cancers results from inheritance of one mutant allele (from either parent) of various tumor-suppressor genes.

      a. In familial cancers associated with tumor-suppressor genes (e.g., retinoblastoma, breast carcinomas, and Wilms' tumor), an individual inherits one mutant allele.

        • Only one somatic mutation, in the remaining normal allele, is required for the cancer to develop.

      b. Sporadic forms of these cancers have a much lower frequency and later onset than familial forms.

Loss-of-function mutations in suppressor genes (e.g., p53) act recessively.

TABLE 10-2:
Selected Human Proto-oncogenes and Tumor-suppressor Genes

Gene Name	Function of Gene Product	Tumors Associated with Mutation
Proto-oncogenes		
BCL-2	Inhibits apoptosis (programmed cell death)	Follicular B cell lymphoma
ERB-B2	Binds epidermal growth factor (cell surface receptor)	Breast, ovarian, stomach cancers
MYC	Activates transcription	Burkitt's lymphoma, neuroblastoma
RAS	Transduces signal from many growth factors (a G protein)	Bladder, lung, colon, and pancreatic cancers
Tumor-suppressor Genes		
APC	Inhibits myc expression	Familial adenomatous polyposis; colorectal carcinoma
BRCA-1, BRCA-2	Involved in DNA repair	BRCA-1: breast, ovary, colon, prostate cancers BRCA-2: male/female breast cancer
NF-1, NF-2	Helps control intracellular signaling	Neurofibromatosis: optic nerve glioma, meningioma, acoustic neuroma, pheochromocytoma
p53	Induces proteins that mediate G_1 arrest or apoptosis of cells with damaged DNA ("guardian of the cell")	Most human cancers; Li-Fraumeni syndrome: breast and brain cancers, leukemia, sarcomas
RB	Induces protein that mediates G_1 arrest	Retinoblastoma, osteosarcoma, breast cancer
WT-1	Represses transcription in developing kidney	Wilms' tumor

TABLE 10-3:
Inherited Diseases Associated with Defective DNA-repair Enzymes

Disease	Type of Cancer Susceptibility	Clinical Features
Ataxia telangiectasia	Lymphomas	Cerebellar ataxia; dilation of blood vessels in skin and eyes; immunodeficiency (B and T cells)
Bloom's syndrome	Carcinomas, leukemias, lymphomas	Facial telangiectasia, growth retardation, immunodeficiency
Fanconi's anemia	Leukemias	Progressive aplastic anemia, pancytopenia, numerous congenital anomalies
Hereditary nonpolyposis colorectal cancer	Colon, ovary	Tumors usually develop before 40 years of age
Xeroderma pigmentosum	Basal cell carcinoma, squamous cell carcinoma, malignant melanomas	Severe skin lesions (absent DNA repair enzymes)

- Two somatic mutations, one in each allele of the involved gene within a given cell lineage, must occur before the disease manifests.

D. Defects in DNA repair systems cause several inherited diseases that are marked by increased cancer susceptibility (Table 10-3).

  1. Patients have increased sensitivity to various agents that damage DNA.
     - Example: Extreme photosensitivity to UV radiation occurs with xeroderma pigmentosum.
  2. Deficiency of appropriate repair enzymes greatly increases the likelihood that somatic cell mutations in other genes are perpetuated, leading to oncogenic transformation (especially in rapidly proliferating tissues such as bone marrow).

Genetic defects in DNA repair enzymes: increased sensitivity to agents that damage DNA, associated with increased cancer risk

Biotechnology

I. Recombinant DNA and DNA Cloning
   A. Cloning is a means of obtaining large quantities of specific DNA fragments for sequencing, genetic engineering, and expression of the encoded proteins.
   B. Target DNA to be cloned is inserted into a cloning vector, forming recombinant DNA, which is introduced (transfected) into rapidly growing cells (e.g., *Escherichia coli* cells) and replicated along with the host cell DNA.
   C. Two methods are commonly used to produce target DNA pieces suitable for cloning: genomic DNA and complementary DNA (cDNA).

   cDNA: double-strand DNA that contains all the coding sequences (exons) corresponding to a single mRNA

   1. Genomic DNA, isolated from cell nuclei, is fragmented with restriction endonucleases, which are enzymes that cleave DNA at specific sites.
      • Genomic DNA fragments may contain all or part of a particular gene and include introns as well as other noncoding sequences.
   2. cDNA is produced from messenger RNA (mRNA) isolated from a particular tissue and does not contain introns.
      a. Reverse transcriptase produces a DNA strand complementary to the mRNA.
      b. After the resulting DNA-mRNA hybrid is denatured, DNA polymerase is used to produce double-strand cDNA from the single-strand DNA copy of the mRNA.
   D. Restriction endonucleases are key to the production of recombinant DNA.

   Restriction endonucleases produce DNA fragments with sticky ends that are used to produce recombinant DNA.

   1. Restriction endonucleases are bacterial enzymes that are highly specific for short nucleotide sequences (restriction sites) and cleave both DNA strands within this region.

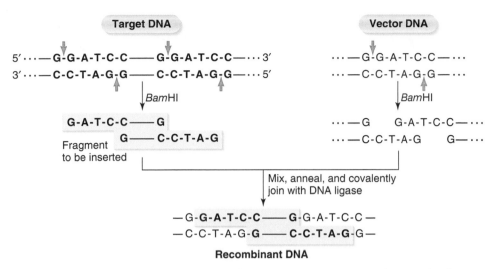

11-1: *Restriction endonucleases and the production of recombinant DNA. Target DNA to be inserted and vector DNA are cleaved with the same restriction enzyme (BamHI), producing complementary sticky ends.*

2. Staggered cuts are made by most restriction enzymes, producing DNA fragments with single-strand ends.
   a. Restriction sites are palindromes; that is, both strands of DNA have the same sequence when read in a 5′ → 3′ direction.
   b. Complementary single-strand sticky ends, which can base-pair, result from a staggered cut in a palindromic sequence.
3. DNA fragments from different sources produced by cleavage with the same restriction enzyme and containing complementary sticky ends will anneal (base-pair) with each other.
4. Joining of the free ends with DNA ligase yields stable recombinant DNA molecules made up of segments from two or more sources (Fig. 11-1).
E. Cloning vectors must possess three essential properties to function in DNA cloning:
   1. Presence of a restriction site, which permits insertion of target DNA
   2. Autonomous replication in a host cell, which permits amplification of target DNA independently of host cell DNA synthesis
   3. Selectable feature that permits transfected host cells containing the vector to be distinguished from cells that do not contain the vector
F. Plasmid vectors are constructed from small, circular, extrachromosomal DNAs (plasmids) that are spontaneously taken up by host bacterial cells.
   1. Target DNA up to 5 kilobases (kb) in length can be inserted into plasmid vectors.
   2. Plasmids used as vectors either naturally contain or are engineered to contain known restriction sites, an origin that permits rapid replication in host cells, and an antibiotic-resistance gene that confers antibiotic resistance on host cells (Fig. 11-2).

Cloning vector: autonomously replicating DNA molecule used to carry a DNA fragment into a host cell

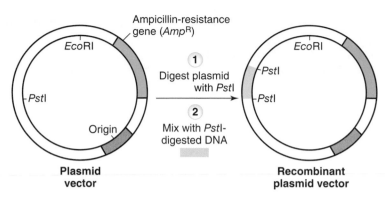

11-2: *Formation of a recombinant plasmid vector. Left, Plasmids used as cloning vectors contain a replication origin (gray), at least one known restriction site, and a selectable gene (dark blue) that confers antibiotic resistance (e.g., Amp^R). Two restriction sites are shown, PstI and EcoRI, at which target DNA could be inserted without disrupting the origin or selectable gene. Right, When plasmids digested with a restriction enzyme (e.g., PstI) are mixed with an excess of target DNA digested with the same enzyme, a large proportion of the plasmids will recombine with target DNA fragments. Host cells that take up a recombinant plasmid will be resistant to ampicillin.*

3. Naturally occurring plasmids, which often carry antibiotic-resistance genes, are readily transferred from one bacterial cell to another, promoting the rapid spread of antibiotic resistance throughout a bacterial population.

G. Other vectors can hold larger DNA fragments and are more efficient than plasmids in transfecting host cells.

    1. Lambda phage vectors, produced from lambda (λ) bacteriophage, can hold DNA fragments up to 20 kb in length.

    2. Yeast artificial chromosomes (YACs) can hold DNA fragments as long as 1000 kb and are easily propagated in yeast cells.

      • YACs have been particularly useful in studying human and other eukaryotic genes, which generally are quite long because of the presence of introns.

H. A summary of basic steps in DNA cloning, which are similar for all types of vectors, is depicted in Fig. 11-3 for a plasmid vector.

    1. Recombinant vectors are transfected into appropriate host cells under conditions that favor incorporation of only one vector per cell.

    2. Each host cell that takes up a plasmid multiplies into a colony of genetically identical cells (a clone), with each cell containing the same recombinant vector.

I. DNA libraries are collections of restriction fragments cloned within suitable host cells.

    1. A genomic DNA library is obtained from restriction enzyme digestion of the entire genome of an organism and theoretically contains all the nuclear DNA sequences.

    2. A cDNA library is obtained from the mixture of mRNAs expressed by a particular tissue under given physiologic conditions.

      • Each clone in a cDNA library carries an intact gene that lacks introns and a promoter region.

Genomic DNA library: each clone contains a fragment of the entire genome of an organism

cDNA library: each clone contains an intact gene

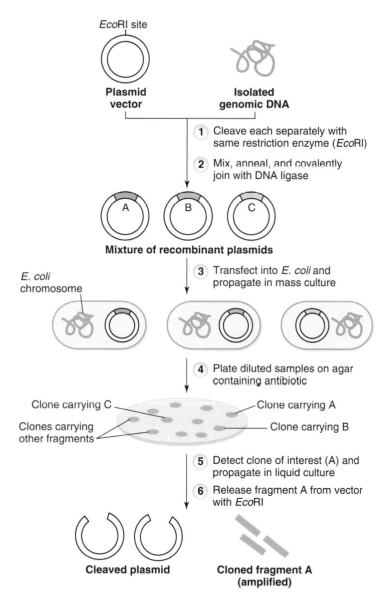

11-3: *Overview of DNA cloning with a plasmid vector. Restriction enzyme digestion of genomic DNA produces multiple fragments with different sequences. Mixing these fragments with cleaved plasmids yields a mixture of recombinant plasmids, each containing a different fragment (e.g., A, B, and C). After growth and plating of transfected E. coli cells on antibiotic-containing agar plates, the fragments are separated physically into different clones. A specific fragment of interest can be identified by hybridization with a complementary probe (see Fig. 11-4) and then isolated from the vector.*

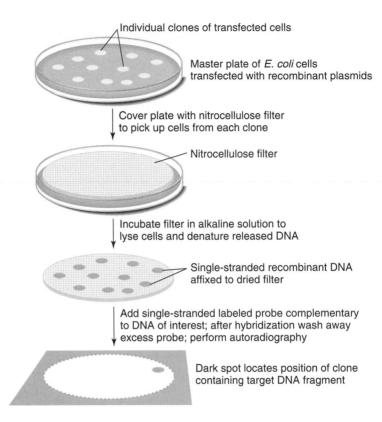

Individual clones of transfected cells

Master plate of *E. coli* cells transfected with recombinant plasmids

Cover plate with nitrocellulose filter to pick up cells from each clone

Nitrocellulose filter

Incubate filter in alkaline solution to lyse cells and denature released DNA

Single-stranded recombinant DNA affixed to dried filter

Add single-stranded labeled probe complementary to DNA of interest; after hybridization wash away excess probe; perform autoradiography

Dark spot locates position of clone containing target DNA fragment

11-4: *Identification of a clone carrying a specific target DNA fragment by membrane hybridization (e.g., fragment A clone in Fig. 11-3). In this technique, a replica of the master plate is transferred to a nitrocellulose filter (blotting) and immobilized on it. Radioactive probe will hybridize only with a recombinant DNA containing a complementary sequence. An autoradiogram is produced by placing an X-ray film over the filter; radioactivity from the labeled probe exposes the film so that a dark spot appears when the film is developed, revealing the location of the target sequence.*

II. Detection of Specific Nucleic Acid Sequences with Probes
   A. Probes are synthetic single-strand oligonucleotides (20 to 30 bases long) that are most often labeled with a radioactive isotope (e.g., ^{32}P) for easy detection.
      • In a mixture of denatured single-strand DNA fragments (or RNAs), a probe will hybridize (base-pair) only with fragments containing a complementary sequence.
   B. Screening of DNA libraries for a specific target DNA fragment can be performed with a membrane hybridization assay using a complementary probe (Fig. 11-4).
   C. Blotting analysis can separate and detect specific nucleic acid sequences or proteins in complex mixtures (Fig. 11-5).
      1. Southern blotting detects DNA with labeled DNA probes.
         • Useful in identifying a specific restriction fragment out of the millions present in a restriction digest of an individual's genomic DNA
      2. Northern blotting detects RNA with labeled DNA probes.

Southern blotting detects DNA; Northern blotting, RNA; Western blotting, proteins; Southwestern blotting, DNA binding proteins. Primers are indicated in black.

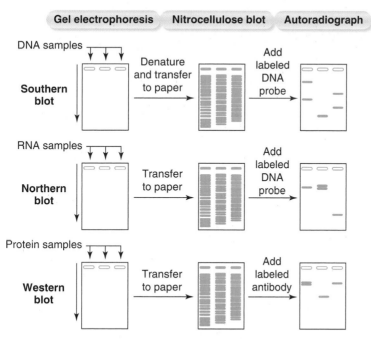

Gel electrophoresis   Nitrocellulose blot   Autoradiograph

11-5: *Blotting analysis for detecting specific DNA sequences (Southern blot), RNA sequences (Northern blot), and proteins (Western blot). After samples from three different sources are separated by gel electrophoresis, the gel is placed on nitrocellulose paper. The nucleic acids or proteins transfer to the paper (blotting) and bind to it, thus maintaining the banding pattern in the gel. The nitrocellulose blot is treated with a radioactive probe that binds to a specific target molecule of interest and then is subjected to autoradiography, eliminating the background interference from all other molecules. In each blot, the three samples exhibit different banding patterns.*

- Useful in determining whether a specific mRNA is expressed in a particular tissue
3. Western blotting detects proteins by using labeled antibodies.
   - Useful confirmatory test for HIV when enzyme-linked immunosorbent assay screening test is positive
4. Southwestern blotting detects DNA binding proteins with labeled DNA probes.
   - Useful in detecting expression of transcription factors that interact with regulatory sequences controlling specific genes

III. Polymerase Chain Reaction
   A. Polymerase chain reaction (PCR) is an *in vitro* enzymatic method for amplifying a target DNA sequence located between two short flanking sites whose sequences are known.
   B. PCR procedure is outlined in Figure 11-6.
      1. Components required in addition to DNA containing the target sequence
         a. Single-strand oligonucleotide primers complementary to the two flanking sites

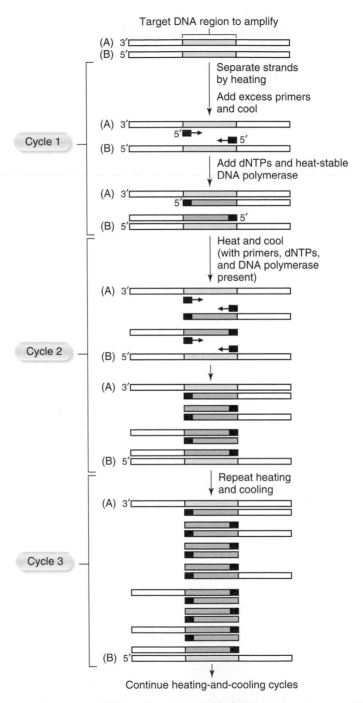

11-6: *Polymerase chain reaction. DNA strands are separated by heating, excess primers are added to begin the replication process, and heat-stable DNA polymerase catalyzes 5′ → 3′ synthesis using deoxyribonucleoside triphosphates (dNTPs). Three cycles of amplification are shown. Note how the strands of the original DNA, labeled A and B, are diluted out, whereas the proportion of new molecules containing only the target DNA region increases rapidly. After 30 cycles, there will be 10^9 target-region molecules for each beginning DNA molecule.*

11-7: *Polymerase chain reaction detection of cystic fibrosis. Use of primers that flank the 3-base deletion in the CFTR gene that causes cystic fibrosis results in different products starting with DNA from normal, carrier, and affected individuals. After samples are amplified, they are analyzed by Southern blotting. The shorter amplification product from the mutant allele 151 base pairs [bp]) moves faster in gel electrophoresis and is easily differentiated from the 154-bp product from the normal allele. The intensity of bands from homozygotes is approximately twice that of bands from the heterozygous carrier.*

     b. Heat-stable DNA polymerase that remains functional throughout the heating phases

     c. All four deoxyribonucleoside triphosphates

  2. Doubling of the target DNA sequence occurs in each heating-cooling cycle.

     • Within a few cycles, nearly all the DNA molecules correspond to the target sequence.

  3. Sensitivity is so great that one target sequence present in a single cell can be amplified and detected.

     • Useful in forensics for identifying DNA from tiny blood, saliva, and semen samples

C. RNA virus infection can be detected with reverse-transcriptase PCR (RT-PCR) at very early stages.

  1. RT is used to convert the viral RNA genome to DNA, which is amplified by PCR and identified by Southern blotting.

  2. HIV, enterovirus, and Norwalk virus infections can be diagnosed with RT-PCR before significant viral replication or detectable antibody production has occurred.

> RT-PCR permits early detection of the RNA viruses HIV, enterovirus, and Norwalk virus.

D. Mutant alleles for certain inherited diseases can be detected by PCR analysis. *Examples:*

  1. Cystic fibrosis is an autosomal recessive disorder caused by a 3-base deletion coding for phenylalanine in the cystic fibrosis transmembrane regulation *(CFTR)* gene (see Chapter 3).

     • DNA from normal, carrier, and affected individuals can be distinguished by PCR analysis using probes that flank the mutated region of *CFTR* (Fig. 11-7).

  2. Other genetic diseases detectable by PCR analysis include familial hypercholesterolemia, hemophilia, Lesch-Nyhan syndrome, lysosomal and glycogen storage diseases, retinoblastoma, sickle cell anemia, β-thalassemia, and von Willebrand's disease.

> Cystic fibrosis: affected, carrier, and normal individuals are distinguished by PCR analysis

IV. Restriction Fragment Length Polymorphisms

  A. DNA polymorphisms are small heritable variations in the DNA sequence found in the general population.

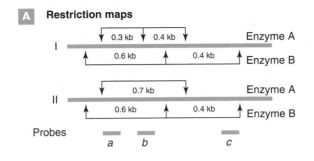

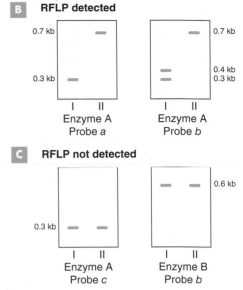

11-8: *RFLP detection depends on restriction enzymes and probes.* **A,** *Restriction maps for enzymes A and B of the same DNA region from two individuals (I and II). Small arrows point to restriction sites. Restriction sites for these individuals differ for enzyme A but not for enzyme B. Oligonucleotide probes a, b, and c are aligned below the DNA sequences with which they hybridize.* **B** *and* **C,** *Southern blots obtained with different enzyme and probe combinations. No polymorphism is detected in this region if the A-digested samples are treated with probe c. Likewise, no polymorphism is detected if the samples are digested only with enzyme B and analyzed with any one of the three probes.*

- These variations occur every 200 to 500 nucleotides in the human genome, but most cause no phenotypic effect because large portions of the human genome do not code for protein.
B. Restriction mapping identifies the restriction sites in a region of DNA and the distance in kilobases between them.
    - The process involves digesting samples of a cloned DNA sequence with different restriction enzymes, detecting the resulting restriction fragments by Southern blotting, and comparing their lengths.
C. Restriction fragment length polymorphisms (RFLPs) lead to variations in the length of DNA fragments produced by a particular restriction enzyme and vary from one individual to another.
D. RFLPs most commonly arise from two sources.
    1. Mutations that create or destroy a restriction site, thus changing the restriction map of the affected DNA region
        - This type of RFLP is the basis for detecting hereditary diseases.
    2. Differences in the number of tandem repeats in repetitive DNA, which is noncoding DNA scattered throughout the genome
        - This type of RFLP is the basis for DNA fingerprinting
E. Detection of RFLPs requires use of the appropriate restriction enzyme and probe for detecting the fragments (Fig. 11-8).
F. RFLP analysis can detect mutant alleles that are consistently associated with a particular polymorphism.

RFLPs: basis for detecting certain genetic diseases and for DNA fingerprinting

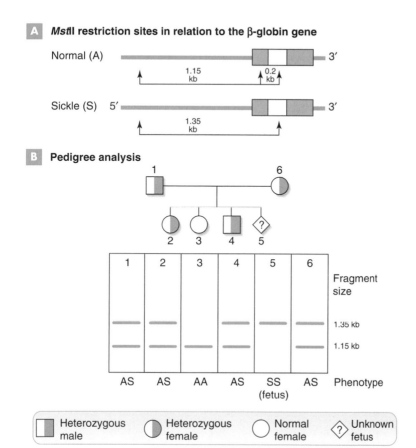

A *Mst*II restriction sites in relation to the β-globin gene

B Pedigree analysis

11-9: *RFLP analysis of sickle cell hemoglobin.* **A,** *Restriction map of a portion of the β-globin gene and an adjacent upstream sequence on chromosome 11. The normal chromosome (A) has three MstII restriction sites, producing two fragments of 1.15 and 0.2 kb on digestion. The sickle cell chromosome (S) lacks the interior MstII site and produces a single 1.35-kb fragment.* **B,** *Southern blots of MstII-digested samples from a family. The parents (1, 6) have two children (2, 4) with sickle cell trait and sought genetic testing regarding a current pregnancy. Homozygotes produce a single band (1.35 kb) and heterozygotes (sickle cell trait) produce two bands (1.15 and 1.35 kb) in the electrophoretic pattern. The single 1.35-kb band produced from fetal DNA (5) indicates that this fetus is homozygous for sickle cell hemoglobin and will develop sickle cell disease following birth.*

1. Sickle cell hemoglobin is an example of a disease-causing mutation that also alters a restriction site within a gene (Fig. 11-9).
   a. Normal, carrier, and affected individuals can be distinguished based on differences in the patterns of restriction fragments.
   b. Because polymorphism arises from the same mutation that causes the disease, the two are always associated.
2. Pedigree analysis may reveal linkage of a RFLP and a disease-producing mutation within a family, even when the nature of the genetic defect or the exact location of the affected gene is unknown.
   • The closer a linked RFLP marker is to the mutation of interest, the more likely that the two will be coinherited and the more accurate diagnosis, based on RFLP analysis, will be.

Sickle cell mutation alters a restriction site so that RFLP analysis can distinguish between affected, carrier, and normal individuals.

Common Laboratory Values

Test	Conventional Units	SI Units
Blood, Plasma, Serum		
Alanine aminotransferase (ALT, GPT at 30°C)	8–20 U/L	8–20 U/L
Amylase, serum	25–125 U/L	25–125 U/L
Aspartate aminotransferase (AST, GOT at 30°C)	8–20 U/L	8–20 U/L
Bilirubin, serum (adult): total; direct	0.1–1.0 mg/dL; 0.0–0.3 mg/dL	2–17 μmol/L; 0–5 μmol/L
Calcium, serum (Ca^{2+})	8.4–10.2 mg/dL	2.1–2.8 mmol/L
Cholesterol, serum	Rec: <200 mg/dL	<5.2 mmol/L
Cortisol, serum	8:00 AM: 6–23 μg/dL; 4:00 PM: 3–15 μg/dL 8:00 PM: ≤50% of 8:00 AM	170–630 nmol/L; 80–410 nmol/L Fraction of 8:00 AM: ≤0.50
Creatine kinase, serum	Male: 25–90 U/L Female: 10–70 U/L	25–90 U/L 10–70 U/L
Creatinine, serum	0.6–1.2 mg/dL	53–106 μmol/L
Electrolytes, serum		
Sodium (Na^+)	136–145 mEq/L	135–145 mmol/L
Chloride (Cl^-)	95–105 mEq/L	95–105 mmol/L
Potassium (K^+)	3.5–5.0 mEq/L	3.5–5.0 mmol/L
Bicarbonate (HCO_3^-)	22–28 mEq/L	22–28 mmol/L
Magnesium (Mg^{2+})	1.5–2.0 mEq/L	1.5–2.0 mmol/L
Estriol, total, serum (in pregnancy)		
24–28 wk; 32–36 wk	30–170 ng/mL; 60–280 ng/mL	104–590 nmol/L; 208–970 nmol/L
28–32 wk; 36–40 wk	40–220 ng/mL; 80–350 ng/mL	140–760 nmol/L; 280–1210 nmol/L
Ferritin, serum	Male: 15–200 ng/mL Female: 12–150 ng/mL	15–200 μg/L 12–150 μg/L

Follicle-stimulating hormone, serum/plasma (FSH)	Male: 4–25 mIU/mL
	Female:
	  Premenopause, 4–30 mIU/mL
	  Midcycle peak, 10–90 mIU/mL
	  Postmenopause, 40–250 mIU/mL
		4–25 U/L
		
		4–30 U/L
		10–90 U/L
		40–250 U/L

Gases, arterial blood (room air)		
pH	7.35–7.45	[H^+] 36–44 nmol/L
P_{CO_2}	33–45 mmHg	4.4–5.9 kPa
P_{O_2}	75–105 mmHg	10.0–14.0 kPa
Glucose, serum	Fasting: 70–110 mg/dL 2 hr postprandial: <120 mg/dL	3.8–6.1 mmol/L <6.6 mmol/L
Growth hormone–arginine stimulation	Fasting: <5 ng/mL Provocative stimuli: >7 ng/mL	<5 μg/L >7 μg/L

Test	Conventional Units	SI Units
Blood, Plasma, Serum—cont'd		
Immunoglobulins, serum		
IgA	76–390 mg/dL	0.76–3.90 g/L
IgE	0–380 IU/mL	0–380 kIU/L
IgG	650–1500 mg/dL	6.5–15 g/L
IgM	40–345 mg/dL	0.4–3.45 g/L
Iron	50–170 µg/dL	9–30 µmol/L
Lactate dehydrogenase, serum	45–90 U/L	45–90 U/L
Luteinizing hormone, serum/	Male: 6–23 mIU/mL	6–23 U/L
plasma (LH)	Female:	
	Follicular phase, 5–30 mIU/mL	5–30 U/L
	Midcycle, 75–150 mIU/mL	75–150 U/L
	Postmenopause, 30–200 mIU/mL	30–200 U/L
Osmolality, serum	275–295 mOsm/kg	275–295 mOsm/kg
Parathyroid hormone, serum,	230–630 pg/mL	230–630 ng/L
N-terminal		
Phosphatase (alkaline), serum	20–70 U/L	20–70 U/L
(p-NPP at 30°C)		
Phosphorus (inorganic), serum	3.0–4.5 mg/dL	1.0–1.5 mmol/L
Prolactin, serum (hPRL)	<20 ng/mL	<20 µg/L
Proteins, serum		
Total (recumbent)	6.0–8.0 g/dL	60–80 g/L
Albumin	3.5–5.5 g/dL	35–55 g/L
Globulin	2.3–3.5 g/dL	23–35 g/L
Thyroid-stimulating hormone,	0.5–5.0 µU/mL	0.5–5.0 mU/L
serum or plasma (TSH)		
Thyroidal iodine (^{123}I) uptake	8–30% of administered dose/24 hr	0.08–0.30/24 hr
Thyroxine (T_4), serum	4.5–12 µg/dL	58–154 nmol/L
Triglycerides, serum	35–160 mg/dL	0.4–1.81 mmol/L
Triiodothyronine (T_3), serum (RIA)	115–190 ng/dL	1.8–2.9 nmol/L
Triiodothyronine (T_3) resin uptake	25–38%	0.25–0.38
Urea nitrogen, serum (BUN)	7–18 mg/dL	1.2–3.0 mmol urea/L
Uric acid, serum	3.0–8.2 mg/dL	0.18–0.48 mmol/L
Cerebrospinal Fluid		
Cell count	0–5 cells/mm³	0–5 × 10⁶/L
Chloride	118–132 mEq/L	118–132 mmol/L
Gamma globulin	3–12% total proteins	0.03–0.12
Glucose	50–75 mg/dL	2.8–4.2 mmol/L
Pressure	70–180 mm H₂O	70–180 mm H₂O
Proteins, total	<40 mg/dL	<0.40 g/L
Hematology		
Bleeding time (template)	2–7 min	2–7 min
Erythrocyte count	Male: 4.3–5.9 million/mm³	4.3–5.9 × 10¹²/L
	Female: 3.5–5.5 million/mm³	3.5–5.5 × 10¹²/L
Erythrocyte sedimentation rate	Male: 0–15 mm/hr	0–15 mm/hr
(Westergren)	Female: 0–20 mm/hr	0–20 mm/hr
Hematocrit (Hct)	Male: 40–54%	0.40–0.54
	Female: 37–47%	0.37–0.47

continued

Test	Conventional Units	SI Units
Hematology—cont'd		
Hemoglobin A_{IC}	≤6%	≤ 0.06%
Hemoglobin, blood (Hb)	Male: 13.5–17.5 g/dL	2.09–2.71 mmol/L
	Female: 12.0–16.0 g/dL	1.86–2.48 mmol/L
Hemoglobin, plasma	1–4 mg/dL	0.16–0.62 mmol/L
Leukocyte count and differential		
Leukocyte count	4500–11,000/mm³	$4.5–11.0 \times 10^9$/L
Segmented neutrophils	54–62%	0.54–0.62
Bands	3–5%	0.03–0.05
Eosinophils	1–3%	0.01–0.03
Basophils	0–0.75%	0–0.0075
Lymphocytes	25–33%	0.25–0.33
Monocytes	3–7%	0.03–0.07
Mean corpuscular hemoglobin (MCH)	25.4–34.6 pg/cell	0.39–0.54 fmol/cell
Mean corpuscular hemoglobin concentration (MCHC)	31–37% Hb/cell	4.81–5.74 mmol Hb/L
Mean corpuscular volume (MCV)	80–100 µm³	80–100 fl
Partial thromboplastin time (activated) (aPTT)	25–40 sec	25–40 sec
Platelet count	150,000–400,000/mm³	$150–400 \times 10^9$/L
Prothrombin time (PT)	12–14 sec	12–14 sec
Reticulocyte count	0.5–1.5% of red cells	0.005–0.015
Thrombin time	<2 sec deviation from control	<2 sec deviation from control
Volume		
Plasma	Male: 25–43 mL/kg	0.025–0.043 L/kg
	Female: 28–45 mL/kg	0.028–0.045 L/kg
Red cell	Male: 20–36 mL/kg	0.020–0.036 L/kg
	Female: 19–31 mL/kg	0.019–0.031 L/kg
Sweat		
Chloride	0–35 mmol/L	0–35 mmol/L
Urine		
Calcium	100–300 mg/24 hr	2.5–7.5 mmol/24 hr
Creatinine clearance	Male: 97–137 mL/min	
	Female: 88–128 mL/min	
Estriol, total (in pregnancy)		
30 wk	6–18 mg/24 hr	21–62 µmol/24 hr
35 wk	9–28 mg/24 hr	31–97 µmol/24 hr
40 wk	13–42 mg/24 hr	45–146 µmol/24 hr
17-Hydroxycorticosteroids	Male: 3.0–9.0 mg/24 hr	8.2–25.0 µmol/24 hr
	Female: 2.0–8.0 mg/24 hr	5.5–22.0 µmol/24 hr
17-Ketosteroids, total	Male: 8–22 mg/24 hr	28–76 µmol/24 hr
	Female: 6–15 mg/24 hr	21–52 µmol/24 hr
Osmolality	50–1400 mOsm/kg	
Oxalate	8–40 µg/mL	90–445 µmol/L
Proteins, total	<150 mg/24 hr	<0.15 g/24 hr

questions

DIRECTIONS: Each numbered item or incomplete statement is followed by options arranged in alphabetical or logical order. Select the best answer to each question. Some options may be partially correct, but there is only **ONE BEST** answer.

1. A pregnant woman spontaneously aborts a fetus at 24 weeks' gestation. The woman and her husband are both of Asian descent, and both have a mild microcytic anemia. Hemoglobin electrophoresis of blood taken from the heart of the fetus has tetramers composed entirely of γ-globin chains. Which of the following types of hemoglobinopathy do the parents most likely have?
   A. Hemoglobin H (HbH) disease
   B. Mild α-thalassemia
   C. Mild β-thalassemia
   D. Sickle cell trait

2. Soon after a 35-year-old African American man begins taking primaquine, his blood studies show a decrease in hemoglobin, an increase in circulating reticulocytes, and hemoglobinuria. Which of the following best explains the decrease in hemoglobin?
   A. Abnormality in the β-globin chain
   B. Defect in α-globin chain synthesis
   C. Deficiency of glucose 6-phosphate dehydrogenase (G6PD)
   D. Deficiency of pyruvate kinase
   E. Increase in glutathione

3. A 48-year-old man with cirrhosis of the liver is not oriented to time or place. After he is placed on a low-protein diet, he experiences some improvement in mental status. Which of the following enzymes is partially responsible for these abnormalities in mental status?

   A. Arginase
   B. Argininosuccinate lyase
   C. Argininosuccinate synthetase
   D. Carbamoyl phosphate synthetase I
   E. Ornithine carbamoyltransferase

4. When exercising, a 19-year-old man develops painful cramps that are associated with acute episodes of myoglobinuria. Administration of oral glucose during the acute episodes does not alleviate the symptoms. Additional studies show that a hemolytic anemia is also present. The patient most likely has a deficiency of which of the following enzymes?
   A. Branching enzyme
   B. Glucose-6-phosphatase
   C. α-Glucosidase
   D. Liver phosphorylase
   E. Phosphofructokinase (PFK)

5. A 57-year-old woman with a recent history of renal calculi is brought to the emergency department because of polydipsia, polyuria, and confusion. She has hypercalcemia and a suspected parathyroid adenoma. Which metabolic consequence often associated with a functioning parathyroid adenoma is decreased?
   A. Absorption of calcium across the intestinal mucosa
   B. Rate of calcium deposition in bone tissue
   C. Synthesis of cholecalciferol from 7-dehydrocholesterol

D. Synthesis of 1,25-dihydroxycholecalciferol from 25-hydroxycholecalciferol

E. Synthesis of 24,25-dihydroxycholecalciferol from 25-hydroxycholecalciferol

6. Which of the following enzymes is believed to be most responsible for the development of cataracts in individuals with diabetes mellitus?
A. Aldolase B
B. Aldose reductase
C. Glucose 6-phosphate dehydrogenase (G6PD)
D. Sorbitol dehydrogenase

7. A 23-year-old woman has just eaten a meal consisting mainly of carbohydrates. Which of the following best describes the activity of capillary lipoprotein lipase and hormone-sensitive lipase in the adipose tissue of this individual?

	Capillary Lipoprotein Lipase	Hormone-Sensitive Lipase
A.	Decreased	Decreased
B.	Decreased	Increased
C.	Increased	Decreased
D.	Increased	Increased

8. Which of the following statements best describes the conditions under which an enzymatic reaction is most likely to occur at maximum velocity (V_{max})?
A. An allosteric activator is present.
B. The amount of enzyme is greater than the amount of substrate.
C. The concentration of the substrate exceeds that of a noncompetitive inhibitor.
D. The enzyme is saturated with substrate.
E. The temperature of the reaction medium is increased.

9. A neonatal nurse notices that the urine produced by a newborn infant has the odor of maple syrup. Which of the following biochemical reactions is most likely defective?
A. Metabolism of aromatic amino acids
B. Metabolism of branched-chain amino acids
C. Metabolism of sulfur-containing amino acids

D. One-carbon transfer reactions
E. Transformation of carbohydrates to amino acids

10. A 1-year-old boy has progressively worsening chronic liver disease and hypotonia. His urine is negative for reducing substances. Which of the following enzymes associated with carbohydrate metabolism is the most likely cause of this child's condition?
A. Aldolase B
B. Galactose 1-phosphate uridyltransferase
C. Glucose 6-phosphatase
D. Glucosyl (4:6) transferase
E. Liver phosphorylase

11. A 28-year-old man has a family history of a disabling disorder that has caused the deaths of his father, grandfather, and two paternal aunts. The father and aunts died at a younger age than did his grandfather, and it appears that the condition progressively worsens with each generation. Which of the following disorders is most likely?
A. Cystic fibrosis
B. Duchenne's muscular dystrophy
C. Huntington's disease
D. Metachromatic leukodystrophy
E. Parkinson's disease

12. A 62-year-old woman whose husband died recently subsists on a diet consisting of cereal and diet cola. She complains of bleeding gums after brushing her teeth and pain in her legs when she walks. Physical examination shows a smooth red tongue, gingivitis, carious teeth, scattered ecchymoses over the trunk, and pinpoint areas of hemorrhage around the hair follicles. The micronutrient deficiency that accounts for these physical findings involves which of the following steps in collagen synthesis?
A. Cleavage of N- and C-terminal propeptide fragments
B. Formation of pro-α-chains
C. Glycosylation of side chain residues

D. Hydroxylation of proline and lysine side chains

E. Triple helix assembly of procollagen

13. The parents of a 3-month-old boy bring the boy to the pediatrician because he is lethargic and has a swollen abdomen. Physical examination shows that the boy has massive hepatomegaly and enlarged kidneys, with a normal spleen and heart. Laboratory studies are notable for hypoglycemia. Biopsy of muscle and liver shows excess glycogen in liver tissue but not in muscle tissue. A glycogen storage disease is suspected. Which of the following best explains the presence of excess glycogen in the liver?

A. Glucokinase absent in liver tissue

B. Glucose 6-phosphatase absent in liver tissue

C. Lack of glycogen synthase in muscle tissue

D. Lack of phosphorylase in liver tissue

14. An inhibitor of the rate-limiting enzyme of cholesterol synthesis would most likely reduce blood cholesterol by which of the following mechanisms?

A. Increasing the conversion of cholesterol to bile acids

B. Inhibiting the formation of HMG CoA

C. Inhibiting the formation of mevalonate

D. Preventing bile acids from being reabsorbed from the intestine

E. Preventing cholesterol from being reabsorbed from the intestine

15. A 52-year-old man with chronic alcoholism has a plasma lipid profile that contains an increase in very low-density lipoprotein (VLDL). The mechanism that best explains the increase in VLDL in both the blood and the liver in chronic alcoholics is

A. Impaired function of apolipoprotein B-100

B. Inactivation of capillary lipoprotein lipase

C. Increased β-oxidation of fatty acids

D. Increased synthesis of glycerol 3-phosphate

16. A healthy adult is placed on a diet that lacks tyrosine but is otherwise balanced. As a result of this diet, nitrogen balance is most likely to

A. Be achieved

B. Become negative

C. Become positive

D. Progress from a negative at equilibrium

E. Progress from a positive at equilibrium

17. A long-distance runner who is planning to run a marathon decides to add fructose to the replacement fluid she will be using during the race. Which of the following statements regarding fructose best describes the fate of this sugar?

A. It enters the glycolytic pathway as fructose 6-phosphate in the liver.

B. It is converted to uridine diphosphate (UDP)-fructose and then epimerized to UDP-glucose.

C. It is metabolized by a pathway other than the glycolytic pathway.

D. It is metabolized in the liver by an aldolase that recognizes fructose 1-phosphate.

E. It is phosphorylated by phosphofructokinase.

18. A 52-year-old man with chronic bronchitis requires continuous supplementary O_2 to maintain an adequate arterial P_{O_2}. Which of the following improves O_2 delivery to this patient's tissues?

A. Decreased arterial pH

B. Decreased red blood cell 2,3-bisphosphoglycerate (2,3-BPG)

C. Decreased temperature

D. Hyperventilation

19. A 25-year-old woman in her second postoperative day after an appendectomy has not eaten since the surgery. Which of the following enzymes is most likely in an inactive state in this patient?

A. Glycogen phosphorylase

B. Glycogen phosphorylase kinase

C. Glycogen synthase

D. Phosphoenolpyruvate carboxykinase

E. Phosphoglucomutase

20. A cell culture of a tumor biopsy is suspected of containing a *ras* oncogene. Which of the

following proteins should be analyzed to confirm this diagnosis?
A. G protein
B. Growth factor
C. Growth factor receptor
D. Nuclear transcription factor

21. A 25-year-old man is found in a semicomatose state and is taken to the emergency department by friends, who say that the man has not eaten for the past 5 days. Which of the following substances has most likely been this patient's primary source of glucose?
A. Amino acids from liver proteins
B. Amino acids from muscle proteins
C. Fatty acids from adipose tissue
D. Glycogen from muscle tissue

22. A 4-year-old child with normal mentation has loss of pigmentation in the skin, hair, and eyes. The patient most likely has a deficiency of which of the following enzymes?
A. Aldolase B
B. Homogentisate oxidase
C. Phenylalanine hydroxylase
D. Tyrosinase

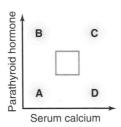

23. A 58-year-old man who has had a total thyroidectomy for a follicular carcinoma of the thyroid complains of muscle twitching. When the patient's blood pressure is being taken, he adducts his thumb into his palm; when his facial nerve is tapped, the muscles of his face twitch. Which of the areas marked on the graph (indicated by the letters A, B, C, and D) represents the most likely levels of parathyroid hormone (PTH) and calcium in this patient?

A. Area A
B. Area B
C. Area C
D. Area D

24. A 19-year-old woman has had to change her prescription for eye glasses three times in the past 6 weeks because of blurry vision that develops soon after she begins wearing the new prescription. She also complains of weight loss, increased appetite, and urinary frequency. Her blood pH is 7.2. Recently, she has noticed a fruity odor to her breath. Which of the following would provide the best information about the cause of this patient's vision problems?
A. Hemoglobin A_{1c}
B. Serum thyroid-stimulating hormone (TSH)
C. Urine dipstick test for glucose
D. Urine dipstick test for ketones

25. A pregnant woman asks her physician about her ability to lactate. She has galactosemia and is unable to consume galactose. Which of the following enzymes would allow the woman to lactate normally?
A. Aldolase B
B. Galactokinase
C. Galactose 1-phosphate uridyltransferase
D. Lactase
E. UDP-hexose epimerase

26. A 3-month-old boy has rapidly progressive central nervous system deterioration, spasticity, and failure to thrive. Physical examination is significant for marked hepatosplenomegaly. Liver biopsy shows an increase of sphingomyelin in the lysosomes. Which of the following enzymes is most likely to be deficient in this infant?
A. Arylsulfatase A
B. Hexosaminidase A
C. Liver phosphorylase
D. Sphingomyelinase

27. In the fasting state, which of the following statements about cAMP best describes its mechanism of action?
A. It activates adenylate cyclase when complexed with the α-subunit of G_S protein.

B. It activates protein kinase A to become a regulator of enzymes by phosphorylation.

C. It binds calcium to activate several cellular enzymes.

D. It binds to receptors on the endoplasmic reticulum, causing calcium to be released into the cytoplasm.

E. It increases the activity of membrane-bound protein kinase C.

28. A 1-year-old child with mental retardation has a deficiency of dihydrobiopterin reductase. This enzyme deficiency is most closely related to which of the following disorders?

A. Galactosemia

B. Maple syrup urine disease

C. Niemann-Pick disease

D. Phenylketonuria (PKU)

E. Wilson's disease

29. A routine physical examination of a 22-year-old woman shows mild splenomegaly. Laboratory studies show a mild normocytic anemia with an increased number of peripheral blood reticulocytes, red blood cells (RBCs) with no central areas of pallor, and an increased mean corpuscular hemoglobin concentration. This patient most likely has an RBC defect that involves which of the following RBC proteins?

A. Actin

B. β-Amyloid

C. Hemoglobin

D. Spectrin

30. A 24-year-old woman with poorly controlled type 1 diabetes mellitus prematurely delivers a large-for-gestational-age infant. Within 6 hours, the newborn develops respiratory difficulties associated with tachypnea and cyanosis. The mechanism for the newborn's increased size at birth is primarily a result in an increase in which of the following hormones?

A. Growth hormone

B. Insulin

C. Prolactin

D. Thyroxine

31. A 28-year-old contractor builds fences using wood treated with a preservative that prevents the wood from rotting and deters infestation by termites. He is currently experiencing muscle weakness and generalized fatigue. The physician finds that the man has been handling wood treated with pentachloro-phenol. Which of the following is the target for this chemical?

A. ATP synthase

B. Cytochrome oxidase

C. Mitochondrial proton pump

D. NADH dehydrogenase

E. Succinate dehydrogenase

32. A 25-year-old woman sees her physician because of exhaustion and diarrhea. Physical examination shows that she has low blood pressure, and blood studies show that she is anemic. Other studies show that she has a tumor of the pituitary gland. An intravenous drip of adrenocorticotropic hormone (ACTH) fails to increase the concentration of urine 17-hydroxycorticoids. The rate-limiting step stimulated by ACTH involves the formation of

A. Cortisol from cholic acid

B. 7-Dehydrocholesterol from cholesterol

C. Mevalonate from HMG CoA

D. Pregnenolone from cholesterol

E. Progesterone from pregnenolone

33. A 24-year-old body builder sees his physician because of a rash, abdominal discomfort, and diarrhea. When questioned about his diet, he admits that he eats approximately 20 raw eggs per day. Which of the following enzymes is most likely dysfunctional?

A. Alanine aminotransferase

B. Lactate dehydrogenase

C. Malate dehydrogenase

D. Pyruvate carboxylase

E. Pyruvate kinase

34. Which of the following groups of enzymes is most involved in the disposal of excess nitrogen from protein in the diet?

A. Amino acid oxidases and arginase

B. Argininosuccinate lyase and cytosolic carbamoyl phosphate synthetase II
C. Glutaminase and amino acid oxidases
D. Glutamine synthetase and urease
E. Transaminases and glutamate dehydrogenase

35. A 5-year-old boy is deaf and has a history of multiple fractures since birth. Physical examination shows a bluish discoloration of the sclera. The patient most likely has a deficiency of
A. Fibrillin
B. α-L-Iduronidase
C. Type I collagen
D. Type III collagen

36. A 3-year-old girl, who is listless approximately 4 hours after eating, is found to have a deficiency of carnitine. Which of the following substrates is the child's primary energy source?
A. Branched-chain amino acids
B. Fatty acids
C. Fructose
D. Glucose
E. Ketone bodies

37. A 28-year-old prisoner decides to go on a hunger strike, and after 1 week a guard notices that the woman's breath has a fruity odor. Which of the following compounds is the rate-limiting enzyme for the process that accounts for the peculiar odor on this woman's breath?
A. Citrate synthase
B. HMG CoA reductase
C. HMG CoA synthase
D. β-Ketothiolase
E. Pyruvate carboxylase

38. A 24-year-old man who recently came to the United States from China complains of shortness of breath. Physical examination shows bibasilar rales, neck vein distention, dependent pitting edema, and footdrop. A chest radiograph shows generalized cardiomegaly and diffuse pulmonary infiltrates. Which of the following enzymes is most likely dysfunctional?
A. Aspartate aminotransferase
B. Isocitrate dehydrogenase

C. Pyruvate carboxylase
D. Transaldolase
E. Transketolase

39. A 28-year-old woman with Cushing's syndrome has hyperglycemia. Which of the following enzymes is most likely causing the hyperglycemia?
A. Aspartate aminotransferase
B. Capillary lipoprotein lipase
C. Phosphoenolpyruvate carboxykinase
D. Pyruvate carboxylase
E. Pyruvate dehydrogenase

40. A 55-year-old man has significantly reduced reabsorption of bile salts resulting from the action of bile salt-binding resins. This is expected to lead to a significant decrease in which of the following steroid compounds?
A. Aldosterone
B. Cholesterol
C. Cortisol
D. Pregnenolone
E. Progesterone

41. A 42-year-old man who works in a battery factory complains of fatigue, headaches, abdominal pain, and chronic diarrhea. Laboratory studies show a hemoglobin of 10 g/dL and a mean corpuscular volume (MCV) of 75 μm^3. A peripheral blood smear shows hypochromic RBCs with coarse basophilic stippling. Which of the following is an additional expected laboratory finding?
A. Decreased serum ferritin
B. Decreased zinc RBC protoporphyrin
C. Increased hemoglobin A_2 (HbA$_2$) and hemoglobin F (HbF)
D. Increased urinary δ-aminolevulinic acid (ALA)

42. A 5-year-old African American girl with sickle cell disease has been treated with hydroxyurea in an attempt to increase the concentration of hemoglobin F in her RBCs. Increased hemoglobin F would most likely act in which of the following ways?

A. Bind more oxygen than sickle β-globin chains

B. Bind more tightly to 2,3-bisphosphoglycerate than sickle β-globin chains

C. Form nonpolymerizing tetramers

D. Prevent the formation of linear aggregates with sickle cell tetramers

43. A 3-month-old boy has progressive hepatomegaly and mild fasting hypoglycemia. Laboratory studies show that when the boy is fasting, lactic acidosis is absent. A biopsy of liver tissue shows that the glycogen granules have an abnormal structure. The patient most likely has a deficiency of which of the following enzymes?

A. Branching enzyme

B. Debranching enzyme

C. Glucose 6-phosphatase

D. α-Glucosidase

E. Liver phosphorylase

44. A 38-year-old woman with chronic alcoholism has been homeless for the past year. Her diet consists primarily of starchy processed "junk" foods, in addition to alcoholic beverages. Physical examination shows noticeably thickened skin and the presence of hyperkeratotic hair follicles. The conjunctivae are dry, and tear production is reduced. Which of the following findings might also be expected?

A. Bleeding gums

B. Hemolytic anemia

C. Impaired night vision

D. Osteomalacia

E. Pain in the long bones

45. A 25-year-old man who has been homeless for several months is admitted to the hospital in a state of starvation. He has not eaten anything in the past week. He is started on a diet in which 60% of the calories come from carbohydrates. This diet would most likely increase the activity of which of the following enzymes?

A. Carnitine acyltransferase

B. Citrate synthase

C. Glucokinase

D. Glucose 6-phosphatase

E. HMG CoA synthase

46. Routine blood studies on an infant show turbid plasma with markedly elevated levels of triacylglycerol. A sample of plasma that has been left in a refrigerator overnight has cream-colored material floating on top. The underlying plasma is clear. Which type of hyperlipoproteinemia is most likely present in this infant?

A. Type I

B. Type IIa

C. Type IIb

D. Type III

E. Type IV

47. A 1-year-old male child is brought to the pediatrician because his parents have noticed that the boy is mutilating himself by chewing on his lips. On examination, the child is found to be mentally retarded and manifesting signs of gouty arthritis. Which of the following enzymes involved in nucleoside metabolism is most likely deficient in this child?

A. Adenosine deaminase

B. Hypoxanthine-guanine phosphoribosyltransferase (HGPRT)

C. Phosphoribosylpyrophosphate synthase

D. Thymidine kinase

E. Xanthine oxidase

48. A 43-year-old man with chronic renal failure who requires hemodialysis complains of generalized bone pain. Physical examination shows bowing of the legs and a sallow complexion. When the man's blood pressure is taken, his thumb flexes into his palm. A radiograph of the bones shows generalized osteopenia. The patient most likely has a deficiency of which of the following vitamins?

A. Niacin

B. Thiamine

C. Vitamin A

D. Vitamin D

E. Vitamin K

49. A 3-year-old child shows signs of mental deterioration and skeletal deformities. Microscopic and laboratory analyses show enlarged lysosomes and increased levels of lysosomal enzymes in the serum. These findings are most likely caused by a defect in which of the following processes?

A. Gene amplification
B. Mannose 6-phosphate attachment
C. Nuclear localization signal
D. Transferrin receptor mRNA

50. A 4-year-old girl has a mild chronic hemolytic anemia that is also present in other family members of both sexes, including cousins, aunts, and uncles. Determination of the P_{50} for hemoglobin shows an oxygen-binding curve with a pronounced right shift (see figure). Which of the following enzymes is most likely to be deficient in this patient?

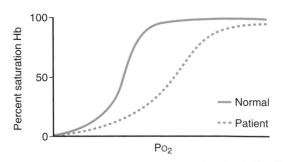

A. Glucose 6-phosphate dehydrogenase (G6PD)
B. Phosphoglucomutase
C. Pyruvate dehydrogenase
D. Pyruvate kinase

answers

1. **B** (mild α-thalassemia) is correct. The fetus died of hemoglobin Bart's disease. Hemoglobin Bart's is composed of tetramers of γ-globin chains because the formation of $\alpha_2\gamma_2$ tetramers is prevented. In Asians, the cause of most microcytic anemias is α-thalassemia, an autosomal recessive disorder. Both parents must have had two gene deletions for α-globin chain synthesis on the same chromosome, resulting in a fetus with no genes for α-globin chains.

   A (hemoglobin H disease) is incorrect. HbH disease is associated with a severe hemolytic anemia; neither of the parents have had this anemia. Individuals with HbH disease have a deletion of three of the four genes necessary for normal α-globin chain synthesis. HbH is composed entirely of β_4 tetramers.

   C (mild β-thalassemia) is incorrect. β-Thalassemia, an autosomal recessive disease, primarily affects Italians, Greeks, and African Americans. It is associated with a decrease in β-globin chain synthesis and is most often caused by defects in DNA splicing. In mild β-thalassemia, HbA is decreased $(\alpha_2\beta_2)$, allowing the excess α-globin chains to combine with δ-globin chains to form HbA_2 and with γ-globin chains to form HbF.

   D (sickle cell trait) is incorrect. Sickle cell trait and sickle cell disease rarely, if ever, affect Asians. Sickle cell trait does not produce anemia, whereas sickle cell disease produces a severe normocytic anemia.

2. **C** (deficiency of glucose 6-phosphate dehydrogenase) is correct. G6PD catalyzes the first step in the pentose phosphate pathway, which is a major source of NADPH in many cells and the sole source of NADPH in RBCs. NADPH is used to regenerate glutathione, particularly in times of oxidative stress. Such stress often occurs with the administration of certain drugs (e.g., primaquine and dapsone). Administration of these drugs to a patient with G6PD deficiency results in severe oxidant damage to the hemoglobin in erythrocytes (formation of Heinz bodies), leading to hemolytic anemia and hemoglobinuria.

   A (abnormality in the β-globin chain) is incorrect. This feature is characteristic of several diseases, including sickle cell disease or sickle cell trait, hemoglobin C disease, and β-thalassemia. These hemolytic diseases are typically not caused by the use of medications.

   B (defect in α-globin chain synthesis) is incorrect. This feature describes α-thalassemia, a hemolytic disease that can vary in severity depending on the number of hemoglobin α genes affected. No form of the disease, regardless of severity, is particularly exacerbated by exposure to drugs.

   D (deficiency of pyruvate kinase) is incorrect. Pyruvate kinase is responsible for the conversion of phosphoenolpyruvate to pyruvate, an irreversible step in glycolysis. A deficiency of this enzyme would result in a halt of all glycolysis, the only source of

ATP for the erythrocytes. A hemolytic anemia, which is not exacerbated by drugs, develops.

E (increase in glutathione) is incorrect. Glutathione is consumed in times of oxidative stress, such as those induced by the administration of primaquine. This patient has insufficient levels of glutathione (none regenerated) to prevent oxidative damage to the erythrocytes by peroxide and peroxide free radicals.

3. **D** (carbamoyl phosphate synthetase I) is correct. This patient is suffering from hepatic encephalopathy, which is most likely induced by a high-protein diet. The excess nitrogen waste from protein is usually handled by the liver (urea cycle), which is damaged in this patient. The ammonia from protein degradation by urease-producing organisms in the bowel is converted to urea in the liver via the urea cycle. The rate-limiting step is the synthesis of carbamoyl phosphate from NH_3 and CO_2, which is catalyzed by carbamoyl phosphate synthetase I. Because the urea cycle is dysfunctional, blood NH_3 levels increase and blood urea nitrogen decreases. A low-protein diet decreases the amount of NH_3 that the urea cycle must metabolize.

A (arginase) is incorrect. Arginase helps cleave arginine to produce ornithine and urea.

B (argininosuccinate lyase) is incorrect. Argininosuccinate lyase catalyzes the conversion of argininosuccinate to arginine and fumarate.

C (argininosuccinate synthetase) is incorrect. Argininosuccinate synthetase catalyzes the condensation of aspartate and citrulline to form argininosuccinate.

E (ornithine carbamoyltransferase) is incorrect. Ornithine transcarbamoylase catalyzes the condensation of ornithine and carbamoyl phosphate to form citrulline.

4. **E** (phosphofructokinase) is correct. PFK, the rate-limiting enzyme of glycolysis, converts fructose 6-phosphate to fructose 1,6-bisphosphate. Deficiency of PFK mimics the painful cramps seen in patients with McArdle's disease. The disease is caused by a deficiency of muscle phosphorylase and inability to generate glucose from glycogen, thus depriving the muscle of an energy source and leading to rhabdomyolysis with concomitant myoglobinuria during exercise. Deficiency of PFK does not alter glycogenolysis. However, the glucose that is produced cannot be used for energy; the muscle reacts during exercise in a similar fashion to McArdle's disease. In general, enzyme deficiencies involving glycolysis lead to hemolytic anemias. Red blood cells rely on anaerobic glycolysis for ATP and therefore hemolyze.

A (branching enzyme) is incorrect. A deficiency of branching enzyme leads to Andersen's disease, a glycogen storage disease. The characteristic abnormal branching pattern is believed to lead to cirrhosis of the liver. Affected patients typically present with failure to thrive within the first 18 months of life and die by 5 years of age.

B (glucose 6-phosphatase) is incorrect. A deficiency of glucose 6-phosphatase, a gluconeogenic enzyme, leads to von Gierke's disease, a glycogen storage disease that affects the liver and kidneys. Children with this disease typically present at 3 or 4 months of age with massive hepatorenomegaly and fasting hypoglycemia.

C (α-glucosidase) is incorrect. A deficiency of α-glucosidase, a lysosomal enzyme that degrades glycogen, leads to Pompe's disease, a lysosomal glycogen storage disease. This disorder is generalized to all tissues, with the heart being the most vulnerable organ. Different manifestations of this disease are characteristic of different age groups. The prognosis is usually worse if the onset of symptoms occurs at an earlier age.

D (liver phosphorylase) is incorrect. A deficiency of liver phosphorylase leads to Hers' disease, a rare glycogen storage disease that initially manifests in childhood as hepatomegaly, growth retardation, and fasting hypoglycemia. Symptoms improve with age and typically disappear by puberty.

5. **B** (rate of calcium deposition in bone tissue) is correct. Parathyroid hormone (PTH) helps maintain normal calcium levels in extracellular fluid by mobilizing calcium from bone. In the kidneys, PTH stimulates the synthesis of 1,25-dihydroxycholecalciferol, which increases calcium absorption across the intestinal mucosa. PTH also increases reuptake of calcium from urine in the distal nephrons. Increased levels of PTH exaggerate both these processes.

A (absorption of calcium across the intestinal mucosa) is incorrect. PTH stimulates the uptake of calcium by the intestine indirectly by triggering the production of 1,25-dihydroxychole-calciferol in the kidneys.

C (synthesis of cholecalciferol from 7-dehydro-cholesterol) is incorrect. The exposure of skin to sunlight triggers synthesis of 7-dehydro-cholesterol. Hormones do not regulate its production.

D (synthesis of 1,25-dihydroxycholecalciferol from 25-hydroxycholecalciferol) is incorrect. PTH stimulates the action of 1-α-hydroxylase in the kidneys, which produces 1,25-dihydroxycholecalciferol from 25-hydroxycholecalciferol. Therefore, serum levels of this substance should increase in this patient.

E (synthesis of 24,25-dihydroxycholecalciferol from 25-hydroxycholecalciferol) is incorrect. PTH stimulates synthesis of 24,25-dihydroxycholecalciferol from 25-

hydroxycholecalciferol indirectly, primarily via increased levels of 1,25-dihydroxycholecal-ciferol. This action likely serves as a means of controlling levels of the active form of vitamin D.

6. **B** (aldose reductase) is correct. Aldose reductase catalyzes the conversion of glucose to sorbitol, which is normally converted to fructose under the influence of sorbitol dehydrogenase. The rate of sorbitol synthesis is increased in the ocular lenses of patients with diabetes mellitus; glucose can readily diffuse into the eye without the need for insulin. The increase in sorbitol concentration in the lens has a strong osmotic effect and "pulls" water into cells, causing them to swell. This action leads to alterations in the refractive index and eventually to formation of cataracts.

A (aldolase B) is incorrect. Aldolase B is responsible for the decondensation of fructose 1-phosphate to glyceraldehyde and dihydroxyacetone phosphate. A deficiency of the enzyme results in hereditary fructose intolerance.

C (glucose 6-phosphate dehydrogenase) is incorrect. G6PD catalyzes the first and irreversible step of the pentose phosphate pathway (i.e., conversion of glucose 6-phosphate to 6-phosphogluconate). A deficiency of G6PD results in a hemolytic anemia.

D (sorbitol dehydrogenase) is incorrect. Sorbitol dehydrogenase catalyzes the conversion of sorbitol to fructose. It is present in the seminal vesicles to provide fructose for spermatozoa.

7. **C** (increased capillary lipoprotein lipase; decreased hormone-sensitive lipase) is correct. In the well-fed state, insulin stimulates the synthesis of capillary lipoprotein lipase, and apolipoprotein C-II activates the enzyme.

These actions result in hydrolysis of circulating chylomicrons derived from the diet and VLDL synthesized in the liver, causing the release of fatty acids and monoglycerides. Insulin inactivates hormone-sensitive lipase in adipose tissue by activating phosphatase, which dephosphorylates the enzyme.

A (both capillary lipoprotein lipase and hormone-sensitive lipase are decreased) and **D** (both capillary lipoprotein lipase and hormone-sensitive lipase are increased) are incorrect. Neither type of lipase in the adipose tissue of this individual is decreased or increased at the same time since capillary lipoprotein lipase is associated with fat storage and hormone-sensitive lipase is associated with fat mobilization.

B (decreased capillary lipoprotein lipase and increased hormone-sensitive lipase) is incorrect. In the fasting state, capillary lipoprotein lipase activity is decreased, whereas hormone-sensitive lipase is increased via activation by epinephrine and the absence of insulin. This releases fatty acids and glycerol into the circulation.

8. **D** (the enzyme is saturated with substrate) is correct. This is the theoretical explanation for the definition of maximal velocity (V_{max}): The V_{max} of a catalyzed reaction is observed at constant enzyme concentration and with increased substrate concentration. Typically, the V_{max} of a reaction is observed for some given concentration of substrate at which all catalytic sites are occupied. Increases beyond that substrate concentration do not lead to further increases in reaction velocity.

A (an allosteric activator is present) is incorrect. An allosteric activator, a substance that binds to an enzyme at a site other than the active site, may increase the affinity with which the enzyme binds the substrate, the rate of substrate turnover, or both. Unless the concentration of substrate is high enough,

however, enzymatic reactions occur at less than V_{max}.

B (the amount of enzyme is greater than the amount of substrate) is incorrect. As noted in the discussion for option A, an enzymatic reaction occurs at V_{max} when the enzyme is fully saturated with substrate.

C (the concentration of substrate exceeds that of a noncompetitive inhibitor) is incorrect. A noncompetitive inhibitor binds an enzyme at a site other than the active site and prevents a reaction from occurring. V_{max} is always decreased with noncompetitive inhibitors, whereas the K_m remains the same. It is important to note that (1) increasing the concentration of substrate does not return the reaction velocity to its original V_{max}, and (2) substrate concentration and inhibitor concentration are totally independent, meaning that the ratio of substrate to inhibitor has no bearing on the substrate concentration required for the reaction to attain its new, lower V_{max}.

E (the temperature of the reaction medium is increased) is incorrect. The rate of enzymatic activity is increased by an increase in temperature, as is V_{max}. Thus, unless the substrate concentration is sufficient to reach V_{max} before the increase in temperature, the reaction still occurs at less than V_{max}.

9. **B** (metabolism of branched-chain amino acids) is correct. A defect in the oxidation of the branched-chain amino acids valine, leucine, and isoleucine (all of which are essential amino acids) leads to a buildup of the corresponding α-keto acids. The accumulation of these acids in the urine leads to its pathognomonic maple syrup odor.

A (metabolism of aromatic amino acids) is incorrect. The aromatic amino acids phenylalanine, tyrosine, and tryptophan, which are primarily increased in chronic liver disease, contribute to the mental status abnormalities associated with hepatic encephalopathy. Branched-chain amino acids are used to reduce the effect of the aromatic amino acids in patients with chronic liver disease.

C (metabolism of sulfur-containing amino acids) is incorrect. This action would be more likely with homocystinuria, which is caused by a deficiency of cystathionine synthetase. Homocystinuria is characterized by mental retardation, osteoporosis, and lens dislocation.

D (one-carbon transfer reactions) is incorrect. This is seen most often in cases of folate deficiency. Tetrahydrofolate transfers methylene groups ($-CH_2-$) to serine to produce 5,10-methylene tetrahydrofolate, which in turn transfers the methylene group to deoxyuridine monophosphate to produce deoxythymidine monophosphate for DNA synthesis.

E (transformation of carbohydrates to amino acids) is incorrect. The urine of individuals with this wide variety of deficiencies does not have the characteristic odor of maple syrup.

10. **D** (glucosyl [4:6] transferase) is correct. This child is exhibiting symptoms of type IV glycogen storage disease known as Andersen's disease, a condition related to a deficiency of the glycogen branching enzyme glucosyl (4:6) transferase. This deficiency classically causes cirrhosis of the liver or cardiac tissue damage, usually with death occurring within the first 1 or 2 years of life.

A (aldolase B) is incorrect. Deficiency of aldolase B, the enzyme that cleaves fructose 1-phosphate, causes hereditary fructose intolerance and leads to fructose (a reducing sugar) in the urine.

B (galactose 1-phosphate uridyltransferase) is incorrect. Deficiency of this enzyme, which is responsible for galactosemia, leads to the presence of galactose (a reducing sugar) in the urine.

C (glucose 6-phosphatase) is incorrect. Deficiency of glucose 6-phosphatase leads to type I glycogen storage disease, or von Gierke's disease. Key features of this condition include a massively enlarged liver (although usually without cirrhosis), severe hypoglycemia, and failure to thrive.

E (liver phosphorylase) is incorrect. Deficiency of liver phosphorylase causes the rare type VI glycogen storage disease, or Hers' disease. The presenting symptoms of type VI disease are much like those of type I disease, but typically the course of this condition is milder.

11. **C** (Huntington's disease) is correct. Huntington's disease is an example of a triplet repeat disorder with an amplification of the CAG trinucleotide in the translated region of the gene. More triplet repeats occur with each generation, leading to earlier appearance of the disease (anticipation). The disorder is autosomal dominant and affects both men and women.

A (cystic fibrosis) is incorrect. Cystic fibrosis is caused by a defective protein known as cystic fibrosis transmembrane conductance regulator. The condition has an autosomal recessive pattern of inheritance; it is not a trinucleotide repeat disorder.

B (Duchenne's muscular dystrophy) is incorrect. Duchenne's muscular dystrophy is caused by an absence or defect of the protein dystrophin, which is a membrane protein important in maintaining the integrity of the muscle fiber. Duchenne's muscular dystrophy has an X-linked pattern of inheritance; it is not a trinucleotide repeat disorder.

D (metachromatic leukodystrophy) is incorrect. The primary cause of metachromatic leukodystrophy is the absence of lysosomal arylsulfatase A activity, resulting in an accumulation of sulfolipids in lysosomes. The condition has an autosomal recessive pattern of inheritance; it is not a trinucleotide repeat disorder.

E (Parkinson's disease) is incorrect. Parkinson's disease is caused by loss of the neurons that generate dopamine in the substantia nigra. Some forms of the disease are autosomal dominant, but none has yet shown a tendency to occur prior to the expected onset.

12. D (hydroxylation of proline and lysine side chains) is correct. Vitamin C as well as molecular O_2 and α-ketoglutarate are the requirements for the proper function of prolyl hydroxylase, the enzyme responsible for hydroxylation of the proline side chains in collagen. Collagen lacking such side chain hydroxyl groups cannot be stabilized by interchain hydroxyl groups. This lowers the melting point of collagen and weakens the connective tissues that contain it, leading to hemorrhage.

A (cleavage of N- and C-terminal propeptide fragments) is incorrect. This process occurs extracellularly, yielding the collagen molecule (monomer). The monomers later associate and are further cross-linked by lysyl oxidase for stability while in the extracellular matrix. The cleavage process occurs via propeptidases and does not depend on vitamin C.

B (formation of pro-α-chains) is incorrect. This step, which involves translation of the mRNA to form the peptide chains found in the endoplasmic reticulum, does not depend on vitamin C.

C (glycosylation of side chain residues) is incorrect. This step, which involves the addition of glucose and galactose sugars to selected proline and lysine residues, does not depend on vitamin C.

E (triple helix assembly of procollagen) is incorrect. This spontaneous process, which occurs in the Golgi apparatus, yields a procollagen molecule and does not require vitamin C.

13. B (glucose 6-phosphatase absent in liver tissue) is correct. Normal hepatic (and renal) tissue contains glucose 6-phosphatase, which releases glucose into the circulation for consumption by peripheral tissues. Peripheral tissues, including muscle, lack this gluconeogenic enzyme. A deficiency of glucose 6-phosphatase leads to an accumulation of glucose 6-phosphate and therefore an accumulation of glycogen, which enlarges the liver and the kidney; this condition is known as von Gierke's disease. Other tissues do not show the same accumulation.

A (glucokinase absent in liver tissue) is incorrect. The liver contains glucokinase, which distinguishes it from peripheral tissues (which contain hexokinase). However, a lack of glucokinase would be expected to decrease the capacity of the liver to trap dietary glucose.

C (lack of glycogen synthase in muscle tissue) is incorrect. Like liver tissue, muscle tissue also possesses glycogen synthase, the rate-limiting enzyme in glycogen synthesis, not degradation.

D (lack of phosphorylase in liver tissue) is incorrect. The liver and muscle both contain phosphorylase, which hydrolyzes glycogen to glucose 1-phosphate. A lack of liver-specific phosphorylase (type VI glycogen storage disease, or Hers' disease) would lead to the hepatomegaly observed in this patient, but the hypoglycemia would be milder because hepatic gluconeogenesis would compensate for reduced glycogenolysis.

14. C (inhibiting the formation of mevalonate) is correct. HMG CoA reductase inhibitors ("statins") reduce blood cholesterol by blocking the conversion of HMG CoA to mevalonate. Examples of the statin drugs are lovastatin, pravastatin, and simvastatin.

A (increasing the conversion of cholesterol to bile acids) is incorrect. HMG CoA reductase inhibitors (statins) do not affect the conversion of cholesterol to bile acids.

B (inhibiting the formation of HMG CoA) is incorrect. HMG CoA reductase inhibitors (statins) reduce blood cholesterol by inhibiting the conversion of HMG CoA to mevalonate, thereby decreasing liver production of cholesterol.

D (preventing bile acids from being reabsorbed from the intestine) is incorrect. Cholestyramine reduces blood cholesterol by preventing bile acids from being reabsorbed from the intestine. This action shunts cholesterol into the bile acid pathway and decreases the amount of cholesterol that the liver sends into the bloodstream.

E (preventing cholesterol from being reabsorbed from the intestine) is incorrect. A low-fat diet helps reduce blood cholesterol by decreasing cholesterol consumption.

15. **D** (increased synthesis of glycerol 3-phosphate) is correct. Ethanol is metabolized in the liver and eventually forms acetate, with NADH as another major product. Chronic consumption of ethanol causes a shift in the cytosolic balance between NAD^+ and NADH in favor of NADH. The altered NAD^+/NADH ratio causes less effective operation of the citric acid cycle, halts efficient oxidation of fatty acids, and causes a shift from dihydroxyacetone phosphate to glyceraldehyde 3-phosphate and eventually to glycerol 3-phosphate. The abundance of glycerol and free fatty acids results in an increased production of triacylglycerol, with increased export from the liver as VLDL, and a fatty liver. These conditions are often seen in chronic alcoholics.

A (impaired function of apolipoprotein B-100) is incorrect. Alcohol consumption alone does not cause impairment of the function of any of the apolipoproteins.

However, this impairment, which occurs in abetalipoproteinemia, does result in fatty liver.

B (inactivation of capillary lipoprotein lipase) is incorrect. Alcohol consumption has not been shown to inhibit the activity of peripheral tissue lipoprotein lipase. Such inhibition leads to an increase in triacylglycerol levels in the plasma; it is a stimulus for hepatic production of VLDL.

C (increased β-oxidation of fatty acids) is incorrect. The reducing environment in the cell from the excess $NADH^+$ leads to a decrease in the oxidation of fatty acids, as stated in the discussion of option D.

16. **A** (be achieved) is correct. A state of nitrogen balance exists when the amount of nitrogen excreted is equal to the amount ingested. This is seen in healthy adults whose intake of dietary protein is adequate. Tyrosine, a nonessential amino acid, is synthesized from phenylalanine in the diet. Failure to include tyrosine in the diet would not affect the nitrogen balance in this individual, who should experience no adverse effects from the diet.

B (become negative) is incorrect. A negative nitrogen balance exists when more nitrogen is excreted than is ingested. This occurs when the protein intake is insufficient or of low quality (e.g., the diet does not provide the correct amounts of all the essential amino acids) or during catabolic states.

C (become positive) is incorrect. A positive nitrogen balance exists when more nitrogen is ingested than is excreted. This occurs primarily in anabolic states (e.g., during a "growth spurt").

D (progress from a negative at equilibrium) and **E** (progress from a positive at equilibrium) are incorrect. Transitional stages of nitrogen balance are not common (whether the end state is positive or negative) because the conditions that lead to a nitrogen imbalance are chronic in nature. For example, a negative nitrogen balance is common following surgery, during advanced stages of cancer, or in individuals with starvation syndromes (e.g., kwashiorkor).

17. **D** (it is metabolized in the liver by an aldolase that recognizes fructose 1-phosphate) is correct. Aldolase B converts fructose 1-phosphate to glyceraldehyde and dihydroxyacetone phosphate. Deficiency of aldolase B results in hereditary fructose intolerance, which leads to profound hypoglycemia on ingestion of moderate amounts of fructose.

A (it enters the glycolytic pathway as fructose 6-phosphate in the liver) is incorrect. Fructose is converted directly to fructose 1-phosphate, not fructose 6-phosphate, by fructokinase. In glycolysis, fructose 6-phosphate is produced from glucose 6-phosphate by the action of phosphohexose isomerase.

B (it is converted to UDP-fructose and then epimerized to UDP-glucose) is incorrect. Galactose, not fructose, is converted to a UDP intermediate, which is then epimerized to UDP-glucose.

C (it is metabolized by a pathway other than the glycolytic pathway) is incorrect. Fructose carbons enter the glycolytic pathway as dihydroxyacetone phosphate and glyceraldehyde 3-phosphate.

E (it is phosphorylated by phosphofructokinase) is incorrect. Phosphofructokinase, the rate-limiting enzyme of glycolysis, phosphorylates fructose 6-phosphate to produce fructose 1,6-bisphosphate.

18. **A** (decreased arterial pH) is correct. Hemoglobin exists in two forms: the relaxed, or R form, which has high O_2 affinity, and the taut, or T form, which has low O_2 affinity. By stabilizing the T form, acidosis decreases the affinity of hemoglobin for O_2 (i.e., it causes a right shift of the O_2 binding curve), thus releasing more O_2. This action is referred to as the Bohr effect.

B (decreased red blood cell 2,3-bisphosphoglycerate) is incorrect. The T form of hemoglobin is stabilized by 2,3-BPG, encouraging hemoglobin to release its O_2 load. Decreased red blood cell 2,3-BPG increases the affinity of hemoglobin for O_2, causing a left shift of the O_2 binding curve.

C (decreased temperature) is incorrect. Elevated temperatures stabilize the T form of hemoglobin. Therefore, decreased temperatures (hypothermia) increase the affinity of hemoglobin for O_2, causing the O_2 binding curve to shift to the left.

D (hyperventilation) is incorrect. Hyperventilation increases the loss of CO_2, causing respiratory alkalosis and a left shift of the O_2 binding curve.

19. **C** (glycogen synthase) is correct. In the fasting state, glucagon causes a wave of phosphorylation through liver cells to begin shifting their metabolism to energy mobilization. Glycogen synthase, the rate-controlling enzyme of glycogenesis, is converted to the less active, glucose 6-phosphate-dependent D form by phosphorylation.

A (glycogen phosphorylase) is incorrect. Glycogen phosphorylase hydrolyzes glycogen to release free glucose 1-phosphate moieties. This enzyme is activated in the fasting state to meet the body's glucose needs.

B (glycogen phosphorylase kinase) is incorrect. Glycogen phosphorylase kinase adds a phosphate group to the phosphorylase enzyme, thereby activating it. The kinase is activated in the fasting state by protein kinase A.

D (phosphoenolpyruvate carboxykinase) is incorrect. Phosphoenolpyruvate carboxykinase, an enzyme in the gluconeogenic pathway, is responsible for converting oxaloacetate to phosphoenolpyruvate. This enzyme is activated in the fasting state.

E (phosphoglucomutase) is incorrect. Phosphoglucomutase catalyzes the reversible conversion of glucose 1-phosphate to glucose 6-phosphate and operates in either direction. It is neither activated nor inactivated in the fed or the fasting state.

20. **A** (G protein) is correct. *Ras* is a mutated G protein that has lost its "off" switch, which is a GTPase. The increase in signaling that results from a permanently activated G protein leads to generation of a "growth" signal and unregulated growth of the cell line, which often leads to cancer.

    B (growth factor) is incorrect. An altered growth factor (e.g., platelet-derived growth factor) is a product of a mutated gene for that growth factor, leading to overproduction (e.g., *sis* oncogene), which may result in an astrocytoma or osteogenic sarcoma.

    C (growth factor receptor) is incorrect. An altered growth factor receptor (e.g., epidermal-derived growth factor, which is a mutated *erb-B2* oncogene) produces a receptor that is active in the absence of the growth factor. Altered growth factor may result in breast cancer.

    D (nuclear transcription factor) is incorrect. A mutated nuclear transcription factor (e.g., a mutated *myc* oncogene) may result in Burkitt's lymphoma or neuroblastoma.

21. **B** (amino acids from muscle proteins) is correct. The patient is in a starvation state. Although gluconeogenesis is markedly reduced in starvation, RBCs still require glucose for energy. The brain uses ketone bodies for fuel in a starvation state. The majority of amino acids come from muscle breakdown; muscle is the most abundant source of amino acids. Alanine and aspartate are both used as substrates for gluconeogenesis. Via transamination, alanine is converted to pyruvate and aspartate is converted to oxaloacetate.

    A (amino acids from liver proteins) is incorrect. The liver, which is not a large repository of proteins, is usually spared even in starvation, primarily because of its central role in the control of gluconeogenesis.

    C (fatty acids from adipose tissue) is incorrect. Fatty acids cannot be converted to glucose, although they do supply the energy required for gluconeogenesis via conversion to acetyl CoA and shuttling through the citric acid cycle.

    D (glycogen from muscle tissue) is incorrect. Muscle has stores of glucose as glycogen; however, it lacks the phosphatase necessary to release glucose into the circulation. Glucose 6-phosphatase, a gluconeogenic enzyme, is found only in hepatic and renal tissues.

22. **D** (tyrosinase) is correct. The patient has the outward signs of albinism, which is caused by defective production of melanin; melanocytes are present, but they do not form melanin. Albinism is most often caused by a lack of tyrosinase (tyrosine hydroxylase), the enzyme that converts tyrosine to dihydroxyphenylalanine.

    A (aldolase B) is incorrect. Aldolase B is required for the metabolism of fructose. A deficiency of aldolase B causes hereditary fructose intolerance.

    B (homogentisate oxidase) is incorrect. Homogentisate oxidase is involved in the catabolism of phenylalanine and tyrosine. A deficiency of homogentisate oxidase causes alkaptonuria. The urine of patients with this condition turns very dark on standing when exposed to free air as a result of the oxidation of homogentisic acid.

C (phenylalanine hydroxylase) is incorrect. Phenylalanine hydroxylase is the enzyme responsible for conversion of phenylalanine to tyrosine. A lack of phenylalanine hydroxylase causes phenylketonuria (PKU). Individuals with PKU must consume a phenylalanine-restricted diet until adulthood.

23. **A** (area A) is correct. The signs of tetany (carpopedal spasm and Chvostek's sign) most likely result from decreased serum calcium levels due to primary hypoparathyroidism, a complication resulting from the patient's previous thyroid surgery. During the repair process following surgery, the blood vessels to the parathyroid glands are often trapped in scar tissue, leading to infarction of the parathyroid glands.

B (area B) is incorrect. Increased PTH and decreased serum calcium are compatible with secondary hyperparathyroidism, such as vitamin D deficiency that causes hypocalcemia in chronic renal failure. Hypocalcemia is the normal stimulus for increased synthesis of PTH.

C (area C) is incorrect. Increased PTH and increased serum calcium are associated with primary hyperparathyroidism resulting from a functioning parathyroid adenoma. Hypercalcemia normally suppresses PTH synthesis.

D (area D) is incorrect. Decreased PTH and increased serum calcium are compatible with all other causes of hypercalcemia (e.g., cancer-induced sarcoidosis). Hypercalcemia normally suppresses PTH synthesis.

24. **A** (hemoglobin A_{1c}) is correct. Hemoglobin A_{1c}, glycosylated hemoglobin, is an excellent indicator of glycemic control during the previous 4 to 8 weeks. The patient, who has type 1 diabetes mellitus, has developed diabetic ketoacidosis, as indicated by her below normal pH. The cause of the patient's blurry vision is alteration of the refractive index of her lens caused by conversion of glucose into sorbitol by aldose reductase. Sorbitol is osmotically active; it draws water into the lens, causing changes that vary with the glucose level in the blood.

B (serum thyroid-stimulating hormone) is incorrect. Signs and symptoms of Graves' disease include weight loss, increased appetite, and eye abnormalities. Graves' disease is diagnosed by determining serum TSH. Urinary frequency and a fruity odor to the breath (ketone bodies) are not features of this disease.

C (urine dipstick test for glucose) is incorrect. The patient would very likely have glucose in the urine. However, this finding does not provide the most information about the patient's diabetic control and cause of her vision problems because the renal threshold for glucose varies.

D (urine dipstick test for ketones) is incorrect. The patient would very likely have ketones in the urine. However, this finding would not provide any information about the cause of her blurry vision, but it does correlate with the fruity odor on her breath.

25. **E** (UDP-hexose epimerase) is correct. This enzyme reversibly converts UDP-glucose to UDP-galactose, which can then combine with glucose to form lactate and permit both normal lactation and normal development in individuals with galactosemia.

A (aldolase B) is incorrect. Aldolase B splits fructose 1-phosphate into glyceraldehyde and dihydroxyacetone phosphate. A deficiency of aldolase B results in hereditary fructose intolerance; it is not involved in lactose synthesis.

B (galactokinase) is incorrect. Galactokinase is responsible for the conversion of galactose to galactose 1-phosphate. Although a deficiency of galactokinase causes a form of galactosemia, the enzyme is not directly involved in the synthesis of lactose.

C (galactose 1-phosphate uridyltransferase) is incorrect. A deficiency of galactose 1-phosphate uridyltransferase causes a form of galactosemia, but it is not involved directly in the synthesis of lactose.

D (lactase) is incorrect. Lactase, an enzyme found primarily in the brush border of the intestine, is responsible for the conversion of lactose to its constituent monosaccharides, glucose and galactose. A deficiency of lactase is responsible for lactose intolerance, which usually causes diarrhea in affected individuals who ingest large amounts of lactose-containing foods (e.g., dairy products).

26. **D** (sphingomyelinase) is correct. A deficiency of sphingomyelinase causes Niemann-Pick disease, an autosomal recessive disease that results in the accumulation of sphingomyelin in the lysosomes. Signs of the disorder include an enlarged liver and spleen and mental retardation of rapid onset, usually within the first 6 months of life.

A (arylsulfatase A) is incorrect. A deficiency of arylsulfatase A, which results in the accumulation of a sulfate-containing ceramide in the lysosomes, causes metachromatic leukodystrophy, an autosomal recessive disease. Mental retardation and demyelination are typical in patients with this deficiency.

B (hexosaminidase A) is incorrect. A deficiency of hexosaminidase A results in the accumulation of GM_2 ganglioside, which is

seen in patients with Tay-Sachs disease and Sandhoff's disease. Mental retardation and blindness are associated with both disorders, but they progress more rapidly in patients with Sandhoff's disease.

C (liver phosphorylase) is incorrect. A deficiency in liver phosphorylase causes Hers' disease, an autosomal recessive disease that results in the inability of the liver to mobilize glucose from glycogen. Hepatomegaly is present, but there are no symptoms of central nervous system deterioration or failure to thrive, nor is sphingomyelin increased in lysosomes.

27. **B** (it activates protein kinase A to become a regulator of enzymes by phosphorylation) is correct. In the fasting state, glucagon activates adenylate cyclase, causing an increase in cAMP. This monophosphate acts as a second messenger by activating protein kinase A and binding to its regulatory subunits. Further action of protein kinase A may regulate enzymes, ion channels, and DNA-binding proteins.

A (it activates adenylate cyclase when complexed with the α-subunit of G_S protein) is incorrect. GTP binds to the α-subunit of G_S protein when the G_S protein interacts with a stimulated hormone receptor. The G_S protein-GTP complex then activates adenylate cyclase, which increases the intracellular concentration of cAMP.

C (it binds calcium to activate several cellular enzymes) is incorrect. Calmodulin binds four molecules of calcium, causing its activation through a conformational change. The calcium-calmodulin complex in turn activates various enzymes, including kinases, cyclases, and phosphodiesterase.

D (it binds to receptors on the endoplasmic reticulum, causing calcium to be released into the cytoplasm) is incorrect. Inositol 1,4,5-triphosphate (IP_3) is produced when hormones stimulate the action of phospholipase C to break down phosphatidylinositol 1,4,5-IP$_3$. IP$_3$ causes rapid release of calcium from intracellular stores, which allows it to perform its "second messenger" function both by combination with calmodulin and by direct stimulation of protein kinase C.

E (it increases the activity of membrane-bound protein kinase C) is incorrect. The action of phospholipase C on phosphatidylinositol 1,4,5-IP$_3$ also produces diacylglycerol. This glycerol increases the activity of membrane-bound protein kinase C, which in turn regulates other proteins through a phosphorylation mechanism.

28. **D** (phenylketonuria) is correct. The secondary form of PKU results from an inability to regenerate tetrahydrobiopterin. This lack of tetrahydrobiopterin affects not only the conversion of phenylalanine to tyrosine but also the hydroxylation of tyrosine and tryptophan, leading to deficiencies of neurotransmitters and additional central nervous system effects. Dietary restriction of phenylalanine is not sufficient to reverse the neurologic effects. Control of the primary form of PKU, which is caused by phenylalanine hydroxylase deficiency, involves dietary restriction of phenylalanine and tyrosine supplementation.

A (galactosemia) is incorrect. Galactosemia, which may present as mental retardation, is caused by a deficiency in galactose 1-phosphate uridyltransferase. The enzyme does not require tetrahydrobiopterin as a cofactor.

B (maple syrup urine disease) is incorrect. The cause of maple syrup urine disease is a deficiency of branched-chain α-keto acid dehydrogenase. This enzyme does not require tetrahydrobiopterin as a cofactor.

C (Niemann-Pick disease) is incorrect. The cause of Niemann-Pick disease, which also presents as mental retardation with hepatosplenomegaly, is a defect in the lysosomal hydrolytic enzyme sphingomyelinase. This enzyme does not require tetrahydrobiopterin as a cofactor.

E (Wilson's disease) is incorrect. The cause of Wilson's disease is a defect in the excretion of copper into the bile. Excess copper in the liver leads to chronic liver disease and decreased synthesis of ceruloplasmin, a copper-binding protein. Excess copper in the blood leads to deposits in the eye (Kayser-Fleischer rings) and the lenticular nuclei in the brain, resulting in movement disorders. Ceruloplasmin does not require tetrahydrobiopterin as a cofactor.

29. **D** (spectrin) is correct. The woman has congenital spherocytosis, a disease caused by a defect in spectrin, which is responsible for maintaining the structural integrity of the RBC membrane. This autosomal dominant disorder is associated with destruction of the spherocytes by macrophages in the spleen.

A (actin) is incorrect. Actin interacts with spectrin but has not been identified in a defective form.

B (β-amyloid) is incorrect. β-Amyloid, which accumulates in plaque in Alzheimer's disease, is not found in RBCs.

C (hemoglobin) is incorrect. Hemoglobin is not defective in congenital spherocytosis. Alterations in globin chain synthesis (e.g., sickle cell anemia and β-thalassemia) cause hemoglobinopathies.

30. **B** (insulin) is correct. Pregnancy is a relatively insulin-resistant state that is somewhat exacerbated in some females to the point at which gestational diabetes develops. This condition leads to a hypersecretion of insulin, which acts as a growth hormone by increasing amino acid uptake in muscle. In addition, it increases the deposition of triacylglycerol in adipose tissue. Pregnant females with gestational diabetes are at increased risk for giving birth to large-for-gestational-age infants, with increased muscle mass and body fat.

A (growth hormone) is incorrect. Although growth hormone may account for large-for-gestational-age infants, it is not the most likely mechanism responsible for the development of such infants in females with gestational diabetes. Hyperglycemia inhibits the release of growth hormone.

C (prolactin) is incorrect. Although the secretion of prolactin is increased in lactating females, it is not responsible for growth stimulation of the fetus. However, the hormone does increase the synthesis of surfactant.

D (thyroxine) is incorrect. Thyroxine levels usually are not altered in pregnancy or in diabetes, and growth of the fetus is typically independent of the amount of thyroxine. However, the synthesis of surfactant does increase the levels of this hormone.

31. **C** (mitochondrial proton pump) is correct. This patient is suffering from a decreased production of ATP, with symptoms of muscle weakness and fatigue. The ATP synthase in the mitochondrion depends on a proton gradient to function. Pentachlorophenol acts like the uncoupling agent dinitrophenol and causes the inner mitochondrial membrane to become permeable to protons. This action destroys the proton gradient and decreases ATP synthesis.

A (ATP synthase) is incorrect. ATP synthase is a target for chemicals that act like oligomycin. In this case, the proton gradient exists, but the synthase is unable to function. An excessive proton gradient is generated, thereby

halting the electron transport chain by the law of mass action.

B (cytochrome oxidase) is incorrect. Cytochrome oxidase is a target for a substance such as cyanide or carbon monoxide. Inhibition of this terminal component of the electron transport chain halts all prior electron transport. Because generation of the proton gradient depends on concomitant electron transport, the gradient dissipates and ATP synthesis ceases.

D (NADH dehydrogenase) is incorrect. NADH dehydrogenase is a target for a chemical that acts like rotenone or amobarbital (Amytal). As explained in the discussion of option B, the cessation of electron transport halts the concomitant proton transport and thus halts ATP synthesis.

E (succinate dehydrogenase) is incorrect. Succinate dehydrogenase is a target for a chemical that acts like malonate, which halts the citric acid cycle and consumption of acetyl CoA. Anaerobic glycolysis continues unabated.

32. **D** (pregnenolone from cholesterol) is correct. The patient has signs of pituitary hypofunction (exhaustion, diarrhea, low blood pressure, and anemia) and is diagnosed with a tumor of the pituitary gland, in the sella turcica. Formation of pregnenolone from cholesterol is the rate-limiting step in the synthesis of steroid compounds. It is regulated by the action of ACTH on the cytochrome P450 side chain cleavage enzyme.

A (cortisol from cholic acid) is incorrect. Cholic acid, a bile salt, is not found in the steroid pathway.

B (7-dehydrocholesterol from cholesterol) is incorrect. The sterol 7-dehydrocholesterol is an intermediate substance in the conversion of lanosterol to cholesterol. It accumulates in the skin as a precursor to cholecalciferol (vitamin D_3).

C (mevalonate from HMG CoA) is incorrect. HMG CoA reductase is the rate-limiting step in cholesterol synthesis, not steroid hormone synthesis.

E (progesterone from pregnenolone) is incorrect. Formation of progesterone from pregnenolone is not rate-limiting.

33. **D** (pyruvate carboxylase) is correct. This man has classic signs of biotin deficiency. Consumption of more than 20 raw eggs per day leads to increased binding of the vitamin by the protein avidin, which is found in high concentrations in raw eggs. Biotin is a cofactor for pyruvate carboxylase, which is a gluconeogenic enzyme that adds CO_2 to pyruvate to form oxaloacetate. The excess pyruvate results in an increase in its conversion to lactic acid.

A (alanine aminotransferase) is incorrect. Alanine aminotransferase, which converts alanine to pyruvate during the alanine cycle, requires pyridoxine (vitamin B_6).

B (lactate dehydrogenase) is incorrect. Lactate dehydrogenase, which converts lactate to pyruvate in the Cori cycle, requires niacin (as NAD^+).

C (malate dehydrogenase) is incorrect. Malate dehydrogenase, which transports carbon from the mitochondria to the cytoplasm for gluconeogenesis, requires niacin (as NAD^+).

E (pyruvate kinase) is incorrect. Pyruvate kinase is responsible for the conversion of phosphoenolpyruvate to pyruvate, with concomitant conversion of ADP to ATP. It does not require biotin as a cofactor.

34. **E** (transaminases and glutamate dehydrogenase) is correct. A transaminase first transfers the amino groups of most amino acids to α-ketoglutarate, producing glutamate plus an α-keto acid corresponding to the original amino acid. Glutamate dehydrogenase then acts on glutamate to produce free NH_3 (oxidative deamination), which is metabolized in the urea cycle in the liver.

A (amino acid oxidases and arginase) is incorrect. The enzyme D-amino acid oxidase metabolizes D-amino acids in the diet, but no such enzymes exist for the metabolism of the L-amino acids present in the tissues of humans and other animals. Arginase is an enzyme whose activity is restricted to cleavage of urea from arginine in the urea cycle of the liver.

B (argininosuccinate lyase and cytosolic carbamoyl phosphate synthetase II) is incorrect. Argininosuccinate lyase is a part of the urea cycle, where it catalyzes the cleavage of argininosuccinate to arginine and fumarate. Cytosolic carbamoyl phosphate synthetase II is not part of the urea cycle. Instead, it is active in utilizing free ammonia for pyrimidine synthesis.

C (glutaminase and amino acid oxidases) is incorrect. Glutaminase functions primarily in the kidneys and the intestine to remove free ammonia from glutamine. In the kidney, NH_3 acidifies the urine. In the intestine, NH_3 is transported directly to the liver, where it enters the urea cycle.

D (glutamine synthetase and urease) is incorrect. Glutamine synthetase joins free ammonia to glutamate to provide glutamine needed for protein synthesis and to detoxify excess ammonia in the brain and the liver. Urease is a bacterial (and plant) enzyme that cleaves urea to CO_2 and NH_3. Bacterial urease also degrades amino acids in the diet, causing the release of NH_3, which is either excreted in stool or delivered to the urea cycle in the liver by the portal vein. Excess urea, which travels to the intestine and, therefore, to the intestinal flora during kidney failure, can contribute to hyperammonemia.

35. **C** (type I collagen) is correct. This patient most likely has osteogenesis imperfecta, which is usually inherited as an autosomal dominant trait. There is a substitution of another amino acid for glycine near the carboxy terminal of α_1 collagen chains. This defect inhibits correct folding and assembly of tropocollagen. Because bone is primarily composed of type I collagen, fractures in patients with this disorder are common. Decreased amounts of type I collagen in the sclera allow the bluish discoloration of the underlying choroidal veins to manifest. Deafness is due to malformation of the auditory ossicles.

A (fibrillin) is incorrect. Fibrillin defects are associated with Marfan syndrome. Fibrillin, a component of elastic tissue, is not present in bone or sclera, which explains the absence of bone fractures and blue sclera.

B (α-L-iduronidase) is incorrect. The enzyme α-L-iduronidase is deficient in Hurler"s syndrome. Skeletal deformities are apparent, but there is no bone fragility or blue sclera.

D (type III collagen) is incorrect. Type III collagen defects (e.g., Ehlers-Danlos syndrome) lead to vascular weakness because the connective tissue is rich in this type of collagen.

36. **D** (glucose) is correct. This child is lethargic, although the mobilization of free fatty acids from adipose tissue and β-oxidation in the liver is occurring. The lack of carnitine causes the carnitine shuttle, which transports fatty acids from the cytosol to the mitochondrial matrix, to be inoperative. Therefore, 12 ATP derived from acetyl CoA, 3 ATP from NADH, and 2 ATP from $FADH_2$ are not available. Hence, the child is subsisting primarily on glucose derived from glycogenolysis as the primary source of energy for all tissues. Gluconeogenesis is suppressed because it relies on fatty acid catabolism as an energy source. This condition produces hypoglycemia. Treatment often involves fatty acids that contain less than 12 carbons, which can pass directly into the mitochondria without the carnitine shuttle.

A (branched-chain amino acids) is incorrect. The metabolism of branched-chain amino acids supplies succinyl CoA for gluconeogenesis. However, without the ATP supplied by fatty acid oxidation, gluconeogenesis cannot operate optimally.

B (fatty acids) is incorrect. Without carnitine, fatty acids with more than 12 carbons cannot enter the mitochondria to be oxidized to acetyl CoA; therefore, they provide no energy.

C (fructose) is incorrect. The body does not store fructose in appreciable quantities to supply energy during fasting conditions.

E (ketone bodies) is incorrect. Ketone bodies are produced from large excesses of acetyl CoA (i.e., from oxidation of fatty acids). Because carnitine is not available to shuttle fatty acids into the mitochondrion, no ketone bodies are produced in the liver.

37. **C** (HMG CoA synthase) is correct. The woman has developed ketonemia because long-term starvation leads to excessive conversion of acetyl CoA (derived from the β-oxidation of fatty acids) to ketone bodies in the liver. HMG CoA synthase catalyzes the formation of HMG CoA from acetoacetyl CoA and acetyl CoA. The fruity odor on the woman's breath signifies the volatile ketone body acetone, which is released in the breath.

A (citrate synthase) is incorrect. Citrate synthase catalyzes the formation of citrate from acetyl CoA and oxaloacetate.

B (HMG CoA reductase) is incorrect. HMG CoA reductase is the rate-limiting enzyme in the synthesis of cholesterol that produces mevalonic acid from HMG CoA.

D (β-ketothiolase) is incorrect. β-Ketothiolase, which is involved in the β-oxidation of fatty acids, catalyzes the production of acetyl CoA that serves as a precursor for ketone bodies.

E (pyruvate carboxylase) is incorrect. Pyruvate carboxylase is a gluconeogenic enzyme that catalyzes the synthesis of oxaloacetate from pyruvate.

38. **E** (transketolase) is correct. The man is deficient in thiamine (vitamin B_1), most likely from eating rice with the outer hull removed. He has symptoms of both wet and dry forms of beriberi, a disease caused by thiamine deficiency. Wet beriberi involves both a left-sided heart failure (pulmonary edema) and a right-sided heart failure (neck vein distention and pitting edema); dry beriberi involves peripheral neuropathy (footdrop caused by peroneal nerve palsy). In patients with beriberi, the enzyme transketolase, which requires thiamine pyrophosphate as a cofactor, does not function normally. Pyruvate dehydrogenase, which also requires thiamine as a cofactor, is also dysfunctional.

A (aspartate aminotransferase) is incorrect. Aspartate aminotransferase catalyzes the conversion of aspartate to oxaloacetate with transfer of the amino group to α-ketoglutarate to form glutamate. It requires pyridoxine (vitamin B_6) as a cofactor.

B (isocitrate dehydrogenase) is incorrect. Isocitrate dehydrogenase, which catalyzes the conversion of isocitrate to α-ketoglutarate, requires niacin in the form of NAD^+.

C (pyruvate carboxylase) is incorrect. Pyruvate carboxylase catalyzes the conversion of pyruvate to oxaloacetate. Like most of the carboxylases, it requires biotin as a cofactor.

D (transaldolase) is incorrect. Transaldolase, which catalyzes the transfer of three-carbon moieties in the pentose phosphate pathway, does not require a vitamin cofactor.

39. **C** (phosphoenolpyruvate carboxykinase) is correct. In states of hypercortisolism, such as Cushing's syndrome, patients develop diabetes mellitus because of increased gluconeogenesis. Cortisol, a gluconeogenic hormone, acts along with glucagon in the synthesis of glucose. Phosphoenolpyruvate carboxykinase is a gluconeogenic enzyme.

A (aspartate aminotransferase) is incorrect. Aspartate aminotransferase catalyzes the conversion of aspartate to oxaloacetate, with the transfer of the amino group to α-ketoglutarate to form glutamate. The enzyme is not affected by glucocorticoids.

B (capillary lipoprotein lipase) is incorrect. The amount of hormone-sensitive lipase, not capillary lipoprotein lipase, is increased by glucocorticoids.

D (pyruvate carboxylase) is incorrect. Pyruvate carboxylase catalyzes the conversion of pyruvate to oxaloacetate. The enzyme is not affected by glucocorticoids.

E (pyruvate dehydrogenase) is incorrect. Pyruvate dehydrogenase catalyzes the irreversible conversion of pyruvate to acetyl CoA. Enzyme activity is increased in response to insulin but not glucocorticoids.

40. **B** (cholesterol) is correct. Cholestyramine and other bile salt-binding resins cause increased excretion of bile salts in the stool. Because bile salts derive from conversion of cholesterol to bile salts in the liver, an upregulation of low-density lipoprotein (LDL) receptors in hepatocytes results in the extraction of cholesterol (primarily carried by LDL) out of the blood and the synthesis of more bile salts. Cholestyramine is used therapeutically to lower cholesterol levels in patients with hypercholesterolemia.

A (aldosterone), **C** (cortisol), **D** (pregnenolone), and **E** (progesterone) are incorrect. None of these compounds are used to synthesize bile salts. Although aldosterone is synthesized in the adrenal cortex from cholesterol, its reduction does not result in a significant decline in concentration.

41. **D** (increased urinary δ-aminolevulinic acid) is correct. The patient has lead poisoning, which commonly occurs in battery factory employees. Elevation of ALA is usually a clue that lead poisoning is present because lead denatures ALA dehydratase, which converts ALA to porphobilinogen. Increased levels of ALA, along with lead, produce demyelination in the brain and increased vessel permeability leading to cerebral edema. Lead poisoning often results in a microcytic anemia, with characteristic coarse basophilic stippling of RBCs because of denaturation of ribonuclease, the enzyme that degrades ribosomes.

A (decreased serum ferritin) is incorrect. Serum ferritin, a circulating soluble protein storage form of iron, correlates with iron stores in the bone marrow macrophages. It is elevated in lead poisoning, where iron accumulates in the mitochondria in developing nucleated RBCs and produces ringed sideroblasts, which contain iron-laden mitochondria surrounding the nucleus. When the sideroblasts die in bone marrow, the iron is stored in macrophages, leading to an increase in iron stores in the marrow as well as iron in the blood.

B (decreased zinc RBC protoporphyrin) is incorrect. In lead poisoning, denaturation of ALA dehydratase and ferrochelatase reduces the amount of zinc protoporphyrin in the RBCs that is available to combine with iron to form heme. In the past, zinc RBC protoporphyrin levels were used to screen for lead poisoning. However, these values are also increased in other conditions (e.g., iron deficiency), which limits the usefulness of the test. Currently, the blood lead level is used as

the screening and confirmatory test for lead poisoning.

C (increased hemoglobin A_2 and hemoglobin F) is incorrect. Lead denatures enzymes involved in hemoglobin synthesis (e.g., ALA dehydratase and ferrochelatase) and in the degradation of ribosomes (e.g., ribonuclease); it does not interfere with globin chain synthesis. Mild β-thalassemia minor is characterized by an increase in HbA_2 and HbF. In this condition, there is a decrease in β-globin chain synthesis, leading to a decrease in HbA (2α, 2β) and a corresponding increase in HbA_2 (2α, 2δ) and HbF (2α, 2γ).

42. **D** (prevent the formation of linear aggregates with sickle cell tetramers) is correct. Hemoglobin F (HbF), or fetal hemoglobin, is a tetramer composed of $\alpha_2\gamma_2$ globin chains. γ-Globin chains prevent the formation of sickle linear aggregates because they do not have the valine substitution that attaches to the sticky spot on adjacent tetramers.

A (bind more oxygen than sickle β-globin chains) is incorrect. Sickle β-globin binds oxygen normally.

B (bind more tightly to 2,3-bisphosphoglycerate than sickle β-globin chains) is incorrect. Sickle β-globin chains do not bind 2,3-bisphosphoglycerate more tightly than HbF.

C (form nonpolymerizing tetramers) is incorrect. γ-Globin chains combine only with α-globin chains to form HbF.

43. **B** (debranching enzyme) is correct. Debranching enzyme deficiency leads to Cori's disease, which is characterized by hepatomegaly and hypoglycemia. Debranching enzyme is required for the proper metabolism of glycogen near its branch points. Without it, glycogenolysis ceases when all terminal chains are at branch points, and no further hydrolysis of glucose residues is possible. The absence of lactic acidosis implies that pyruvate is not being generated because of the slow operation of the glycolytic pathway. Treatment of Cori's disease, a glycogen storage disease, involves avoidance of fasting and liberal access to dietary protein for gluconeogenesis.

A (branching enzyme) is incorrect. Deficiency of branching enzyme leads to Andersen's disease. The abnormal branching pattern (lack of branches) in the glycogen molecule is believed to result in cirrhosis of the liver. Affected patients typically present with failure to thrive within the first 18 months of life and die by 5 years of age.

C (glucose 6-phosphatase) is incorrect. Deficiency of glucose 6-phosphatase leads to von Gierke's disease, which affects the liver and kidneys. Children with this enzyme deficiency typically present at 3 or 4 months of age with massive hepatorenomegaly and fasting hypoglycemia.

D (α-glucosidase) is incorrect. Deficiency of α-glucosidase leads to Pompe's disease, a lysosomal glycogen storage disease. This condition is generalized to all tissues; the heart is the most vulnerable organ.

E (liver phosphorylase) is incorrect. Liver phosphorylase deficiency leads to Hers' disease. This rare disease initially manifests in childhood as hepatomegaly and fasting hypoglycemia. Both symptoms improve with age and typically disappear by puberty.

44. **C** (impaired night vision) is correct. This patient shows signs of vitamin A deficiency (thick skin, follicular hyperkeratosis, and dry eyes), which are probably caused by a diet lacking in sources of vitamin A (retinol) such as vegetables. Other than keratotic thickening of the epithelium, a major symptom of this vitamin deficiency is impaired night vision as a result of the reduced synthesis of visual purple.

A (bleeding gums) is incorrect. A deficiency of vitamin C leads to defective collagen formation and causes bleeding gums. This condition is often manifested by weakened mucous membranes. Vitamin C (ascorbic acid) is found in citrus fruits, broccoli, tomatoes, and strawberries.

B (hemolytic anemia) is incorrect. Vitamin E deficiency causes hemolytic anemia. Vitamin E prevents lipid peroxidation of cell membranes; its deficiency damages red blood cell membranes. Vitamin E (tocopherol) is found in vegetable oils and wheat germ.

D (osteomalacia) is incorrect. Vitamin D deficiency causes osteomalacia, or softening of the bones, a condition that leads to decreased mineralization of bone. Vitamin D (calcitriol) is found in fortified milk or is manufactured in the body from 7-dehydrocholesterol.

E (pain in the long bones) is incorrect. Vitamin A overdose or vitamin D deficiency may cause pain in the long bones, with associated osteomalacia and an increase in pathologic fractures. Sources of vitamin A (retinol) are liver and yellow and dark green leafy vegetables.

45. **C** (glucokinase) is correct. The restoration of ample carbohydrate to the diet would increase insulin concentrations. Glucokinase, located in liver and pancreatic cells, is increased in concentration and activity by insulin. Hexokinase, which is located in extrahepatic cells, is not regulated by insulin.

A (carnitine acyltransferase) is incorrect. Carnitine acyltransferase is already maximally increased in order to oxidize fatty acids released during starvation.

B (citrate synthase) is incorrect. Citrate synthase is already maximally increased in order to metabolize the acetyl CoA from fatty acid oxidation.

D (glucose 6-phosphatase) is incorrect. Glucose 6-phosphatase is already maximally increased in order to release glucose produced in the liver via gluconeogenesis into the bloodstream.

E (HMG CoA synthase) is incorrect. To adapt to starvation, HMG CoA synthase, the rate-limiting enzyme in ketogenesis, is already maximally increased in order to form ketone bodies.

46. **A** (type I) is correct. Type I hyperlipoproteinemia, a disease most commonly seen in children, is associated with a deficiency of either capillary lipoprotein lipase or apolipoprotein C-II in VLDL. This condition leads to an accumulation of chylomicrons, which are the least dense of all the lipoproteins; these cells float on the surface of plasma when left in a refrigerator overnight.

B (type IIa) is incorrect. Type IIa hyperlipoproteinemia is typically associated with a deficiency of LDL receptors and an attendant increase in plasma LDL levels. Affected patients have a tendency to develop early, severe atherosclerosis and coronary artery disease.

C (type IIb) is incorrect. The cause of type IIb hyperlipoproteinemia is unknown. However, in addition to elevated levels of LDL, like those found in patients with type IIa hyperlipoproteinemia, plasma levels of triacylglycerol are also increased. Affected patients have an increased risk of developing both atherosclerosis and coronary artery disease.

D (type III) is incorrect. Type III hyperlipoproteinemia is associated with a deficiency of apolipoprotein E, which leads to an accumulation of intermediate-density lipoprotein and chylomicron remnants. Affected patients typically form xanthomas and suffer from atherosclerosis in the peripheral and coronary arteries.

E (type IV) is incorrect. Type IV hyperlipoproteinemia is associated with the overproduction or reduced clearance of VLDL in the liver in individuals with glucose intolerance. The incidence of atherosclerosis is increased.

47. **B** (hypoxanthine-guanine phosphoribosyltransferase) is correct. This child is manifesting signs and symptoms of Lesch-Nyhan syndrome, an X-linked recessive disorder. A complete deficiency of HGPRT causes this condition. HGPRT is responsible for the salvage of purines by converting hypoxanthine and guanine to their monophosphated forms. Lack of this enzyme leads to destruction of free hypoxanthine and guanine, increased uric acid levels, and ensuing mental retardation and, less important, gout. The cause of the self-mutilatory behavior in Lesch-Nyhan syndrome is unknown.

A (adenosine deaminase) is incorrect. Adenosine deaminase catalyzes the conversion of adenosine to inosine in the degradation pathway of adenosine. A deficiency of this enzyme leads to a form of severe combined immunodeficiency disease.

C (phosphoribosylpyrophosphate synthase) is incorrect. Phosphoribosylpyrophosphate synthase catalyzes the rate-limiting step in the synthesis of purine nucleotides and plays an important role in many other pathways. The most common alteration of this synthase is overactivity, which leads to an overproduction of purines and ensuing hyperuricemia and gout.

D (thymidine kinase) is incorrect. Thymidine kinase is an enzyme in the salvage pathway for pyrimidines (specifically thymine) that converts thymidine to TMP. Drugs such as acyclovir, used primarily to treat herpes, inhibit viral versions of this enzyme.

E (xanthine oxidase) is incorrect. Xanthine oxidase, the terminal enzyme in the degradation pathway of purines, converts xanthine to uric acid. This enzyme can be inhibited by allopurinol, which reduces the production of uric acid and abates the occurrences of gout in individuals prone to attacks.

48. **D** (vitamin D) is correct. Patients with chronic renal failure often have small, shriveled kidneys with little, if any, viable parenchyma. Because one of the functions of the kidneys is to carry out the 1-α-hydroxylation of 25-hydroxycholecalciferol, they cannot form active vitamin D, or 1,25-dihydroxycholecalciferol, which leads to hypocalcemia and signs of tetany. Hypocalcemia stimulates the secretion of parathyroid hormone (secondary hyperparathyroidism), leading to increased mobilization of calcium from bone and the bone problems observed in this patient.

A (niacin) is incorrect. Niacin is the precursor to NAD^+ and NADH; thus, it is required in a number of important reactions in the body. Niacin deficiency (pellagra), which is characterized by diarrhea, dermatitis, and dementia, is not directly involved in bone or calcium metabolism.

B (thiamine) is incorrect. Thiamine is a cofactor for several enzymes, such as pyruvate dehydrogenase and transketolase. Thiamine deficiency, which is characterized by heart failure, peripheral neuropathy, and memory problems, is not involved in bone resorption or calcium metabolism.

C (vitamin A) is incorrect. Vitamin A, which is dependent on fat absorption for uptake from the intestine, is required for adequate vision and proper keratinization but not for bone maintenance or calcium homeostasis. Vitamin A deficiency is characterized by dry skin and night blindness.

E (vitamin K) is incorrect. Vitamin K plays a prominent role in the coagulation cascade because it is responsible for the terminal carboxylation of several key clotting factors. Vitamin K deficiency is not directly involved in bone resorption or calcium homeostasis.

49. **B** (mannose 6-phosphate attachment) is correct. This patient has I cell (inclusion cell) disease (also known as mucolipidosis II), which is caused by defective shuttling of lysosomal enzymes into lysosomes. Enzymes destined for lysosomes normally receive a mannose 6-phosphate marker in the Golgi apparatus. In I cell disease, the enzymatic ability to phosphorylate mannose in the Golgi apparatus is lacking, and enzymes are targeted at extracellular sites other than lysosomes. Because the lysosomes lack enzymes, undegraded molecules accumulate in the lysosomes and form inclusion bodies.

A (gene amplification) is incorrect. Gene amplification is the process of simultaneously activating multiple copies of DNA fragments that code for the same RNA, thus leading to a drastic increase in the concentration of the final product. This process occurs during both the development of resistance to methotrexate (via amplification of the dihydrofolate reductase gene) and the early stages of development in the ovum (primarily for ribosomal RNA needs). It does not play a role in the targeting of lysosomal enzymes.

C (nuclear localization signal) is incorrect. The nuclear localization signal, which is a sequence that contains five positively charged amino acids (usually lysine residues), directs proteins into the nucleus. It does not influence the targeting of lysosomal enzymes.

D (transferrin receptor mRNA) is incorrect. Transferrin, a protein, is responsible for the shuttling of iron in the body. The level of iron in cells directly influences the transcription of the transferrin receptor gene. Therefore, low levels of iron lead to an increased expression of the receptor and, hence, an increased uptake of iron via transferrin endocytosis. However, transferrin receptor mRNA is not related to the targeting of lysosomal enzymes.

50. **D** (pyruvate kinase) is correct. The patient has a deficiency of pyruvate kinase, which converts phosphoenolpyruvate to pyruvate and regenerates two molecules of ATP. This deficiency is an autosomal recessive disorder. The cause of the associated mild chronic hemolytic anemia is the reduction of ATP produced from glycolysis. The anemia is mild because of the increase in 2,3-bisphosphoglycerate (2,3-BPG), which is proximal to the blockage in the glycolytic pathway. An increase in 2,3-BPG shifts the O_2 binding curve to the right; therefore, less hemoglobin is necessary to release O_2 to tissue. In the peripheral blood, the reduced supply of ATP causes RBCs to lose water and have a spiculated appearance.

A (glucose 6-phosphate dehydrogenase) is incorrect. G6PD deficiency, which has an X-linked pattern of inheritance, does not affect the O_2 binding curve.

B (phosphoglucomutase) is incorrect. Phosphoglucomutase catalyzes the reversible conversion of glucose 6-phosphate to glucose 1-phosphate for glycogen synthesis. It is not present in RBCs because it does not synthesize glycogen.

C (pyruvate dehydrogenase) is incorrect. Pyruvate dehydrogenase is not an RBC enzyme; it occurs in the mitochondria, which are not present in mature RBCs.

DIRECTIONS: Each numbered item or incomplete statement is followed by options arranged in alphabetical or logical order. Select the best answer to each question. Some options may be partially correct, but there is only **ONE BEST** answer.

1. A 23-year-old African American woman complains of fatigue and exhaustion from exercise. Physical examination shows conjunctival pallor. When asked, she tells the physician that her menstrual flow is heavy. A complete blood cell count shows moderately severe anemia with a low mean corpuscular volume (MCV). Which of the following laboratory tests is most useful in determining the cause of the anemia?
   A. Hemoglobin electrophoresis
   B. Serum ferritin level
   C. Serum iron level
   D. Serum total iron-binding capacity (TIBC)

2. A 2-month-old female infant has coarse facial features, mental retardation, corneal clouding, and hepatomegaly. Analysis of fibroblasts cultured from the patient most likely shows a deficiency in which of the following enzymes?
   A. Glucosidase
   B. Hexosaminidase
   C. α-L-Iduronidase
   D. Phosphotransferase
   E. Sphingomyelinase

3. A comatose 4-year-old child has a blood glucose level of 600 mg/dL, glucosuria, and a serum bicarbonate level of 10 mEq/L. Which of the following enzymes is most responsible for the mobilization of fatty acids in this patient?
   A. Carnitine acyltransferase
   B. Hormone-sensitive lipase
   C. Lipoprotein lipase

   D. Pancreatic lipase
   E. Phospholipase D

4. A 68-year-old man with a 50-year history of cigarette smoking develops weight loss, jaundice, and light-colored stools. Findings on physical examination include a palpable gallbladder. The total bilirubin is 10 mg/dL, and the unconjugated bilirubin is 8 mg/dL. CT scan shows a mass in the head of the pancreas. Urinalysis is most likely to yield which of the following results?

	Urine Bilirubin	Urine Urobilinogen
A.	0	0
B.	0	+2
C.	+2	0
D.	+2	+2

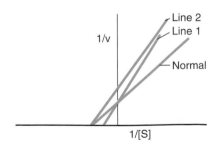

5. Investigation of a recently identified metabolic enzyme under different experimental conditions produces the results shown in the figure. Which of the following conditions best explains line 1?

A. Addition of a competitive inhibitor
B. Addition of a noncompetitive inhibitor
C. Change in pH
D. Change in temperature
E. Increased ionic strength

6. A 52-year-old man complains of progressive loss of energy, numbness and tingling in his toes, loss of balance, and a sore tongue. Laboratory studies show the patient's serum level of vitamin B_{12} is 30% that of the normal concentration. Which of the following best describes the role that folate plays in this patient's symptoms?
A. *S*-Adenosylmethionine is substituting for methyltetrahydrofolate (methyl-FH_4) as a methyl donor.
B. Conversion of methyl-FH_4 to dihydrofolate is being blocked.
C. Folate deficiency is creating a vitamin B_{12} deficiency.
D. Methyl-FH_4 is being used for conversion of glycine to serine.
E. Methylene-FH_4 conversion to another form of FH_4 is being blocked.

7. A 48-year-old woman with type 2 diabetes mellitus complains of intermittent problems with blurry vision. Physical examination shows a normal lens and mild diabetic retinopathy. Which of the following would best evaluate the possibility that chronically elevated glucose levels contribute to this patient's condition?
A. Blood glucose (fasting)
B. Blood ketones
C. Hemoglobin A_{1c} concentration
D. Serum C-peptide

8. A 23-year-old woman who has had diabetes mellitus since the age of 10 is unconscious when admitted to the emergency department. Physical examination shows a blood pressure of 80/40 mmHg; heart rate of 124 beats/minute, and respiratory rate of 35 breaths/minute. She has poor skin turgor and a fruity odor to her breath. Her blood glucose level is 750 mg/dL. Which of the following enzymes is most likely responsible

for the presence of a fruity odor on this patient's breath?
A. Acetyl CoA carboxylase
B. Citrate lyase
C. HMG CoA reductase
D. HMG CoA synthase
E. Pyruvate dehydrogenase

9. A 38-year-old woman with diabetic ketoacidosis has blurry vision and severe epigastric pain that radiates to her back. Physical examination shows yellow papular lesions scattered over her trunk and limbs and turbidity of the retinal vessels. Lipid studies show an elevation of both chylomicrons and very low-density lipoprotein (VLDL). Which of the following mechanisms most likely accounts for these clinical and laboratory findings?
A. Absence of LDL receptors
B. Congenital absence of lipoprotein lipase
C. Deficiency of apolipoprotein C-II (apoC-II)
D. Deficiency of functional apolipoprotein E (apoE)
E. Increased liver synthesis of triacylglycerol (TG)

10. A 3-month-old infant is brought to the pediatrician because of unremitting diaper rash and worsening cough. Physical examination is notable for a child below the 5th percentile on all growth curves and with diaper rash and oral thrush. A chest radiograph shows an infiltrate consistent with *Pneumocystis carinii* pneumonia. A complete blood cell count shows a complete lack of lymphocytes. Which of the following enzymes is most likely deficient in this infant?
A. Adenosine deaminase
B. Hypoxanthine-guanine phosphoribosyltransferase (HGPRT)
C. Phosphoribosylpyrophosphate synthase
D. Thymidine kinase
E. Xanthine oxidase

11. A 1-year-old boy has had progressive psychomotor retardation associated with chronic lactic acidosis since birth. Blood glucose and hemoglobin concentration are both normal. The boy most likely has a deficiency of which of the following enzymes?

A. Phosphoenolpyruvate carboxykinase
B. Phosphofructokinase
C. Pyruvate dehydrogenase
D. Pyruvate kinase

12. A 25-year-old man complains of a dragging sensation in his abdomen. Physical examination shows massive hepatosplenomegaly. Cytologic examination of bone marrow shows numerous macrophages with a fibrillar-appearing cytoplasm. The patient most likely has a deficiency of which of the following enzymes?

A. β-Galactosidase
B. Glucocerebrosidase
C. Hexosaminidase A
D. Sphingomyelinase

13. In one form of severe combined immunodeficiency disease (SCID), a buildup of one particular purine leads to the inhibition of synthesis of others by inhibiting the rate-limiting step in purine biosynthesis. Which of the following enzymes catalyzes the rate-limiting step in purine biosynthesis?

A. Adenosine deaminase
B. Hypoxanthine-guanine phosphoribosyltransferase (HGPRT)
C. Phosphoribosylpyrophosphate (PRPP) synthase
D. Thymidine kinase
E. Xanthine oxidase

14. A 24-year-old man returns from a trip to India and has profuse, watery diarrhea and a feeling of lightheadedness when he stands. Gram's stain of stool shows comma-shaped gram-negative organisms and an absence of an inflammatory reaction. Which of the following most accurately describes the biochemical alterations underlying this patient's diarrhea?

A. Activation of a G_q protein
B. Activation of a G_s protein
C. Inactivation of a G_i protein
D. Inhibition of a Cl^- channel
E. Stimulation of guanylyl cyclase activity

15. A 42-year-old woman with severe rheumatoid arthritis begins taking an immunosuppressive drug. A few weeks later, she develops moderately severe macrocytic anemia, with pancytopenia and hypersegmented neutrophils. The most likely mechanism underlying this drug-induced anemia involves inhibition of

A. Dihydrofolate reductase
B. Intestinal conjugase
C. Production of intrinsic factor
D. Reabsorption of folate

16. Researchers are developing a new drug to treat type IV hyperlipoproteinemia. The drug would be most useful in treating this disorder if it acted in which of the following ways?

A. Increased apolipoprotein B-100 (apoB-100) synthesis
B. Increased leptin synthesis
C. Inhibited apolipoprotein E (apoE) synthesis
D. Inhibited capillary lipoprotein lipase
E. Inhibited cholesterol ester transfer protein

17. A 45-year-old man comes to the emergency department complaining of an inability to walk because his foot hurts. The patient says that the previous evening he consumed a rather sumptuous meal and drank a large amount of alcohol. Physical examination is notable for an exquisitely tender and erythematous left first metatarsophalangeal joint. The patient has been taking a medication for this condition but is given a new medication to help prevent future occurrences of such attacks. Which of the following enzymes involved in nucleotide metabolism is most likely to be the target of the new drug?

A. Adenosine deaminase
B. Hypoxanthine-guanine phosphoribosyltransferase (HGPRT)
C. Phosphoribosylpyrophosphate synthase
D. Thymidine kinase
E. Xanthine oxidase

18. A clinical laboratory is developing a blood test for prostate cancer, and researchers are investigating an enzyme believed to be unique to

the prostate. An assay for the enzyme (E) involves the following reactions:

$$A + ATP + kinase \rightarrow B \sim P$$
$$B \sim P + E + NAD^+ \rightarrow C \sim P + E + NADH$$

To measure the amount of E that is released into the blood, which of the following conditions must be met?

A. ATP must be present in excess.
B. Enzyme E must be present in excess.
C. Kinase must be proportional to E.
D. NAD$^+$ must be rate-limiting.
E. Reactant A must be rate-limiting.

19. A 9-month-old infant is brought to the pediatrician because of incessant coughing with posttussive emesis. The child has had no immunizations. Physical examination shows an infant in acute distress, continually coughing, and with a characteristic inspiratory whoop after a bout of coughing. A chest radiograph shows no evidence of epiglottitis. Which of the following most accurately describes the biochemical basis for the clinical findings?

A. Activation of a G_q protein
B. Activation of a G_s protein
C. Inactivation of a G_i protein
D. Inhibition of a Cl$^-$ channel
E. Stimulation of guanylyl cyclase activity

20. A 24-year-old obese man has been following a popular weight loss diet for several weeks. He reports that his breath has a peculiar odor. A urine dipstick test would be expected to be positive for which of the following molecules?

A. Acetoacetate
B. Bilirubin
C. Glucose
D. β-Hydroxybutyrate
E. Nitrite

21. During a checkup of a 5-month-old infant, the physician notices that the infant's urine has a mousy odor. The infant has a decreased attention to his surroundings and a noticeable twitch. Laboratory studies show that his serum

phenylalanine hydroxylase is 2% that of the normal level. Which of the following metabolic intermediates is unable to be synthesized at normal levels in this patient?

A. Dihydroxyphenylalanine (DOPA)
B. Phenylalanine
C. Phenyllactic acid
D. Phenylpyruvate
E. Tyrosine

22. A 48-year-old man, who was born and raised in Mexico, complains of chronic diarrhea. His diet consists mainly of corn and corn-related products. He has a raised, hyperpigmented rash around his neck and on the back of both hands and forearms. Which of the following vitamins is most likely deficient in this patient?

A. Niacin
B. Pyridoxine
C. Thiamine
D. Vitamin A
E. Vitamin C

23. A 25-year-old woman complains of chest pain. On physical examination, a mid-systolic click is audible, followed by late systolic murmur, indicating a valvular disease. Which of the following glycosaminoglycans is associated with the valvular lesion?

A. Chondroitin sulfate
B. Dermatan sulfate
C. Heparan sulfate
D. Hyaluronic acid
E. Keratan sulfate

24. A 59-year-old man is brought to the emergency department with complaints of chest pain for the past hour. When asked about his current medications, he says he is taking a drug for his blood pressure and one for his angina but cannot remember their names. He does remember that he was told that any time he has chest pain to take the angina pill by holding it under his tongue until it dissolves. His physician told him it helps open the blood vessels. Which of the following best explains the biochemical mechanism of action of the angina medication?

A. Activation of a G_q protein
B. Activation of a G_s protein
C. Inactivation of a G_i protein
D. Inhibition of a Cl^- channel
E. Stimulation of guanylyl cyclase activity

25. During a physical examination of a 24-year-old man who is mentally retarded, the physician notices clumsiness and spasticity of the patient's limbs, emotional lability, and decreased visual-spatial discrimination. Laboratory studies show spherical granular masses in urinary sediment that stain positive with PAS and Alcian blue. The patient most likely has a deficiency of which of the following enzymes?
A. Arylsulfatase A
B. β-Glucosidase
C. Hexosaminidase A
D. Muscle phosphorylase
E. Sphingomyelinase

26. A 3-month-old infant develops cardiomegaly, leading to both left-sided and right-sided heart failure. Physical examination shows muscular atrophy without hypotonia. Which enzyme is most likely deficient in this infant?
A. Branching enzyme
B. Glucose 6-phosphatase
C. α-Glucosidase
D. Liver phosphorylase
E. Phosphofructokinase (PFK)

27. A 27-year-old man complains of genital sores. On questioning, the physician learns that the patient recently had an unsafe sexual contact. A Tzanck smear is positive for multinucleated giant cells with intranuclear inclusions. The physician initiates therapy with an antiviral agent. Which of the following enzymes is inhibited by the antiviral agent?
A. Adenosine deaminase
B. Hypoxanthine-guanine phosphoribosyltransferase (HGPRT)
C. Phosphoribosylpyrophosphate (PRPP) synthase
D. Thymidine kinase
E. Xanthine oxidase

28. A 35-year-old woman with type 1 diabetes mellitus is snowbound at a ski resort and is unable to take insulin for 3 days. Laboratory studies show hyperglycemia and increased anion gap metabolic acidosis. Which of the following biochemical pathways is mainly responsible for providing the substrate for this patient's acid-base disorder?
A. Catabolism of branched-chain amino acids
B. Citric acid cycle
C. Gluconeogenesis
D. Glycogenolysis
E. β-Oxidation of fatty acids

29. Oligomycin interferes with the synthesis of high-energy compounds by which of the following mechanisms?
A. Blocking the transfer of electrons from cytochrome b to cytochrome c
B. Closing the proton channel in the stalk of ATP synthase
C. Inhibiting adenine nucleotide carriers in the inner mitochondrial membrane
D. Inhibiting the oxidation of NADH
E. Uncoupling electron transport from oxidative phosphorylation

30. A 3-year-old child has ambiguous genitalia, diffuse pigmentation, and hypertension. Laboratory studies show an increase in plasma adrenocorticotropic hormone, a decrease in serum cortisol, and an increase in urine 17-ketosteroids. Chromosome analysis shows an XX genotype. Which of the following enzymes involved in adrenal steroid synthesis is most likely deficient in this patient?
A. 11-β-Hydroxylase
B. 17-α-Hydroxylase
C. 18-Hydroxylase
D. 21-α-Hydroxylase

31. A 22-year-old woman with poorly controlled gestational diabetes delivers a large-for-gestational-age infant at 24 weeks. Within 6 hours, the newborn has respiratory difficulties associated with tachypnea and cyanosis. Which of the following substances is most likely deficient in this newborn?

A. Cardiolipin
B. Ceramide
C. Dipalmitoyl phosphatidylcholine
D. Ganglioside
E. Sphingomyelin

32. A 1-year-old boy has a history of recurrent bacterial and fungal infections. Serum protein electrophoresis shows a flat γ-globulin region. Further testing shows increased concentrations of dATP in white blood cells. Which of the following is the most likely diagnosis?
A. Adenosine deaminase deficiency
B. Bruton's agammaglobulinemia
C. Lesch-Nyhan syndrome
D. Oroticaciduria
E. Purine-nucleoside phosphorylase deficiency

33. A 48-year-old woman complains of heart palpitations that keep her awake at night. Findings on physical examination include bilateral exophthalmos, thyromegaly, sinus tachycardia, and pretibial myxedema. Which of the following glycosaminoglycans accounts for the pretibial myxedema?
A. Chondroitin sulfate
B. Dermatan sulfate
C. Heparan sulfate
D. Hyaluronic acid
E. Keratan sulfate

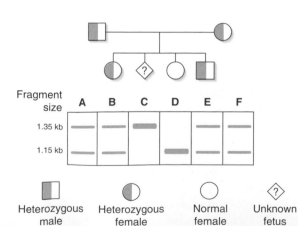

Fragment size

| | A | B | C | D | E | F |
1.35 kb
1.15 kb

Heterozygous male   Heterozygous female   Normal female   Unknown fetus

34. The pedigree in the preceding figure describes a family with a history of sickle cell trait. The mother (F), who is pregnant with her fourth child (C), wants to know whether the fetus she is carrying is normal or has either sickle cell disease or sickle cell trait. The results of six Southern blot tests using Mst-II endonuclease-digested DNA samples from each family member are shown below the corresponding symbol on the pedigree. Based on restriction fragment length polymorphism analysis, which of the following correctly characterizes the hematologic status of the fetus?
A. Normal
B. Sickle cell disease
C. Sickle cell trait

35. A 62-year-old woman complains of a sore tongue and generalized weakness. Physical examination indicates atrophy of the papillae on the tongue, pallor of the conjunctivae, and absent vibratory sensations in both lower extremities. A complete blood cell count shows a severe macrocytic anemia with hypersegmented neutrophils and pancytopenia. A bone marrow aspirate shows hypercellularity and markedly enlarged, immature nuclei in all nucleated cells. Which of the following is the most likely cause of this patient's symptoms?
A. Decreased activity of dihydrofolate reductase
B. Decreased activity of thymidylate synthetase
C. Decreased concentration of N^5-methyltetrahydrofolate
D. Decreased synthesis of deoxyribose thymidine monophosphate
E. Decreased synthesis of deoxyribose uridine monophosphate

36. A 20-year-old man of Greek descent has normocytic anemia and hemoglobinuria that occur following infections and the administration of quinoline drugs. Which of the following alterations in red blood cells (RBCs) is most likely present in this patient?
A. Decreased cellular glucose 6-phosphate concentrations
B. Decreased total NAD and NADH pools

C. Decreased total NADP and NADPH pools
D. Increased glucose 6-phosphate dehydrogenase
    activity
E. Increased oxidation of membrane lipids

37. A 65-year-old man with a known history of
chronic alcoholism complains of severe chest pain
that radiates down the inside of his left arm. An
ECG shows a prior acute anterior myocardial
infarction (MI). A complete blood cell count
shows a macrocytic anemia with hypersegmented
neutrophils and mild pancytopenia. No
neurologic abnormalities are evident. The plasma
homocysteine level is increased. Which of the
following best explains the increase in plasma
homocysteine in this patient?
A. Decreased level of cystathionine synthase
B. Decreased level of dihydrofolate reductase
C. Decreased level of thymidylate synthetase
D. Decreased serum folate
E. Decreased serum vitamin B_{12}

38. A full-term male infant begins to show
irritability and lethargy 36 hours after birth.
Laboratory studies show a plasma ammonia level
that is 60 times normal and a urinary orotate
level that is 100 times normal. Which enzyme is
most likely defective in this infant?
A. Arginase
B. Carbamoyl-phosphate synthetase II
C. Ornithine transcarbamoylase
D. Serine hydroxymethyltransferase

39. A 25-year-old man has hypovolemic shock
secondary to blood loss from fractures of the
pelvis and right femur. He must receive blood
compatible in type with his own to prevent a
hemolytic transfusion reaction. This patient
should be transfused with which of the following
blood types?
A. Type A
B. Type AB
C. Type B
D. Type O

40. A 46-year-old woman with rheumatoid arthritis
complains to her physician of having a bad taste

in her mouth and a rash near her mouth.
The rash has resisted treatment with topical
hydrocortisone. She recently had a basal cell
carcinoma surgically removed from her face, and
the wound is not healing properly. The patient
most likely has a deficiency of which of the
following nutrients?
A. Chromium
B. Copper
C. Vitamin C
D. Vitamin E
E. Zinc

41. A 20-year-old man develops markedly elevated
serum lactate concentrations and hypoglycemia
under fasting conditions. Which of the following
enzymes may be defective or absent in this
patient?
A. Glucose 6-phosphate dehydrogenase (G6PD)
B. Glycogen phosphorylase
C. Phosphoenolpyruvate carboxykinase
D. Pyruvate kinase

42. A 75-year-old man develops urinary retention.
Findings on physical examination include an
enlarged, soft prostate gland and a bladder that is
distended to the height of the umbilicus. A renal
ultrasound shows enlargement of the bladder,
both ureters, and the calyceal system of both
kidneys. The hormone responsible for the
enlarged prostate is directly produced by which
of the following enzymes?
A. Aromatase
B. 17-α-Hydroxylase
C. 21-α-Hydroxylase
D. Oxidoreductase
E. 5-α-Reductase

43. A 4-day-old infant has physiologic jaundice of
the newborn. She receives phototherapy with
blue light to reduce the level of bilirubin in her
blood and eliminate jaundice in her skin. Which
of the following mechanisms best explains the
manner in which phototherapy reduces
jaundice?
A. Increases conjugating enzymes in the liver
B. Increases synthesis of vitamin D in the skin

C. Metabolizes bilirubin into biliverdin

D. Oxidizes bilirubin into a water-soluble form

44. A medication is prescribed for a 79-year-old man who complains of difficulty in starting to urinate and in completely emptying his bladder. One week after the patient begins taking the medication, he returns to his physician complaining of dizziness on rising from a seated or reclining position. He says that he even fainted once upon quickly arising from bed. Which of the following processes is a normal biochemical signaling method that is being disrupted by this medication?

A. Activation of a G_q protein

B. Activation of a G_s protein

C. Inactivation of a G_i protein

D. Stimulation of guanylyl cyclase

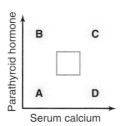

45. A 62-year-old woman has a recurrent history of calculi and peptic ulcer disease. A radionuclide scan of the parathyroid glands shows a well-circumscribed mass in the right inferior parathyroid gland. Which of the areas marked on the graph (indicated by the letters A, B, C, and D) represents the most likely levels of parathyroid hormone (PTH) and calcium in this patient?

A. Area A

B. Area B

C. Area C

D. Area D

46. A 21-year-old man has a history of intermittent jaundice since birth. Physical examination shows conjunctival pallor and mild splenomegaly.

Laboratory studies show a slightly increased unconjugated (indirect) bilirubin and a normocytic anemia with an increased peripheral blood reticulocyte count. Numerous spiculated RBCs are apparent in the peripheral smear. The patient most likely has a deficiency of which one of the following enzymes?

A. Glucose 6-phosphatase

B. Glucose 6-phosphate dehydrogenase (G6PD)

C. Pyruvate dehydrogenase

D. Pyruvate kinase

47. A 2-year-old child suffers from a rare genetic disease that is characterized by fat malabsorption, spinocerebellar degeneration, hemolytic anemia, and pigmented retinopathy. Total cholesterol and triacylglycerol levels are extremely low, and levels of chylomicrons, VLDL, and LDL are not detectable. The patient most likely has an abnormality associated with which of the following apolipoproteins?

A. Apolipoprotein A (apoA)

B. Apolipoprotein B (apoB)

C. Apolipoprotein C-II (apoC-II)

D. Apolipoprotein E (apoE)

48. A 28-year-old woman has an intermittent history of severe abdominal pain that typically occurs after she has consumed a few glasses of wine or after she has been on "crash diets." In visits to many different physicians during the past few years, she has undergone several laboratory tests (e.g., complete blood cell count and electrolytes), barium studies, and laparoscopic examinations, none of which has revealed the cause of her pain. Her physician now orders a urine specimen for culture. The woman collects the specimen and leaves it near a window for approximately 30 minutes, when she notices that the urine color has changed from pale yellow to wine red. Which of the following compounds is most likely responsible for the color change?

A. Hemoglobin

B. Myoglobin

C. Porphobilin

D. Urobilin

E. Uroporphyrin I

49. A 58-year-old man who has smoked for the past 30 years is experiencing seizures. X-rays show a small cell carcinoma of the lung. MRI shows generalized cerebral edema; however, there is no evidence of metastatic disease. His plasma osmolality is 250 mOsm/kg. Which of the following minerals is most likely responsible for these signs and symptoms in this patient?

A. Calcium
B. Magnesium
C. Phosphorus
D. Potassium
E. Sodium

50. A febrile 45-year-old man, who has been an alcoholic for the past 3 years, complains of severe pain in the right metatarsophalangeal joint of the big toe. Findings on physical examination include erythema and heat over the joint. A complete blood cell count shows an absolute neutrophilic leukocytosis with more than 10% band neutrophils in a 100 cell count. Synovial fluid shows needle-shaped crystals that have been phagocytosed by neutrophils. Which of the following findings best describes the pathophysiologic process underlying these findings?

A. Decreased activity of hypoxanthine-guanine phosphoribosyltransferase (HGPRT)
B. Decreased activity of xanthine oxidase
C. Decreased renal excretion of uric acid
D. Increased activity of phosphoribosylpyrophosphate synthetase

answers

1. **B** (serum ferritin level) is correct. This patient has a microcytic anemia (low MCV), most likely due to iron deficiency anemia resulting from menorrhagia (excessive menstrual flow). Serum ferritin is the most sensitive screening test for all the iron-related disorders. A fraction of circulating ferritin closely correlates with the amount of iron stored in the macrophages in bone marrow. Hence, in iron deficiency anemia, serum ferritin levels are decreased and correspond to absent iron stores in bone marrow. Increased serum ferritin indicates increased iron stores in bone marrow (e.g., anemia of chronic disease and hemochromatosis).

   A (hemoglobin electrophoresis) is incorrect. Hemoglobin electrophoresis is indicated only if thalassemia (globin chain deficiency) or abnormal hemoglobin (e.g., hemoglobin S and hemoglobin C) is suspected as a cause of the anemia. The patient's history of menorrhagia and microcytic anemia is more highly predictive of iron deficiency than of a genetic disorder such as thalassemia (microcytic anemia) or sickle cell disease (normocytic anemia).

   C (serum iron level) is incorrect. Serum iron levels are not as sensitive or as specific a test as serum ferritin in the diagnosis of iron deficiency. Serum iron levels do not always reflect iron stores in bone marrow. For example, in anemia of chronic disease, which also results in microcytic anemia, serum iron is decreased and serum ferritin is increased. Iron levels vary with the time of day the blood sample is taken, thus reducing the test's sensitivity.

   D (serum total iron-binding capacity) is incorrect. In the diagnosis of iron deficiency anemia, serum TIBC, like serum iron, is not as sensitive and specific a test as serum ferritin. Serum TIBC (the binding protein of iron) reflects the amount of transferrin that is present in the blood. Iron stores in bone marrow are inversely related to transferrin synthesis. For example, when iron stores are decreased (in iron deficiency anemia), transferrin synthesis is increased, thus increasing serum TIBC. When iron stores are increased (in anemia of chronic disease or hemochromatosis), serum transferrin synthesis is decreased, which decreases serum TIBC. Furthermore, serum TIBC is not always increased in iron deficiency anemia, hence reducing its sensitivity.

2. **C** (α-L-iduronidase) is correct. The infant has the classic features of Hurler's syndrome, an autosomal recessive lysosomal storage disease caused by a deficiency of the enzyme α-L-iduronidase. This condition, which is classified as a mucopolysaccharidosis, leads to an accumulation of dermatan and heparan sulfate. Analysis of fibroblast cultures provides evidence for the presence or absence of many enzymes.

   A (glucosidase) is incorrect. A deficiency of β-glucosidase causes Gaucher's disease, an autosomal recessive condition that leads to the accumulation of glucocerebroside in reticuloendothelial cells (Gaucher cells). This disorder is the most frequent form of the sphingolipidoses and is characterized by splenomegaly, increased skin pigmentation, and bone lesions.

B (hexosaminidase) is incorrect. A deficiency of hexosaminidase A results in the accumulation of GM_2 ganglioside, which is seen in patients with Tay-Sachs disease and Sandhoff's disease. Mental retardation and blindness are associated with both disorders, but they progress more rapidly in patients with Sandhoff's disease.

D (phosphotransferase) is incorrect. Loss of a phosphotransferase that tags lysosomal enzymes for compartmentation in lysosomes causes I cell disease. Affected individuals have mental deterioration, skeletal deformities, and elevated lysosomal enzymes in the plasma and urine.

E (sphingomyelinase) is incorrect. A deficiency of sphingomyelinase causes Niemann-Pick disease, an autosomal recessive disorder that leads to the accumulation of sphingomyelin. Signs of this disorder include an enlarged liver and spleen and mental retardation of rapid onset, usually within the first 6 months of life (type A disease).

3. **B** (hormone-sensitive lipase) is correct. This child is most likely suffering from a first presentation of type 1 diabetes mellitus. Hormone-sensitive lipase hydrolyzes triacylglycerol in adipose tissue to release free fatty acids. The lack of insulin and the presence of glucagon lead to the activation of hormone-sensitive lipase, which allows for increased release of free fatty acids and glycerol from adipose tissue.

A (carnitine acyltransferase) is incorrect. This enzyme couples free fatty acids to carnitine so that they are transported into the mitochondria and oxidized to provide fuel for the cells. It is not responsible for release of free fatty acids.

C (lipoprotein lipase) is incorrect. This enzyme is responsible for the hydrolysis of triacylglycerol in chylomicrons and VLDL to release free fatty acids for their uptake into extrahepatic tissues (primarily adipose).

D (pancreatic lipase) is incorrect. This digestive enzyme hydrolyzes dietary triacylglycerols present in the small intestine to facilitate their uptake.

E (phospholipase D) is incorrect. This enzyme is found in plants and animals. In mammals, it is responsible for hydrolysis of phosphatidylcholine.

4. **C** (urine bilirubin +2, urine urobilinogen 0) is correct. Normally, the results would be urine bilirubin 0 and urine urobilinogen +1. This patient has carcinoma of the head of the pancreas, which is caused most commonly by carcinogens in cigarette smoke. The common bile duct, which passes through the head of the pancreas, is completely obstructed by the mass, leading to distention of the gallbladder and reflux of bile containing conjugated bilirubin back into the liver. Conjugated (direct) bilirubin is water soluble, so any bilirubin in the urine is conjugated. In the blood, more than 50% of the total bilirubin is conjugated. Obstruction of bile flow, the most common cause of absence of urobilinogen in the urine, results in light-colored stools because of the absence of urobilinogen in the stool. Urobilin, the oxidation product of urobilinogen, is responsible for the brown color of stool and the yellow color of urine.

A (urine bilirubin 0, urine urobilinogen 0) is incorrect. In most patients, conjugated bilirubin is normally present in trace amounts in the urine. Obstruction of bile flow is the most common cause of absence of urobilinogen in the urine.

B (urine bilirubin 0, urine urobilinogen +2) is incorrect. These findings occur when an increase in unconjugated (indirect) bilirubin is presented to the liver for conjugation. This mainly occurs in hemolytic anemias in which there is macrophage destruction of RBCs, leading to an increase in unconjugated (indirect) bilirubin. Examples include congenital spherocytosis, sickle cell anemia, ABO and/or Rh incompatibility resulting in hemolytic disease of the newborn, and a type of autoimmune hemolytic anemia.

D (urine bilirubin +2, urine urobilinogen +2) is incorrect. These findings occur primarily in hepatitis, in which disruption of bile ductules in the liver occurs, leading to increased conjugated bilirubin in the blood and decreased recycling of urobilinogen by the inflamed liver. The result is increased amounts of urobilinogen in the urine.

5. **A** (addition of a competitive inhibitor) is correct. Line 1 illustrates a competitive inhibitor with an increase in the Michaelis-Menten constant (K_m) and no change in the maximal velocity (V_{max}). The X-intercept equals $-1/K_m$, and the Y-intercept equals $1/V_{max}$.

B (addition of a noncompetitive inhibitor) is incorrect. A noncompetitive inhibitor decreases V_{max} by decreasing the number of active enzyme molecules available. It does not affect the K_m of the remaining active molecules. Line 2 represents the action of a noncompetitive inhibitor.

C (change in pH) is incorrect. A change in pH has the potential to alter the charge distribution within the active site, with dramatic effects on both K_m and V_{max}. Both intercepts of line 1 would have been affected.

D (change in temperature) is incorrect. An increase in temperature above the optimum increases K_m and decreases V_{max} as a result of denaturation of the enzyme. Both intercepts of line 1 would have been affected.

E (increased ionic strength) is incorrect. Increased ionic strength increases K_m and decreases V_{max} as a result of denaturation of the enzyme. Both intercepts of line 1 would have been affected.

6. **B** (conversion of methyl-FH_4 to dihydrofolate is being blocked) is correct. Pernicious anemia is caused by a lack of intrinsic factor, which is the protein required for proper absorption of vitamin B_{12}. Vitamin B_{12} reduces the conversion of methyl-FH_4 to dihydrofolate. This traps all of the folate as methyl-FH_4, a form that cannot participate in any other folate-requiring reactions because the oxidation state of the single carbon is important.

A (*S*-adenosylmethionine is substituting for methyl-FH_4 as a methyl donor) is incorrect. Methyl-FH_4 is required for the conversion of homocysteine to methionine, a precursor of *S*-adenosylmethionine. Reactions that require *S*-adenosylmethionine do not use methyl-FH_4.

C (folate deficiency is creating a vitamin B_{12} deficiency) is incorrect. A vitamin B_{12} deficiency creates a folate deficiency because the available folate is in the form of methyl-FH_4, which is not used in DNA synthesis.

D (methyl-FH_4 is being used for conversion of glycine to serine) is incorrect. Methyl-FH_4 must be used for conversion of homocysteine to methionine. Serine hydroxymethyltransferase uses 5,10-methylene-FH_4 for conversion of glycine to serine.

E (methylene-FH_4 conversion to another form of FH_4 is being blocked) is incorrect. Interconversion between carbon-FH_4 oxidation states does not require vitamin B_{12}.

7. **C** (hemoglobin A_{1c} concentration) is correct. Blurry vision in this patient most likely results from poor glycemic control and the effect of glucose conversion to sorbitol by aldose reductase in the lens. Sorbitol, which is osmotically active, causes water to move into the lens, with subsequent alteration in its refraction to light. Hemoglobin A_{1c} measures the average level of glucose in the blood over the previous 4 to 8 weeks; it is the product of a concentration-dependent nonenzymatically catalyzed condensation of glucose and hemoglobin.

A (blood glucose) is incorrect. Blood glucose only provides information about insulin levels over the previous 4 to 6 hours.

B (blood ketones) is incorrect. Blood ketones are not an indicator of glycemic control. They are an indication that insulin levels are very low or absent.

D (serum C-peptide) is incorrect. C-peptide levels are an indicator of endogenous insulin release by the β islet cells, not of glycemic control.

8. D (HMG CoA synthase) is correct. HMG CoA synthase, the rate-limiting step in the production of ketones from acetyl CoA, accounts for the fruity odor. The smell of acetone on the breath, the signs of volume depletion (poor skin turgor), and the hyperglycemia indicate that the patient is in a state of diabetic ketoacidosis. Lack of insulin leads to elevated levels of free fatty acids and increased fatty acid oxidation in the liver, with concomitant ketogenesis.

A (acetyl CoA carboxylase) is incorrect. Acetyl CoA carboxylase, the enzyme that forms malonyl CoA, is the rate-limiting enzyme in the biosynthesis of fatty acids. Fatty acid oxidation is occurring, and fatty acid synthesis is inhibited.

B (citrate lyase) is incorrect. Citrate lyase converts citrate to oxaloacetate and acetyl CoA, generating cytosolic acetyl CoA for the synthesis of fatty acids. This system is inactive during times of fatty acid oxidation.

C (HMG CoA reductase) is incorrect. HMG CoA reductase is related to cholesterol metabolism and not to ketone metabolism. It converts HMG CoA to mevalonate.

E (pyruvate dehydrogenase) is incorrect. This patient's symptoms are the result of excessive ketone production, which decreases the activity of this enzyme. Acetyl CoA inhibits pyruvate dehydrogenase.

9. E (increased liver synthesis of triacylglycerol) is correct. This patient has hyperchylomicronemia syndrome, which is classically seen in diabetic ketoacidosis. The excess TG causes the eruptive xanthomas. The epigastric pain results from acute pancreatitis, and the retinal findings are indicative of lipemia retinalis.

A (absence of LDL receptors) is incorrect. The absence of LDL receptors causes familial hypercholesterolemia, in which plasma levels of LDL are elevated but TG levels are usually normal. Affected patients may present with xanthomas; pancreatitis is rare.

B (congenital absence of lipoprotein lipase) and C (deficiency of apolipoprotein C-II) are incorrect. Although the patient's symptoms are typical of both these deficiencies, these disorders usually manifest in infancy or childhood, not in middle age.

D (deficiency of functional apolipoprotein E) is incorrect. In dysbetalipoproteinemia, serum levels of intermediate-density lipoproteins (IDLs) and chylomicron remnants are elevated. Affected patients may present with xanthomas and early onset peripheral vascular disease.

10. A (adenosine deaminase) is correct. This child is manifesting common signs and symptoms of SCID as a result of a deficiency of the enzyme adenosine deaminase. This enzyme is responsible for the conversion of adenosine to inosine in the degradation pathway of adenosine. The deficiency leads to an accumulation of adenosine (which is toxic to lymphocytes) and dATP (which inhibits ribonucleotide reductase). The inhibition of

the ribonucleotide reductase results in a decreased supply of deoxynucleotides for DNA synthesis and decreased production of both B and T cell precursors.

B (hypoxanthine-guanine phosphoribosyltransferase) is incorrect. HGPRT is responsible for the salvage of purines by converting hypoxanthine and guanine to their monophosphated forms. Lack of HGPRT leads to destruction of free hypoxanthine and guanine, increased uric acid levels, and ensuing mental retardation and, less important, gout.

C (phosphoribosylpyrophosphate synthase) is incorrect. Phosphoribosylpyrophosphate synthase catalyzes the rate-limiting step in the synthesis of purine nucleotides and plays an important role in many other pathways. The most common alteration of this synthase is overactivity, which leads to an overproduction of purines and ensuing hyperuricemia and gout.

D (thymidine kinase) is incorrect. Thymidine kinase is an enzyme in the salvage pathway for pyrimidines (specifically thymine) that converts thymidine to TMP. Drugs such as acyclovir, which are used primarily to treat herpes, inhibit viral versions of this enzyme.

E (xanthine oxidase) is incorrect. Xanthine oxidase, the terminal enzyme in the degradation pathway of purines, converts xanthine to uric acid. This enzyme can be inhibited by allopurinol, which reduces the production of uric acid and abates the occurrences of gout in individuals prone to attacks.

11. C (pyruvate dehydrogenase) is correct. The patient most likely has a deficiency of pyruvate dehydrogenase, which is inherited as an autosomal recessive trait. Pyruvate dehydrogenase is responsible for the conversion of pyruvate to acetyl CoA, which then enters the citric acid cycle. A deficiency

of this enzyme results in an accumulation of pyruvate with concomitant formation of lactate. The low ATP yield per glucose molecule in the absence of the citric acid cycle and oxidative phosphorylation leads to central nervous system dysfunction.

A (phosphoenolpyruvate carboxykinase) is incorrect. A deficiency of phosphoenolpyruvate carboxykinase, a gluconeogenic enzyme, results in hypoglycemia; this patient has a normal fasting blood glucose.

B (phosphofructokinase) is incorrect. A deficiency of phosphofructokinase leads to cessation of glycolysis in all cells. The primary source of ATP is β-oxidation of fatty acids; lactic acidosis is not present in this patient.

D (pyruvate kinase) is incorrect. A deficiency of pyruvate kinase produces a hemolytic anemia; this patient has a normal hematocrit. Lactic acidosis is not a characteristic of this enzyme deficiency.

12. B (glucocerebrosidase) is correct. The man has Gaucher's disease, an autosomal recessive lysosomal storage disease characterized by a deficiency of glucocerebrosidase (β-glucosidase), leading to an accumulation of glucocerebroside in macrophages throughout the body. Type I (the adult type) is marked by hepatosplenomegaly, erosion of the long bones, and an elevation of total acid phosphatase. The macrophages have a fibrillar appearance because of the accumulation of glucocerebroside in the lysosomes.

A (β-galactosidase) is incorrect. Krabbe's disease, which is characterized by β-galactosidase deficiency, leads to mental retardation.

C (hexosaminidase A) is incorrect. Tay-Sachs disease, which is characterized by a deficiency of hexosaminidase A, leads to mental retardation and blindness at an early age. A cherry-red macula is a characteristic retinal finding.

D (sphingomyelinase) is incorrect. Niemann-Pick disease, which is characterized by a deficiency in sphingomyelinase, leads to an enlarged liver and spleen. Macrophages have a foamy appearance as a result of an accumulation of sphingolipid in the lysosomes. The disorder is fatal in early life.

13. C (phosphoribosylpyrophosphate synthase) is correct. PRPP synthase catalyzes the formation of phosphoribosylpyrophosphate from ribose 5-phosphate and ATP, the rate-limiting step in the synthesis of purine nucleotides. PRPP synthase also plays an important role in many other pathways. The most common alteration of PRPP synthase is overactivity, which leads to an overproduction of purines and the development of hyperuricemia and gout. The enzyme also plays a role in pyrimidine synthesis by supplying PRPP, the source of the ribose moiety in pyrimidine nucleosides.

A (adenosine deaminase) is incorrect. Adenosine deaminase is responsible for the conversion of adenosine to inosine in the degradation pathway of adenosine. A deficiency of this enzyme also leads to SCID.

B (hypoxanthine-guanine phosphoribosyltransferase) is incorrect. HGPRT is responsible for the salvage of purines by converting hypoxanthine and guanine into their monophosphated forms. A lack of this enzyme leads to destruction of free hypoxanthine and guanine, increased uric acid levels, ensuing mental retardation, and, less important, gout.

D (thymidine kinase) is incorrect. Thymidine kinase participates in the salvage pathway for pyrimidines (specifically thymine) that converts thymidine to thymidine monophosphate. Agents such as acyclovir, which are primarily used to treat herpes, exploit the action of viral versions of this enzyme, converting aycyclovir to an activated

triphosphate form. This activated form can then inhibit viral DNA synthesis.

E (xanthine oxidase) is incorrect. Xanthine oxidase, a terminal enzyme in the degradation pathway of purines, helps convert xanthine to uric acid. Allopurinol inhibits this enzyme, decreasing the production of uric acid as well as the frequency of gout in individuals prone to attacks.

14. B (activation of a G_s protein) is correct. The history and stool findings of this patient are characteristic of cholera caused by *Vibrio cholerae*. The cholera toxin acts on the intestinal mucosa and produces diarrhea by covalently modifying a G_s protein by ADP ribosylation. This is effective in permanently turning the protein "on," thus elevating intracellular levels of cAMP. This action stimulates the opening of chloride channels, resulting in a secretory diarrhea. Cholera is a toxin-induced disease and has no inflammatory component. Treatment involves fluid and electrolyte replacement to prevent dehydration (manifested as orthostatic symptoms in this case) and electrolyte imbalance.

A (activation of a G_q protein) is incorrect. G_q proteins activate phospholipase C, which cleaves phosphatidylinositol diphosphate to diacylglycerol and inositol triphosphate, in turn raising intracellular calcium concentrations. Examples of G_q receptors are type 1 muscarinic cholinergic receptors (M_1) and α_1-adrenergic receptors in the autonomic nervous system.

C (inactivation of a G_i protein) is incorrect. G_i proteins, when activated, inhibit the formation of cAMP. Permanent inactivation of the G_i protein, which leads to elevated levels of cAMP, is the mechanism of action of the pertussis toxin in respiratory epithelium.

D (inhibition of a Cl^- channel) is incorrect. The Cl^- channel, the final step in the generation of secretions from part of the intestines, is activated in this patient. Inhibition of the channel leads to a lack of secretions; this condition is often seen in patients with defective channels (e.g., with cystic fibrosis).

E (stimulation of guanylyl cyclase activity) is incorrect. Guanylyl cyclase, which produces cGMP from GTP, is part of the mechanism of action of a number of molecules, including the atrial natriuretic peptides and all agents that produce nitric oxide for vasodilation. Drugs such as sildenafil inhibit the breakdown of cGMP, thereby increasing cGMP concentrations and producing vasodilatory effects.

15. **A** (dihydrofolate reductase) is correct. The patient is most likely taking methotrexate, which is a competitive inhibitor of dihydrofolate reductase. The lack of dihydrofolate reductase leads to a lack of tetrahydrofolate and therefore inhibits the conversion of dUMP to TMP. This process stops proper DNA synthesis and occurs primarily in rapidly dividing cells, which are cells of hematopoietic origin.

B (intestinal conjugase) is incorrect. Intestinal conjugase is responsible for the conversion of the polyglutamate form of folate to the more readily absorbed monoglutamate form. Inhibition of intestinal conjugase is not a known side effect of immunosuppressive agents.

C (production of intrinsic factor) is incorrect. Intrinsic factor is secreted by the parietal cells of the stomach and binds to vitamin B_{12} in foodstuffs. Intrinsic factor is required for proper absorption of vitamin B_{12} in the terminal ileum. Lack of vitamin B_{12} can lead to a macrocytic anemia, but it would be unlikely to do so within a few weeks. Furthermore, methotrexate does not interfere with the production of intrinsic factor.

D (reabsorption of folate) is incorrect. Alcohol and oral contraceptives are known to interfere with absorption of the monoglutamate form of folate in the jejunum (methotrexate is not).

16. **B** (increased leptin synthesis) is correct. Type IV hyperlipoproteinemia is characterized by an increase in synthesis or a decrease in catabolism of VLDLs. VLDLs are synthesized in the liver and are the primary vehicle for carrying endogenously synthesized triacylglycerol (TG), which is synthesized from excess carbohydrate in the diet. Leptin is an appetite suppressant produced by adipose tissue that would curtail both obesity and excessive consumption of carbohydrate, both of which are associated with this type of hyperlipidemia.

A (increased apolipoprotein B-100 synthesis) is incorrect. ApoB-100 is already elevated in type IV hyperlipoproteinemia because it is attached to VLDLs in the liver.

C (inhibited apolipoprotein E synthesis) is incorrect. ApoE is required to clear the circulation of both IDLs, which are derived from VLDLs, and chylomicron remnants. A deficiency of apoE leads to an increase in these lipid fractions and would not be expected to lower VLDL levels. An agent that inhibits the synthesis of apoE would produce a dysbetalipoproteinemia (type III hyperlipoproteinemia).

D (inhibited capillary lipoprotein lipase) is incorrect. An agent that inhibits lipoprotein lipase would increase both chylomicrons and VLDL levels, causing the disease to worsen.

E (inhibited cholesterol ester transfer protein) is incorrect. An agent that inhibits cholesterol ester transfer protein would be useful in increasing the concentration of high-density lipoprotein (HDL) cholesterol. This protein transfers TG from VLDLs to HDLs in exchange for cholesterol esters. Therefore, blocking the protein keeps TG in VLDLs, causing their serum concentration to increase.

17. **E** (xanthine oxidase) is correct. This patient is manifesting classic signs and symptoms of an acute gouty flare. Gout is caused by deposition of uric acid crystals (monosodium urate) in synovial joint space and often favors the first metatarsophalangeal joint (podagra). The condition can be quite painful and, in its chronic form, is disfiguring. The patient was prescribed allopurinol, a drug that inhibits xanthine oxidase, the terminal enzyme in the degradation pathway of purines that converts hypoxanthine to xanthine and uric acid. This reduces the production of uric acid and decreases the occurrences of gout. Allopurinol is used to treat gout when there is an overproduction of uric acid.

A (adenosine deaminase) is incorrect. Adenosine deaminase catalyzes the conversion of adenosine to inosine in the degradation pathway of adenosine. A deficiency of this enzyme leads to a form of SCID.

B (hypoxanthine-guanine phosphoribosyltransferase) is incorrect. HGPRT is responsible for the salvage of purines by converting hypoxanthine and guanine to their monophosphated forms. Lack of HGPRT leads to destruction of free hypoxanthine and guanine, increased uric acid levels, and ensuing mental retardation and, less important, gout.

C (phosphoribosylpyrophosphate synthase) is incorrect. Phosphoribosylpyrophosphate synthase catalyzes the rate-limiting step in the synthesis of purine nucleotides and plays an important role in many other pathways. The most common alteration of this synthase is overactivity, which leads to an overproduction of purines and ensuing hyperuricemia and gout.

D (thymidine kinase) is incorrect. Thymidine kinase is an enzyme in the salvage pathway for pyrimidines (specifically thymine) that converts thymidine to TMP. Drugs such as acyclovir, which are used primarily to treat herpes, inhibit viral versions of this enzyme.

18. **A** (ATP must be present in excess) is correct. An accurate measurement of E requires that it is functioning at maximal velocity (V_{max}). Conditions that do not permit V_{max} will produce an underestimate of the true amount of enzyme. Recall that the V_{max} of an enzyme-catalyzed reaction is proportional to its concentration. Therefore, to obtain an accurate measurement, all reaction components other than the enzyme must be present in excess to ensure that it remains saturated with substrates.

B (enzyme E must be present in excess) is incorrect. This would produce a reaction in which another reagent is rate-limiting, causing an underestimate of the actual concentration of enzyme.

C (kinase must be proportional to E) is incorrect. The kinase must be present in excess in order to maintain B ~ P in excess to ensure that E is always measured at V_{max}.

D (NAD$^+$ must be rate-limiting) is incorrect. This would produce a reaction in which the actual amount of enzyme would be underestimated.

E (reactant A must be rate-limiting) is incorrect. If A were the rate-limiting reagent, then the concentration of enzyme would be underestimated.

19. **C** (inactivation of a G_i protein) is correct. This infant has classic symptoms of infection with *Bordetella pertussis,* the etiologic agent in whooping cough. One of the toxins secreted by *B. pertussis* covalently modifies the G_i protein in respiratory phagocytes, leading to impaired function of the G_i protein and elevated levels of cAMP. This action leads to ineffective phagocytosis and chemotaxis, and it inhibits lysosomal degradation of the bacteria.

A (activation of a G_q protein) is incorrect. G_q proteins activate phospholipase C, which cleaves phosphatidylinositol diphosphate to diacylglycerol and inositol triphosphate, in turn raising intracellular calcium concentrations. Examples of G_q receptors are type 1 muscarinic cholinergic receptors (M_1) and α_1-adrenergic receptors.

B (activation of a G_s protein) is incorrect. G_s proteins, when activated, stimulate the activity of adenylate cyclase, generating increased concentrations of cAMP in cells. The action of the cholera toxin involves irreversible activation of a G_s protein. Other receptors that operate via G_s proteins include β_1- and β_2-adrenergic receptors.

D (inhibition of a Cl^- channel) is incorrect. The Cl^- channel, the final step in the generation of secretions from part of the intestines, becomes activated in this patient. Inhibition of the channel leads to a lack of secretion, a condition that is often seen in patients with defective channels (e.g., with cystic fibrosis).

E (stimulation of guanylyl cyclase activity) is incorrect. Guanylyl cyclase, which produces cGMP from GTP, is part of the mechanism of action of a number of molecules, including the atrial natriuretic peptides and all agents that produce nitric oxide for vasodilation. Drugs such as sildenafil inhibit the breakdown of cGMP, thereby increasing cGMP concentrations and having vasodilatory effects.

20. **A** (acetoacetate) is correct. The patient's breath has the odor of acetone, which is a sign of ketosis. The ketone urine dipstick contains nitroprusside, which produces a color reaction only with acetoacetic acid. It cannot detect acetone or β-hydroxybutyric acid. This patient is probably following one of the popular low-carbohydrate/high-fat diets, and his body is responding to decreased levels of insulin by increasingly mobilizing fats and producing ketone bodies for fuel.

B (bilirubin) is incorrect. Bilirubin is always abnormal in the urine and is present only in obstructive jaundice or hepatitis. In these

disorders, direct or conjugate water-soluble bilirubin has access to the bloodstream. Only acetoacetate is detected by the ketone urine dipstick test.

C (glucose) is incorrect. Increased glucose, with spilling of glucose into the urine, would be expected to result during diabetic ketoacidosis. Instead, this patient is probably depriving his body of carbohydrates.

D (β-hydroxybutyrate) is incorrect. The ketone urine dipstick test detects only acetoacetate. A different test must be used to detect β-hydroxybutyrate.

E (nitrite) is incorrect. Nitrites are usually present only with urinary tract infections caused by bacteria capable of reducing nitrate to nitrite (e.g., *Escherichia coli*).

21. **E** (tyrosine) is correct. Phenylalanine hydroxylase catalyzes the conversion of phenylalanine to tyrosine. Individuals with phenylketonuria (PKU) have a deficiency of phenylalanine hydroxylase and can neither degrade phenylalanine nor synthesize tyrosine properly; they require phenylalanine as a dietary supplement. The levels of the amino acid must be strictly controlled, with neither too much nor too little being given to patients with PKU, particularly prior to adolescence. Without proper treatment, PKU leads to mental retardation. The mousy odor is caused by the buildup of phenylpyruvate and phenyllactate.

A (dihydroxyphenylalanine) is incorrect. DOPA is synthesized from dietary tyrosine in children with PKU. It is a precursor of dopamine and other catecholamines.

B (phenylalanine) is incorrect. Phenylalanine accumulates in patients with PKU because phenylalanine hydroxylase cannot convert it to tyrosine. The buildup of phenylalanine causes a shunting of metabolism toward phenylketones that appear in the tissue and in blood.

C (phenyllactic acid) is incorrect. Phenyllactic acid synthesis is accelerated in PKU. This acid contributes to the mousy odor of the urine of patients with the disease.

D (phenylpyruvate) is incorrect. Phenylpyruvate synthesis is accelerated in PKU, and the compound is then converted to phenyllactate and phenylacetate. These compounds, which are excreted in the urine, are measurable in patients with PKU who have recently ingested phenylalanine.

22. **A** (niacin) is correct. Niacin (vitamin B_3, nicotinic acid) is required for the synthesis of NAD^+, a cofactor for catabolic reactions, and $NADP^+$, a cofactor for anabolic reactions. Niacin is found in meats, fish, milk, and eggs. In corn, niacin is present in a bound form and cannot be reabsorbed; deficiency of the vitamin is therefore most likely to occur in countries in which corn is the primary source of food. This patient has diarrhea and dermatitis, two of the three symptoms found in niacin deficiency (pellagra). Dermatitis occurs primarily on sun-exposed areas (e.g., the back of hands and neck). Dementia may be a potential complication of niacin deficiency.

B (pyridoxine) is incorrect. Pyridoxine (vitamin B_6) is present in whole-grain cereals, eggs, meats, fish, soybeans, and nuts. It is involved in heme synthesis, transamination reactions, and synthesis of neurotransmitters. Deficiency of pyridoxine is associated with defects in heme synthesis (sideroblastic anemia), peripheral neuropathy, and convulsions. The most common cause of pyridoxine deficiency is isoniazid, a drug used in the treatment of tuberculosis.

C (thiamine) is incorrect. Thiamine (vitamin B_1) is present in enriched and whole-grain cereals, brewer's yeast, meats, legumes, and nuts. It is involved in transketolase reactions and oxidative decarboxylation reactions involving pyruvate dehydrogenase, α-ketoglutarate dehydrogenase, and α-keto acid dehydrogenase reactions. Deficiency is most often due to alcohol excess. Signs and symptoms of thiamine deficiency include Wernicke's encephalopathy, Korsakoff's psychosis, and peripheral neuropathy.

D (vitamin A) is incorrect. Vitamin A is obtained from cod liver oil, dairy products, egg yolk, and dark green leafy and yellow vegetables. It is important in preventing squamous metaplasia, maintaining rhodopsin, wound healing, spermatogenesis, and normal growth in children. Deficiency results in night blindness, blindness resulting from squamous metaplasia of conjunctival epithelium, respiratory infections, and dry skin (follicular hyperkeratosis).

E (vitamin C) is incorrect. Vitamin C is present in fruits and vegetables. It is important in hydroxylation of proline and lysine residues in collagen synthesis, catecholamine synthesis, reduction of iron from the ferric state to the ferrous state, trapping free radicals, and maintaining tetrahydrofolate in its reduced state. Deficiency results in small-vessel instability (ecchymoses), poor wound healing, glossitis, hemarthroses, perifollicular hemorrhage, and loosened teeth.

23. **B** (dermatan sulfate) is correct. This patient has mitral valve prolapse, which is characterized by redundancy of the mitral valve leaflets, causing them to prolapse into the left atrium during systole. This results in a click during prolapse, followed by a short systolic murmur due to mitral regurgitation. The glycosaminoglycan dermatan sulfate is found in valvular tissue in the heart. Glycosaminoglycans, the major components of ground substance in the interstitial tissue, are complexes of branched, negatively charged polysaccharide chains that contain amino sugars (e.g., glucosamine or galactosamine) and acid sugars (iduronic acid or glucuronic

acid). Sections through the mitral valve in a patient with mitral valve prolapse would show myxomatous degeneration involving loss of dermatan sulfate.

A (chondroitin sulfate) is incorrect. This glycosaminoglycan is found primarily in cartilage.

C (heparan sulfate) is incorrect. This glycosaminoglycan is found primarily in the glomerular basement membrane, where it is responsible for the strong negative charge that repels albumin.

D (hyaluronic acid) is incorrect. This glycosaminoglycan is the major component of synovial fluid, where it serves as a joint lubricant.

E (keratan sulfate) is incorrect. This glycosaminoglycan is found in cartilage, where it is associated with chondroitin sulfate.

24. **E** (stimulation of guanylyl cyclase activity) is correct. This patient is most likely taking nitroglycerin pills for his angina. This medication releases nitric oxide (NO) into the bloodstream. In turn, NO stimulates the activity of guanylyl cyclase, increasing the concentration of cGMP in the cell. This leads to vasodilation, especially of arterioles, typically with relief of anginal symptoms in many patients.

A (activation of a G_q protein) is incorrect. G_q proteins activate phospholipase C, which cleaves phosphatidylinositol diphosphate to diacylglycerol and inositol triphosphate, which then raises the intracellular calcium concentration. Examples of G_q receptors are type 1 muscarinic cholinergic receptors (M_1) and α_1-adrenergic receptors.

B (activation of a G_s protein) is incorrect. When activated, G_s proteins stimulate the activity of adenylate cyclase, generating increased concentrations of cAMP in cells. The action of the cholera toxin involves irreversible activation of a G_s protein. Other receptors that operate via G_s proteins include β_1- and β_2-adrenergic receptors.

C (inactivation of a G_i protein) is incorrect. G_i proteins, when activated, inhibit the formation of cAMP. Permanent inactivation of the G_i protein, which leads to elevated levels of cAMP, is the mechanism of action of the pertussis toxin.

D (inhibition of a Cl^- channel) is incorrect. The Cl^- channel, the final step in the generation of secretion from part of the intestines, becomes activated in this patient. Inhibition of the channel leads to a lack of secretion, a condition that is often seen in patients with defective channels (e.g., with cystic fibrosis).

25. **A** (arylsulfatase A) is correct. A deficiency of arylsulfatase results in metachromatic leukodystrophy, which is an autosomal recessive disease. This disorder causes accumulation of a sulfate-containing ceramide (positive PAS and Alcian blue stain) in lysosomes. The most common symptoms are demyelination of nerve cells leading to mental retardation and motor abnormalities.

B (β-glucosidase) is incorrect. A deficiency of β-glucosidase results in Gaucher's disease, an autosomal recessive disease. This disorder is the most frequently occurring form of sphingolipidosis. It causes accumulation of ceramide with an attached glucose moiety and has different staining properties and tissue localization than does metachromatic leukodystrophy. Gaucher cells in the adult form are found in the reticuloendothelial system. Presenting symptoms may include mental retardation, but there are no signs of adverse effects on myelin production.

C (hexosaminidase A) is incorrect. A deficiency of hexosaminidase A results in Tay-Sachs disease, an autosomal recessive disorder, causing the accumulation of GM_2 ganglioside. Symptoms of Tay-Sachs disease include mental retardation and blindness.

D (muscle phosphorylase) is incorrect. A deficiency in muscle phosphorylase results in McArdle's disease, an autosomal recessive disorder. The disease causes the loss of an immediate source of glucose to support muscle contraction, which leads to muscle cramping with exercise (a common presenting symptom).

E (sphingomyelinase) is incorrect. A deficiency in sphingomyelinase results in Niemann-Pick disease, an autosomal recessive disorder. This disorder causes sphingomyelin to accumulate in the lysosomes, which produces symptoms such as liver and spleen enlargement in addition to mental retardation. It is usually fatal early in life.

26. **C** (α-glucosidase) is correct. The infant most likely has Pompe's disease. This lysosomal glycogen storage disease (type II) is characterized by a deficiency of α-glucosidase. An excess amount of normal glycogen accumulates in all tissues, with the heart being the most vulnerable.

A (branching enzyme) is incorrect. Branching enzyme deficiency produces Andersen's disease (type IV glycogen storage disease). The abnormal branching pattern is believed to lead to cirrhosis of the liver. Patients with this disease typically are diagnosed with failure to thrive within the first 18 months of life and die by 5 years of age.

B (glucose 6-phosphatase) is incorrect. Glucose 6-phosphatase deficiency produces von Gierke's disease (type I glycogen storage disease), which affects the liver and kidneys. Children with this disease are diagnosed with massive hepatorenomegaly and fasting hypoglycemia at 3 or 4 months of age.

D (liver phosphorylase) is incorrect. Liver phosphorylase deficiency produces Hers' disease (type VI glycogen storage disease). This is a rare disease that initially manifests in childhood as hepatomegaly and growth retardation. Both symptoms improve with age and typically disappear by puberty.

E (phosphofructokinase) is incorrect. PFK, the rate-limiting enzyme of glycolysis, helps convert fructose 6-phosphate to fructose 1,6-bisphosphate. This process deprives the muscle of an energy source and leads to rhabdomyolysis with concomitant myoglobinuria with exercise. Deficiency of PFK (type VII glycogen storage disease) does not alter glycogenolysis. However, the glucose that is produced cannot be used for energy; therefore, during exercise, the muscle reacts much as it does in McArdle's disease (type V). Red blood cells rely on anaerobic glycolysis for their source of ATP and therefore undergo hemolysis.

27. **D** (thymidine kinase) is correct. This patient has a herpes infection (most likely type 2). The medication prescribed by the physician was probably acyclovir (or a newer recent derivative). This agent mimics a nucleoside and must be phosphorylated by thymidine kinase in order to block viral replication. Notably, some virions of the herpes family have been found that do not contain thymidine kinase; therefore, they are resistant to acyclovir and its congeners.

A (adenosine deaminase) is incorrect. Adenosine deaminase is responsible for the conversion of adenosine to inosine in the degradation pathway of adenosine. A deficiency of this enzyme leads to a form of SCID.

B (hypoxanthine-guanine phosphoribosyl-transferase) is incorrect. HGPRT is responsible for the salvage of purines by converting hypoxanthine and guanine into their monophosphated forms. Lack of HGPRT leads to destruction of free hypoxanthine and guanine, increased uric acid levels, ensuing mental retardation, and, less important, gout.

C (phosphoribosylpyrophosphate synthase) is incorrect. PRPP synthase, which catalyzes the rate-limiting step in the synthesis of purine nucleotides, plays an important role in many other pathways. The most common alteration of PRPP synthase is overactivity, which leads to an overproduction of purines and the development of hyperuricemia and gout.

E (xanthine oxidase) is incorrect. Xanthine oxidase, a terminal enzyme in the degradation pathway of purines, helps convert xanthine to uric acid. Allopurinol, which decreases the production of uric acid as well as the frequency of gout in individuals prone to attacks, may inhibit this enzyme.

28. **E** (β-oxidation of fatty acids) is correct. The patient is currently in diabetic ketoacidosis. This condition is secondary to an increase in acetoacetate and β-hydroxybutyrate, the anions responsible for the increased anion gap metabolic acidosis. Ketogenesis occurs primarily in the liver and requires acetyl CoA derived from the β-oxidation of fatty acids in the mitochondrial matrix.

A (catabolism of branched-chain amino acids) is incorrect. Muscle is the primary tissue that catabolizes branched-chain amino acids (e.g., valine, leucine, and isoleucine). Valine is catabolized to succinyl CoA (glucogenic substrate), leucine to acetyl CoA and acetoacetate (ketogenic substrates), and isoleucine to acetyl CoA and succinyl CoA. An increase in branched-chain keto acids derived from these amino acids occurs in maple syrup urine disease, which results from a deficiency of branched-chain α-keto acid dehydrogenase. These keto acids are not the source of anions in diabetic ketoacidosis.

B (citric acid cycle) is incorrect. In addition to providing NADH, FADH$_2$, and GTP for ATP synthesis, the citric acid cycle also provides substrates for gluconeogenesis (e.g., succinyl CoA). It plays no role in ketogenesis.

C (gluconeogenesis) is incorrect. Gluconeogenesis is primarily responsible for hyper-

glycemia in diabetic ketoacidosis and plays no role in ketogenesis.

D (glycogenolysis) is incorrect. Glycogenolysis is one of the initial causes of hyperglycemia in diabetic ketoacidosis. However, it is self-limited once liver glycogen stores are depleted and plays no role in ketogenesis.

29. **B** (closing the proton channel in the stalk of ATP synthase) is correct. Prevention of the flow of protons through the ATP synthase stalk inhibits ATP synthesis. Normally, the electron transport chain pumps protons out of the mitochondrial matrix, and the return of protons to the matrix "down" the gradient drives the synthesis of ATP by ATP synthase. When oligomycin is present, protons cannot complete this circuit.

A (blocking the transfer of electrons from cytochrome b to cytochrome c) is incorrect. Antimycin A, an antibiotic, blocks the flow of electrons between cytochrome b and cytochrome c.

C (inhibiting adenine nucleotide carriers in the inner mitochondrial membrane) is incorrect. Atractyloside, a plant toxin, inhibits the adenine nucleotide carrier, causing depletion of the ADP pool and the eventual inhibition of ATP synthesis.

D (inhibiting the oxidation of NADH) is incorrect. The drug amobarbital and the insecticide rotenone block proton pumping by inhibiting the transfer of electrons from flavin mononucleotide to coenzyme Q. Thus, they prevent the oxidation of NADH by NADH dehydrogenase and inhibit oxidative phosphorylation.

E (uncoupling electron transport from oxidative phosphorylation) is incorrect. Dinitrophenol uncouples these two processes by permitting protons to diffuse freely back into the matrix. This action results in an uninterrupted flow of electrons that allows protons to circumvent ATP synthase while being pumped out of the mitochondrial matrix. ATP synthase does not produce ATP.

30. A (11-β-hydroxylase) is correct. This child has adrenogenital syndrome, which consists of a group of autosomal recessive conditions that involve enzyme deficiencies in adrenal steroid synthesis, leading to hypocortisolism. A deficiency of 11-β-hydroxylase results in an increase in steroid compounds proximal to the enzyme block and a decrease in those compounds distal to the block. Levels of the 17-ketosteroids dehydroepiandrosterone and androstenedione are increased because they are proximal to the block. Androstenedione is converted to testosterone, which is converted to dihydrotestosterone by 5-α-reductase. Dihydrotestosterone is primarily responsible for producing ambiguous genitalia in females. 11-Deoxycortisol is increased because it is proximal to the enzyme block, and cortisol is decreased because it is distal to the block. There is also an increase in 11-deoxycorticosterone, a weak mineralocorticoid that is responsible for salt retention, leading to hypertension.

B (17-α-hydroxylase) is incorrect. 17-α-Hydroxylase is responsible for the conversion of pregnenolone to 17-hydroxypregnenolone and progesterone to 17-hydroxyprogesterone. Each compound is again converted to 17-ketosteroids. Because the 17-ketosteroids are increased in this patient, 17-α-hydroxylase deficiency is not a possible cause of the symptoms.

C (18-hydroxylase) is incorrect. 18-Hydroxylase, which converts corticosterone to aldosterone, does not cause hypocortisolism or any of the symptoms evident in this patient.

D (21-α-hydroxylase) is incorrect. In 21-α-hydroxylase deficiency, the 17-ketosteroids are increased, but the 17-hydroxycorticoids and the mineralocorticoid compounds (11-deoxycorticosterone, corticosterone, and aldosterone) are decreased. Mineralocorticoid

deficiency leads to the loss of sodium in the urine and retention of potassium in the blood. Sodium loss results in hypotension, not hypertension.

31. C (dipalmitoyl phosphatidylcholine) is correct. The newborn has respiratory distress syndrome (RDS), which is caused by a lack of production of lung surfactant by type II pneumocytes in the lungs. Dipalmitoyl phosphatidylcholine (lecithin), the primary lung surfactant, reduces surface tension, preventing the collapse of alveoli. RDS is very common in premature infants (usually <32 weeks' gestation) because of lung immaturity. In addition, RDS frequently occurs in infants born to diabetic mothers as the result of fetal hyperglycemia and hyperinsulinemia, which delay surfactant production.

A (cardiolipin) is incorrect. Cardiolipins are lipids that occur in high concentration in the inner mitochondrial membrane.

B (ceramide) is incorrect. Ceramide, which is a precursor to sphingomyelin and ganglioside, occurs primarily in the myelin sheath.

D (ganglioside) is incorrect. Gangliosides are cerebrosides that occur in myelin.

E (sphingomyelin) is incorrect. Sphingomyelins occur in nerve tissue and blood.

32. A (adenosine deaminase deficiency) is correct. Adenosine deaminase deficiency leads to an extremely large accumulation of dATP, which inhibits ribonucleotide reductase. The resulting impairment in both T cell (recurrent fungal infections) and B cell function (hypogammaglobulinemia with a flat γ-globulin region) has led to the name severe combined immunodeficiency disease, or SCID.

B (Bruton's agammaglobulinemia) is incorrect. Bruton's agammaglobulinemia is an X-linked recessive disorder in which pre-B cells cannot mature into B cells, causing an isolated hypogammaglobulinemia.

C (Lesch-Nyhan syndrome) is incorrect. Lesch-Nyhan syndrome results from a genetic deficiency in hypoxanthine-guanine phosphoribosyltransferase, which prevents the salvage of both hypoxanthine and guanine. The blocked salvage simultaneously leads to a decrease in the concentrations of inosine monophosphate and guanosine monophosphate (feedback inhibitors of the first step in purine synthesis) and an increase in phosoribosylpyrophosphate (the limiting substrate in the first step of purine synthesis).

D (oroticaciduria) is incorrect. Oroticaciduria results from a deficiency of the enzymes that convert orotate into uridine 5'-monophosphate. The buildup of orotic acid leads to abnormal growth and megaloblastic anemia. Treatment with a uridine-rich diet is successful.

E (purine nucleoside phosphorylase deficiency) is incorrect. Purine nucleoside phosphorylase deficiency results in an accumulation of dGTP and dATP, both of which inhibit ribonucleotide reductase. This causes impairment of T cell function (but not B cell function).

33. **B** (dermatan sulfate) is correct. This patient has Graves' disease, which results from an IgG antibody directed against the thyroid-stimulating hormone receptor. Pretibial myxedema, a nonpitting type of edema, results from excessive deposition of the glycosaminoglycan dermatan sulfate in the interstitial tissue. Glycosaminoglycans, the major components of ground substance in the interstitial tissue, are complexes of branched, negatively charged polysaccharide chains that contain amino sugars (e.g., glucosamine or galactosamine) and acid sugars (iduronic acid or glucuronic acid). The glycosaminoglycan dermatan sulfate is found in skin and in valvular tissue of the heart.

A (chondroitin sulfate) is incorrect. This glycosaminoglycan is found principally in cartilage.

C (heparan sulfate) is incorrect. This glycosaminoglycan is found principally in the glomerular basement membrane, where it is responsible for the strong negative charge that repels albumin.

D (hyaluronic acid) is incorrect. This glycosaminoglycan is the major component of synovial fluid, where it serves as a joint lubricant.

E (keratan sulfate) is incorrect. This glycosaminoglycan is found in cartilage, where it is associated with chondroitin sulfate.

34. **B** (sickle cell disease) is correct. The normal β-globin gene has three Mst-II restriction sites that, after digestion with Mst-II endonuclease, cleave a 1.35-kb fragment into a 1.15-kb fragment and a 0.2-kb fragment. The 1.15-kb fragment is identified by electrophoresis, and the smaller 0.2-kb fragment is lost. The sickle cell gene lacks the interior Mst-II restriction site because the point mutation that produces sickle cell hemoglobin occurs at this same site. Therefore, individuals homozygous for the sickle cell gene (fetus C) have two 1.35-kb fragments (one from each chromosome). Heterozygous individuals (carriers of the sickle cell trait) have one 1.15-kb fragment from the normal chromosome and one 1.35-kb fragment from the chromosome with the sickle cell gene. Female child D is normal and has two 1.15-kb fragments (note that the line is twice as thick).

A (normal) is incorrect. For normal individuals without the sickle cell gene, the 1.35-kb fragments on both chromosomes are cleaved into two 1.15-kb fragments.

C (sickle cell trait) is incorrect. In sickle cell trait, the chromosome with the sickle cell gene is not digested, leaving only a single

1.35-kb fragment. The normal chromosome is digested, producing a single 1.15-kb fragment.

35. D (decreased synthesis of deoxyribose thymidine monophosphate) is correct. The macrocytic anemia with pancytopenia (decrease of all cell lines) and the signs of posterior column disease (decreased vibratory sensation) result from a vitamin B_{12} deficiency. A deficiency of either vitamin B_{12} or folate leads to decreased synthesis of DNA in all nucleated cells. Hence, the nuclear DNA does not mature, and the nucleus remains abnormally enlarged. The large nucleated hematopoietic cells in bone marrow (normoblasts, neutrophils, and megakaryocytes), called megaloblasts, are destroyed by macrophages before they reach the circulation. Thus, pancytopenia (anemia, neutropenia, and thrombocytopenia) develops. Posterior column disease reflects the role of vitamin B_{12} in maintaining nerve cell membrane integrity.

A (decreased activity of dihydrofolate reductase) is incorrect. Dihydrofolate reductase converts oxidized dihydrofolate back to tetrahydrofolate. Inhibition of the enzyme by methotrexate or trimethoprim results in decreased tetrahydrofolate and reduced DNA synthesis. No neurologic abnormalities are associated with folate deficiency.

B (decreased activity of thymidylate synthetase) is incorrect. Inhibition of this enzyme leads to reduced DNA synthesis and a macrocytic anemia with no neurologic abnormalities.

C (decreased concentration of N^5-methyl-tetrahydrofolate) is incorrect. The presence of neurologic disease rules out the diagnosis of folate deficiency.

E (decreased synthesis of deoxyribose uridine monophosphate) is incorrect. The nucleotide dUMP is used to synthesize dTMP.

36. E (increased oxidation of membrane lipids) is correct. The patient has glucose 6-phosphate dehydrogenase (G6PD) deficiency, an X-linked recessive disorder, which is common in individuals of Mediterranean descent. G6PD deficiency leads to a reduced level of glutathione, which makes the RBC membranes vulnerable to the oxidizing effects of drugs such as primaquine and dapsone.

A (decreased cellular glucose 6-phosphate concentrations) is incorrect. Glucose 6-phosphate concentrations do not cause the symptoms of hemolytic anemia described. These concentrations would affect the energy charge of the RBC and cause reduced ability to regulate osmotic balance.

B (decreased total NAD and NADH pools) is incorrect. A decreased pool of NAD and NADH would lead to reduced ability to form lactate and would indirectly reduce the energy charge of the RBC. It would not produce the symptoms of hemolytic anemia described in the patient.

C (decreased total NADP and NADPH pools) is incorrect. The symptoms of hemolytic anemia are not produced by a reduced pool of NADP and NADPH but, rather, by a reduction in the amount of NADPH available.

D (increased glucose 6-phosphate dehydrogenase activity) is incorrect. The patient's symptoms are caused by a deficiency, not an increase, in G6PD.

37. D (decreased serum folate) is correct. Alcoholism is the most common cause of folate deficiency. Alcoholism accompanied by a poor diet leads to decreased liver stores of folate and decreased reabsorption of the monoglutamate form of folate in the jejunum. Vitamin B_{12} (cobalamin) removes the methyl group from N^5-methyltetrahydrofolate (circulating form of folate) to produce methyl-vitamin B_{12} and tetrahydrofolate. The methyl group is then transferred to homocysteine to produce methionine. Therefore, a decrease in either N^5-methyl-tetrahydrofolate or vitamin B_{12} results in increased plasma homocysteine levels. An increase in plasma homocysteine levels leads to damage of endothelial cells and the potential for vessel thrombosis, which may have played a role in this patient's MI.

A (decreased level of cystathionine synthase) is incorrect. Deficiency of cystathionine synthase is present in homocystinuria, a rare autosomal recessive disease. Cystathionine synthase catalyzes the reaction that converts homocysteine to cystathionine. Elevated plasma homocysteine and methionine (regenerated from homocysteine) as well as a propensity for vessel thrombosis are characteristic of this disorder.

B (decreased level of dihydrofolate reductase) is incorrect. Dihydrofolate reductase converts oxidized dihydrofolate back to tetrahydrofolate. The amount of dihydrofolate reductase increases during deficiency of folate by gene amplification.

C (decreased level of thymidylate synthetase) is incorrect. Thymidylate synthetase converts deoxyribose uridine monophosphate to deoxyribose thymidine monophosphate, which is used in DNA synthesis. This enzyme requires folate, and although the amount of enzyme present is not decreased, its activity will be decreased.

E (decreased serum vitamin B_{12}) is incorrect. Vitamin B_{12} deficiency produces neurologic abnormalities in the spinal cord and central nervous system. Because there are no neurologic findings in this case, vitamin B_{12} deficiency is unlikely.

38. **C** (ornithine transcarbamoylase) is correct. Defects of the urea cycle retard the disposal of free NH_3, causing it to accumulate in the bloodstream. The more proximal the enzyme defect in the urea cycle, the more pronounced the increase in NH_3 in the blood. A deficiency of ornithine transcarbamoylase in the mitochondrion blocks the entry of nitrogen into the urea cycle as carbamoyl phosphate by preventing its conversion to citrulline. The carbamoyl phosphate in the mitochondrion eventually leaks into the cytoplasm, where it accelerates the pyrimidine pathway, leading to the appearance of orotic acid in the urine.

A (arginase) is incorrect. Arginase is responsible for cleaving arginine to urea and ornithine; a deficiency of arginase leads to a buildup of arginine. Typically, the metabolism of arginine by other pathways (creatine and nitric acid synthase) or its elimination in the urine prevent this accumulation. In rare instances of excessive protein intake, a deficiency of arginase may lead to a mild to moderate hyperammonemia.

B (carbamoyl-phosphate synthetase II) is incorrect. Carbamoyl-phosphate synthetase II, the cytosolic form of the enzyme, catalyzes one of the initial steps in pyrimidine synthesis. If this enzyme were deficient, the urea cycle, which would have a functional carbamoyl-phosphate synthetase I, would remove any accumulated ammonia.

D (serine hydroxymethyltransferase) is incorrect. Serine hydroxymethyltransferase reversibly transfers a single-carbon unit from methylene tetrahydrofolate to glycine to synthesize serine. A deficiency of this enzyme does not result in hyperammonemia.

39. **D** (type O) is correct. Individuals with type O blood lack A and B antigens (glycoproteins) on the surface of their RBCs. Instead, three antibodies (isohemagglutinins) circulate in their blood: anti-A IgM, anti-B IgM, and anti-A/anti-B IgG. Therefore, these individuals can safely receive only type O blood. Otherwise, antibodies against other blood types would destroy the transfused cells and produce a hemolytic transfusion reaction.

A (type A) is incorrect. Individuals with type A blood have anti-B IgM antibodies. Therefore, they require either type A blood or type O blood (packed RBCs, not whole blood) for transfusion. Because type O blood does not have A or B antigen, it is used to transfuse A, B, and AB patients when blood of the patient's type is not available.

B (type AB) is incorrect. Individuals with type AB blood lack antibodies in their blood. Because they can receive transfusions with blood of any type if blood of their type is not available, they are the so-called "universal recipients."

C (type B) is incorrect. Individuals with type B blood have anti-A IgM antibodies. Therefore, they require either type B blood or type O blood.

40. **E** (zinc) is correct. The patient most likely has a deficiency of zinc, which commonly occurs in patients who have chronic inflammation. Associated signs and symptoms of zinc deficiency are poor wound healing, inability to taste (dysgeusia), inability to smell (anosmia), perioral rash, hypogonadism, and growth retardation. Zinc is a cofactor in many metalloenzymes, including superoxide dismutase, which neutralizes oxygen free radicals; collagenase, which is important in wound remodeling; and alkaline phosphatase, which is important in bone mineralization.

A (chromium) is incorrect. Chromium is a component of glucose tolerance factor, which helps maintain a normal glucose level in blood, and is also a cofactor in insulin. Associated signs of chromium deficiency are glucose intolerance and peripheral neuropathy, neither of which are present in this patient.

B (copper) is incorrect. Copper, like zinc, is a cofactor in metalloenzymes, including ferroxidase, lysyl oxidase, and tyrosinase.

Signs and symptoms of copper deficiency include poor wound healing, which is present in this patient, as well as iron deficiency and a dissecting aortic aneurysm.

C (vitamin C) is incorrect. Vitamin C (ascorbic acid) hydroxylates proline and lysine, reduces ferric iron (Fe^{3+}) to ferrous iron (Fe^{2+}), acts as an antioxidant, and is a cofactor for the enzyme that converts dopamine to norepinephrine. Diets that lack adequate fruits and vegetables can cause vitamin C deficiency. Signs and symptoms of vitamin C deficiency include poor wound healing, which is present in this patient, as well as bleeding diathesis (e.g., ecchymoses, hemarthroses, and bleeding gums) and glossitis.

D (vitamin E) is incorrect. Vitamin E is an antioxidant that protects polyunsaturated fats and fatty acids in cell membranes from lipid peroxidation. Signs and symptoms of vitamin E deficiency include hemolytic anemia, peripheral neuropathy, posterior column degeneration, and myopathy, none of which are present in this patient.

41. **C** (phosphoenolpyruvate carboxykinase) is correct. Phosphoenolpyruvate carboxykinase helps convert oxaloacetate to phosphoenolpyruvate. A deficiency of this enzyme prevents the conversion of pyruvate to glucose via gluconeogenesis under fasting conditions. The buildup of pyruvate leads to increased conversion to lactate, which diffuses into the bloodstream. In general, deficiencies of gluconeogenic enzymes result in fasting hypoglycemia and lactic acidosis.

A (glucose 6-phosphate dehydrogenase) is incorrect. G6PD deficiency inhibits the pentose phosphate pathway and decreases the cellular levels of NADPH, leading to hemolytic anemia precipitated by oxidizing agents (e.g., primaquine).

B (glycogen phosphorylase) is incorrect. Glycogen phosphorylase deficiency does not prevent pyruvate carbons from being converted to glucose, although this deficiency does inhibit glycogenolysis and can cause mild hypoglycemia.

D (pyruvate kinase) is incorrect. Pyruvate kinase deficiency inhibits the conversion of phosphoenolpyruvate to pyruvate, leading to a decreased lactate level at all times.

42. **E** (5-α-reductase) is correct. The enzyme 5-α-reductase converts testosterone to dihydrotestosterone, the hormone that is mainly responsible for benign prostatic hyperplasia (BPH) and prostate cancer. The patient has BPH, which is the most common cause of urinary retention with hydronephrosis in elderly men.

A (aromatase) is incorrect. Aromatase irreversibly converts androgens (e.g., dihydrotestosterone, testosterone, and androstenedione) to estrogens (e.g., estradiol and estrone).

B (17-α-hydroxylase) is incorrect. 17-α-Hydroxylase is important in the conversion of 17-hydroxypregnenolone to dehydroepiandrosterone and 17-hydroxyprogesterone to androstenedione. These two weak androgens (dehydroepiandrosterone and androstenedione), which are also known as 17-ketosteroids, are produced in both the adrenal cortex and Leydig cells in the testes.

C (21-α-hydroxylase) is incorrect. This enzyme is important in the conversion of 17-hydroxyprogesterone to 11-deoxycortisol in steroid synthesis in the adrenal cortex. Neither compound is involved in the pathogenesis of BPH.

D (oxidoreductase) is incorrect. This enzyme converts androstenedione to testosterone in the adrenal cortex and Leydig cells.

43. **D** (oxidizes bilirubin into a water-soluble form) is correct. Water-soluble forms of bilirubin are nontoxic and are excreted in the urine. Phototherapy with blue light causes bilirubin to undergo photooxidation, which produces the water-soluble form.

A (increases conjugating enzymes in the liver) is incorrect. Phototherapy does not increase the synthesis of conjugating enzymes in the liver.

B (increases synthesis of vitamin D in the skin) is incorrect. Ultraviolet light increases vitamin D synthesis in the skin. Vitamin D does not alter the concentration of bilirubin in the skin or blood.

C (metabolizes bilirubin into biliverdin) is incorrect. Biliverdin, which is more water soluble than bilirubin, is converted to bilirubin in macrophages before it is conjugated in the liver. Conversion of biliverdin to bilirubin is an energy-requiring reaction and is not reversed by phototherapy.

44. **A** (activation of a G_q protein) is correct. This patient has signs of benign prostatic hyperplasia. The medication is most likely an α_1-adrenergic antagonist. α_1-Adrenergic receptors work by activating G_q proteins. These proteins then activate phospholipase C, the enzyme that cleaves phosphatidylinositol diphosphate to diacylglycerol and inositol triphosphate, which in turn raises intracellular calcium concentrations. Although such agents decrease tone in the prostate, they also decrease vasomotor tone and lead to orthostasis.

B (activation of a G_s protein) is incorrect. G_s proteins, when activated, stimulate adenylate cyclase, generating increased concentrations of cAMP in the cell. Irreversible activation of a G_s protein is characteristic of the action of cholera toxin. Other receptors that operate via G_s proteins include β_1- and β_2-adrenergic receptors.

C (inactivation of a G_i protein) is incorrect. G_i proteins, when activated, inhibit the formation of cAMP. The mechanism of action of the pertussis toxin involves permanent inactivation of the G_i protein, which leads to elevated levels of cAMP.

D (stimulation of guanylyl cyclase) is incorrect. Guanylyl cyclase produces cGMP from GTP; this is the mechanism of action of several molecules, including the atrial natriuretic peptides and all agents that produce nitric oxide for vasodilation. Drugs such as sildenafil inhibit the breakdown of cGMP, thereby increasing cGMP concentrations to exert their vasodilatory effects.

45. **C** (area C) is correct. The patient has primary hyperparathyroidism resulting from a functioning parathyroid adenoma in the right inferior parathyroid gland. Recurrent calculi are the most common symptomatic presentation of this condition. Stimulation of gastrin release in the pylorus and antrum by calcium leads to peptic ulcer disease.

A (area A) is incorrect. Decreased PTH and decreased serum calcium are compatible with primary hypoparathyroidism since reduced PTH leads to a decrease in plasma calcium.

B (area B) is incorrect. Increased PTH and decreased serum calcium are compatible with secondary hyperparathyroidism (e.g., vitamin D deficiency causing hypocalcemia in chronic renal failure). Hypocalcemia is the normal stimulus for increased synthesis of PTH.

D (area D) is incorrect. Decreased PTH and increased serum calcium are compatible with all other causes of hypercalcemia (e.g., cancer-induced sarcoidosis). Hypercalcemia normally suppresses PTH synthesis.

46. **D** (pyruvate kinase) is correct. The patient has a deficiency of pyruvate kinase, an autosomal recessive disease. Pyruvate kinase, a glycolytic enzyme, catalyzes the conversion of

phosphoenolpyruvate to pyruvate; the reaction produces a net gain of two ATP. Mature RBCs, which require ATP for energizing ion pumps, lack mitochondria and use only glucose for fuel. Loss of ATP results in loss of water from the RBCs, causing them to appear spiculated. Splenic macrophages remove the damaged cells, resulting in an increase in unconjugated bilirubin. Because pyruvate kinase is subsequent to 1,3-biphosphoglycerate (1,3-BPG), there is an increased conversion of 1,3-BPG to 2,3-BPG, which shifts the oxygen binding curve to the right and lessens the severity of the anemia.

A (glucose 6-phosphatase) is incorrect. Glucose 6-phosphatase deficiency is found in von Gierke's disease, which is a glycogenosis associated with a fasting hypoglycemia and increased deposition of glycogen in the liver and kidneys. This deficiency does not result in a hemolytic anemia.

B (glucose 6-phosphate dehydrogenase) is incorrect. G6PD deficiency, an X-linked recessive disease associated with a deficiency of glutathione in RBCs, results in oxidant damage to RBCs by peroxide and peroxide free radicals. This process causes clumping of hemoglobin (Heinz bodies) and damage to the membrane, which results in intravascular hemolysis. Circulating RBCs have parts of their membranes removed by splenic macrophages (bite cells). Splenomegaly is not a feature of the disease.

C (pyruvate dehydrogenase) is incorrect. Pyruvate dehydrogenase deficiency does not cause a hemolytic anemia. RBCs do not contain mitochondria and therefore do not contain pyruvate dehydrogenase.

47. **B** (apolipoprotein B) is correct. The patient has abetalipoproteinemia, a rare autosomal recessive disease characterized by the inability to form chylomicrons or VLDL. ApoB is necessary for the formation of chylomicrons (apoB-48), VLDL (apoB-100), and LDL (apoB-100). The absence of chylomicrons, which carry diet-derived triacylglycerol (TG), and VLDL, which carries endogenously synthesized TG, accounts for the markedly decreased levels of TG in the blood. Furthermore, LDL is the major carrier for cholesterol and is derived from hydrolysis of VLDL, so serum cholesterol levels are also very low. The clinical findings in this patient (like most patients with abetalipoproteinemia) result from vitamin E deficiency. This fat-soluble vitamin is normally reabsorbed with fat. In abetalipoproteinemia, TG and the fat-soluble vitamins cannot be packaged into chylomicrons in the small intestine. TG accumulates in the lamina propria of the villi and prevents the reabsorption of fat and fat-soluble vitamins from the intestinal lumen, which leads to steatorrhea (excess fat in stools). Vitamin E deficiency is associated with spinocerebellar degeneration and hemolytic anemia. Treatment involves megadoses of vitamin E.

A (apolipoprotein A) is incorrect. ApoA is unique to HDL. Deficiency of apoA, a rare disease, is associated with the absence of HDL and a predisposition for premature coronary artery disease.

C (apolipoprotein C-II) is incorrect. ApoC-II is important in the activation of capillary lipoprotein lipase, which hydrolyzes TG and VLDL to release fatty acids and glycerol. ApoC-II is deficient in familial hyperchylomicronemia syndrome (type I hyperlipoproteinemia) and is associated with an increase in chylomicrons that begins in early childhood.

D (apolipoprotein E) is incorrect. ApoE is present on chylomicrons, VLDLs, and IDLs. A mutant form of apoE characterizes familial dysbetalipoproteinemia (type III hyperlipoproteinemia). The apoB and apoE receptors in the liver cannot remove chylomicron remnants and IDLs that have the mutant form of apoE, so these remnants accumulate in the blood and increase TG and cholesterol levels.

48. **C** (porphobilin) is correct. Porphobilinogen, which is excreted in the urine, is colorless, but in the presence of light it is oxidized to porphobilin, which has a wine-red color. The recurrent, neurologically induced abdominal pain precipitated by either drugs that induce the liver cytochrome P450 system or dietary restriction is characteristic of acute intermittent porphyria, an autosomal dominant disease caused by a deficiency of uroporphyrinogen I synthase. This enzyme catalyzes the conversion of porphobilinogen to hydroxymethylbilane, one of the reactions in heme synthesis. Deficiency of the enzyme leads to a proximal accumulation of both porphobilinogen and aminolevulinic acid. Confirmation of the diagnosis involves documentation of the enzyme deficiency in RBCs. Treatment involves carbohydrate loading and infusion of heme, both of which inhibit aminolevulinic acid synthase, the rate-limiting enzyme in heme synthesis.

A (hemoglobin) is incorrect. The presence of hemoglobin in the urine, or hemoglobinuria, occurs primarily with intravascular hemolysis. Hemoglobinuria is characterized by wine-colored urine that does not change color after exposure to light.

B (myoglobin) is incorrect. The presence of myoglobin, or myoglobinuria, occurs primarily after strenuous exercise, leading to rhabdomyolysis (rupture of muscle). Myoglobinuria is characterized by wine-colored urine that does not change color after exposure to light.

D (urobilin) is incorrect. Urobilin, the oxidation product of urobilinogen, is the pigment normally responsible for the yellow color of urine. This substance normally occurs in trace amounts in urine. An increase in urobilin turns the urine dark yellow. It does not turn wine red with exposure to light.

E (uroporphyrin I) is incorrect. Levels of uroporphyrin I are increased in porphyria cutanea tarda, a disorder characterized by a deficiency of uroporphyrinogen decarboxylase. The presence of uroporphyrin I in urine colors it wine red when voided. Porphyria cutanea tarda is associated with photosensitive skin lesions, such as vesicles and bullae; fragile skin; and fine hair on the face.

49. **E** (sodium) is correct. Sodium is the primary mineral that contributes to the plasma osmolality, which refers to the total number of solutes in plasma; plasma glucose and blood urea nitrogen (BUN) are less important contributors. A low plasma osmolality almost always indicates the presence of hyponatremia because blood glucose and BUN cannot be low enough to cause abnormal plasma osmolality. Sodium is limited to the extracellular fluid (ECF) because of the Na^+/K^+ ATPase pump, which keeps sodium in the ECF and potassium in the intracellular fluid (ICF). Alterations in the serum sodium concentration establish an osmotic gradient between ECF and ICF. This osmotic gradient results in the movement of water into the ICF compartment in order to equalize the osmolality in both compartments, which accounts for the cerebral edema that is causing the seizures. Ectopic secretion of antidiuretic hormone (ADH) by the small cell carcinoma of the lung accounts for the hyponatremia. ADH reabsorbs electrolyte free water out of the distal and collecting ducts, resulting in a dilutional hyponatremia.

A (calcium) is incorrect. Calcium is important in the mineralization of bone and teeth; nerve conduction; muscle contraction; binding of vitamin K-dependent coagulation factors in forming clots; and, as a complex with calmodulin, activation of enzymes for signal transduction across membranes (e.g., adenylate cyclase).

B (magnesium) is incorrect. Magnesium is involved in calcium metabolism (controls synthesis and release of parathyroid hormone), muscle contraction (modulates the vasoconstrictive effects of intracellular calcium), and nerve impulse propagation. It also serves as a cofactor for ATPases (e.g., Na^+/K^+ and Ca^{2+} ATPase pumps).

C (phosphorus) is incorrect. Phosphorus is important in the mineralization of bone and teeth, trapping of monosaccharides in cells, activation and deactivation of enzymes, and excretion of acid in the urine (e.g., titratable acidity). It is also an important component of DNA and RNA, ATP, and phosphorylated vitamins (e.g., thiamine and pyridoxine).

D (potassium) is incorrect. Potassium plays only a very minor role in the control of the osmotic pressure in the ECF compartment. Compared to sodium, potassium has a much reduced serum concentration in the ECF compartment.

50. **C** (decreased renal excretion of uric acid) is correct. The patient has classic acute gouty arthritis involving the right big toe. The majority of cases of gout are caused by underexcretion of uric acid in the kidneys resulting from competition for excretion of acids (e.g., lactic acid and keto acids) with uric acid for excretion in the proximal tubules. Alcoholics commonly have both lactic acid and β-hydroxybutyric acid ketoacidosis, the former due to conversion of pyruvate to lactate by excess production of NADH in alcohol metabolism and the latter due to increased ketogenesis related to excess acetyl CoA from alcohol metabolism. Other causes of underexcretion are renal failure and lead poisoning. Hyperuricemia usually occurs in gout, but it is necessary to find monosodium urate crystals in the synovial fluid to confirm the diagnosis.

A (decreased activity of hypoxanthine-guanine phosphoribosyltransferase) is incorrect. This condition is present in Lesch-Nyhan syndrome, which is an X-linked recessive disorder characterized by total deficiency of HGPRT, a salvage enzyme for hypoxanthine and guanine. Loss of the enzyme results in conversion of hypoxanthine and guanine to xanthine, which is converted to uric acid, leading to hyperuricemia. Symptoms include severe mental retardation; patients often must be restrained to prevent self-mutilation.

B (decreased activity of xanthine oxidase) is incorrect. This condition would occur if the patient had been taking allopurinol, which inhibits xanthine oxidase and prevents conversion of hypoxanthine to xanthine to uric acid. Allopurinol is principally used to treat gout associated with deficiency of HGPRT or overactivity of phosphoribosylpyrophosphate synthetase. The hypoxanthine formed is water soluble and more easily excreted by the kidneys.

D (increased activity of phosphoribosylpyrophosphate synthetase) is incorrect. This condition is an uncommon genetic cause of overproduction of uric acid and would most likely have occurred before the patient reached adulthood.

Index

Note: Page numbers followed by f indicate figures; those followed by t indicate tables; and those followed by b indicate boxed material.